YMCA Personal Training Manual

SECOND EDITION

YMCA of the USA

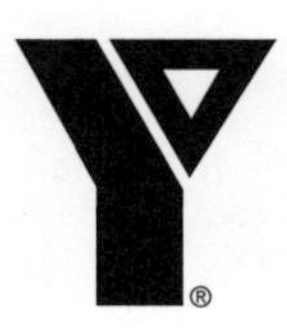

Library of Congress Cataloging-in-Publication Data

YMCA personal training manual / YMCA of the USA.
p. cm.
"Revised edition of YMCA personal training instructor manual, published in 2000."
Includes bibliographical references and index.
ISBN 0-7360-6021-9 (soft cover)
1. Personal trainers--Handbooks, manuals, etc. I. Title: Personal training manual. II. YMCA of the USA.
III. YMCA personal training instructor manual
RC1211.Y63 2005
613.7'1--dc22

2005004384

ISBN: 0-7360-6021-9

Published for the YMCA of the USA by Human Kinetics, Inc.

This book is a revised edition of *YMCA Personal Training Instructor Manual*, published in 2000 by Human Kinetics.

YMCA Project Coordinator: Michael J. Spezzano; **Acquisitions Editor:** Patricia Sammann; **Managing Editor:** Wendy McLaughlin; **Assistant Editor:** Kim Thoren; **Copyeditor:** Annette Pierce; **Proofreader:** Anne Rogers; **Indexer:** Betty Frizzell; **Permission Manager:** Carly Breeding; **Graphic Designer:** Fred Starbird; **Graphic Artist:** Sandra Meier; **Photo Manager:** Dan Wendt; **Cover Designer:** Thom Whitaker; **Photographer (interior):** Dan Wendt unless otherwise noted. Photos on pages 11, 21, 79, 143, 153, 159, and 183 © YMCA of the USA. All other photos © Human Kinetics.; **Art Manager:** Kareema McLendon; **Illustrator:** Argosy; **Printer:** Versa Press

We thank YMCA of Champaign in Champaign, Illinois, for assistance in providing the location for the photo shoot for this book.

Printed in the United States of America

10 9 8 7 6 5 4 3 2 1

Copies of this book may be purchased from the YMCA Program Store, P.O. Box 5076, Champaign, IL 61825-5076, 800-747-0089.

YMCA of the USA does not operate any programs; YMCA of the USA is a not-for-profit corporation that provides advice and guidance, but not rules of compliance, to local YMCAs.

Contents

Preface

Personal training has come a long way since it first became popular in the early 1990s. Since then, the body of knowledge has expanded not only in the area of exercise and physical activity for fitness, but also in the value of exercise in maximizing health and the quality of life. With today's emphasis on promoting physical activity and combating obesity throughout the United States, there has never been a better time to promote safe and effective exercise to the American public.

A professional, high-quality personal training instructor plays an important role in helping people achieve their fitness goals. Of all the variables that can affect exercise compliance, perhaps the most significant is the quality of the exercise instructor. A qualified, enthusiastic professional will prescribe progressive exercise to minimize the chance of injury, ensure variety and fun during the session, help the participant establish realistic goals, provide periodic evaluations, keep accurate records, and recognize participants' accomplishments.

This is one of the reasons why the YMCA of the USA is updating the *YMCA Personal Training Manual* (formerly called the *YMCA Personal Training Instructor Manual)* and the accompanying certification course. As the demand for quality personal training instruction increases, YMCAs and the exercising public demand better qualified and certified instructors. YMCA personal training instructors are expected to be conversant in the information presented in this manual, experienced in the techniques and skills required to implement programs, and up to date on emerging technologies and programs. This manual represents the most current picture of the responsibilities of YMCA personal training instructors and the knowledge and instructional techniques they must master to provide effective exercise instruction to members. It is the required text for the YMCA of the USA's YMCA Personal Training Instructor certification course and focuses on how to lead personal training sessions, covering the following areas:

- The role of personal training instructors in the YMCA movement
- Basic physiological information about the cardiorespiratory and musculoskeletal systems
- Description of cardiorespiratory and muscular strength training programs
- Guidelines and physiology of flexibility training
- Information about health screening and fitness assessment
- Guidelines for developing individual exercise programs
- Basic nutrition information
- Information about motivating participants
- Communication and teaching techniques
- Methods for avoiding, recognizing, and treating various exercise-related injuries
- Suggestions for program administration

The book also includes practical tools in the appendix such as educational topic outlines and health screening forms, as well as a glossary of fitness training terms.

As a YMCA personal training instructor, you have an abundance of information at your fingertips. Your challenge is to learn how to apply it in a way that is effective and enjoyable, brings results, and ensures the long-term success of your participants.

Acknowledgments

The YMCA of the USA would like to acknowledge the contributions of those who played key roles in the development of this manual: Michael J. Spezzano, national health and fitness specialty consultant for the YMCA of the USA, who provided staff leadership for the project; contributing authors Rosemary Lindle, PhD, University of Maryland at College Park, and Wayne Westcott, PhD, South Shore YMCA, Quincy, Massachusetts; editorial reviewers Melissa Davis, director, and Elizabeth Fleck, associate director, Knowledge Publishing and Products, YMCA of the USA, Chicago.

The YMCA of the USA would also like to gratefully acknowledge the contributions and cooperation of the following organizations and the use of their materials and information throughout this manual: the American Council on Exercise (ACE), the National Exercise Trainers Association (NETA, formerly NDEITA), and the American College of Sports Medicine (ACSM).

Credits

This book contains material published by the American Council on Exercise (ACE) in the following manual: *ACE Personal Trainer Manual, Third Edition* (2003). It also contains information from the National Exercise Trainers Association (NETA) from the following manual: *Personal Trainer Manual* (2001).

The YMCA of the USA does not claim any copyright for publications of the American Council on Exercise or the National Exercise Trainers Association that are reprinted with permission in this book.

Copies of this book may be purchased from the YMCA Program Store, P.O. Box 5076, Champaign, IL 61825-5076, 1-800-747-0089.

The YMCA of the USA does not oversee, control, or otherwise operate any health and fitness programs.

CHAPTER 1

Personal Training in the YMCA

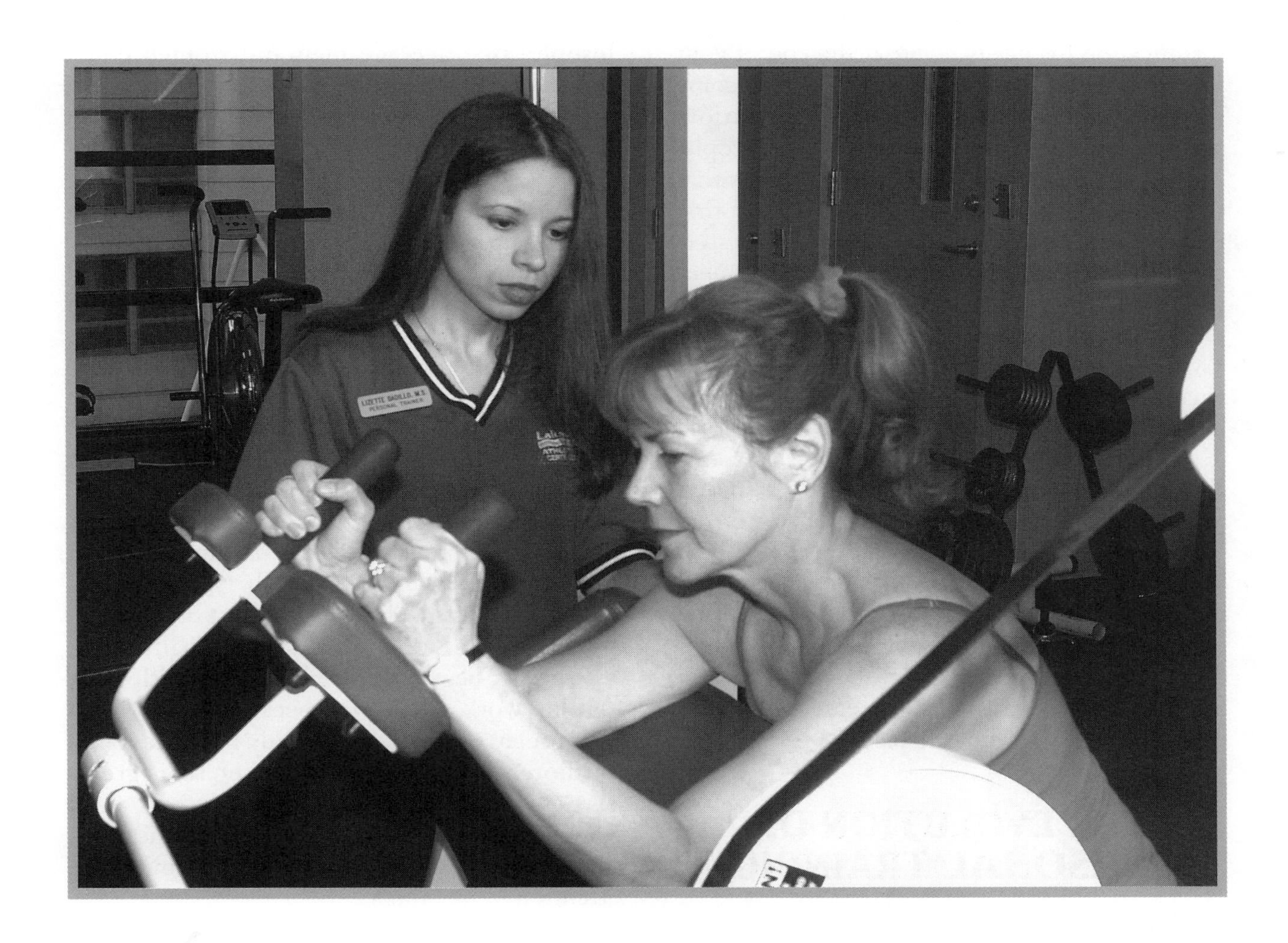

Welcome to the team of dedicated YMCA personal training instructors helping members achieve their personal exercise goals in YMCAs across the nation. You'll soon discover that the members of this team are diverse in age and background. Amid this diversity, however, a common bond exists among successful instructors. Each has accepted the challenge to become the best instructor he or she can be.

You do not acquire the skills to become the best personal training instructor you can be simply by attending a certification workshop, nor does this qualification magically occur at the end of your first training session. Commitment to become your best requires time, energy, motivation, practice, a love of learning, and a love of people. Becoming your best is an ongoing process that begins as you prepare to work with your first member and continues as you polish your style through every training session with every member you teach.

In this chapter we start by explaining how YMCA personal training programs came about, what personal training means at a YMCA, and how personal training programs should be designed to serve all age groups. We then talk about what a good personal trainer should be able to do; how personal training relates to the YMCA's mission, goals, and values; the YMCA code of ethnics, and the YMCA's expectations for personal trainers. Following this, we describe additional YMCA training available to you, then discuss how you can educate your members and use that knowledge and other personal skills to work effectively with participants.

THE EVOLUTION OF PERSONAL TRAINING

In 1876, Boston YMCA gymnasium superintendent Robert J. Roberts introduced a new form of exercise with dumbbell weights that he termed "bodybuilding." By the early 1900s, many YMCA gymnasiums included weight training rooms. This was consistent with the "muscular Christianity" mission of that era, which advocated a strong spirit, a strong mind, and a strong body. Unfortunately, most weight training rooms were dominated by small groups of well-developed men, which was somewhat intimidating to others. As a result, for years weight training was considered an inappropriate physical activity by most adults and definitely off-limits for youth and women.

Throughout the 1970s, the typical YMCA weight room was a small space with unfamiliar equipment, muscular men, and loud noises. It remained an uninviting place. However, as larger strength training facilities were introduced, with convenient new weight training machines and programs based on the philosophy that average men and women could benefit from relatively brief strength training sessions, newcomers were attracted to weight training. Many YMCAs retained the traditional free-weight room for those interested in weightlifting and bodybuilding, and then added a modern strength training facility for those interested in general conditioning and developing better muscular fitness. Far from being a fad, the interest in strength training grew steadily throughout the 1990s and is now one of the most popular forms of exercise in the country.

In the YMCA, the use of personal trainers began almost exclusively with strength training, as more and more members added this new component to their workouts. Because strength training was new to many members, they sought assistance from qualified staff, most often called strength training instructors. Gradually these instructors began helping members with their aerobic workouts as well because many members preferred individual, mostly machine-based cardiorespiratory exercise rather than group exercise classes. As the scope of instructors' work broadened, so did their titles, and many YMCAs now have staff that provide personal training and attention to members.

More and more, YMCA members participating in physical activity seek personal attention, guidance, and coaching from caring, well-trained, and knowledgeable fitness staff. This personal instruction helps members understand the many components of physical fitness and provides them with individualized programs that help them become physically fit. Comprehensive fitness programs include cardiorespiratory, muscular strength, and flexibility exercises.

STRENGTH TRAINING COMES OF AGE

Strength training is not to be confused with lifting extremely heavy weights, as in competitive weightlifting, or building extremely large muscles, as in competitive bodybuilding. Very few people have the genetic capacity to be successful in these sports. Also, some competitive weightlifters and bodybuilders jeopardize their overall health and fitness in their quest for stronger and larger muscles. The main purpose of YMCA strength training programs is to help people improve their overall health and fitness through better muscular development.

Strength training is now universally recognized as an appropriate form of exercise for people of all ages as a means to enhance their overall health and fitness. Performing resistance training exercises can stimulate muscle development for everyone within each person's genetic framework. Few have the potential to build exceptionally large muscles, but people of all ages can increase their muscle strength and physical capacity through regular resistance exercise. In addition to helping people look better, feel better, and function better, strength training reduces injury risk, delays the degenerative effects of aging, and enhances the joy of living.

Although strength training is the best means for developing and maintaining a strong, functional, and injury-resistant musculoskeletal system, it is only one dimension of health-related fitness. YMCA personal training addresses total fitness, with an emphasis on cardiorespiratory conditioning, flexibility, and muscular strength and endurance. Part of the YMCA philosophy is also to encourage people to participate in leisure sports and activities that provide health benefits and fun.

WORKING WITH DIFFERENT AGE GROUPS

Personal training programs can be designed to meet the fitness needs of all age groups. The YMCA personal training programs you create should be developmentally appropriate for people of various ages and for special populations, and they should take into account individual differences. For example, people of different ages have different exercise capacities and should train accordingly. Consider the following age groups, all of whose members can benefit from well-designed personal training programs:

- **Youth.** Preteens (ages 7 through 12) are still growing and maturing. However, in today's society few youth engage in sufficient physical activity, especially progressive resistance exercise. As a result they do not develop the strong muscles, tendons, and bones that should be an integral part of their developmental years. Preteens can benefit greatly from systematic strength exercise, but their training should be basic and brief, focusing on low resistance and high repetitions. They require relatively little resistance exercise to produce excellent strength gains. At this age, strength training should be only one component of a physical activity program. Youth need the opportunity to join in active games with their peers that give them opportunities to use their creativity and have fun. Most youth lose their enthusiasm for exercise when they are confronted with lengthy training sessions. That's why fun and variety are important.
- **Adolescents.** Teenagers (ages 13 through 18) continue to experience physical growth and maturation, with the development of secondary gender characteristics. Particularly pronounced among teenage males is enhanced upper-body size. Most teens are capable of regular and rigorous resistance training that produces high levels of strength and muscularity. This is a time when many teens, both male and female, are interested in their physiques and are willing to spend considerable time and effort to achieve their physical objectives. They may choose to do longer or harder workouts, performing more exercises and more sets than they did as preteens.
- **Young adults.** Young adults include men and women who have attained physical maturity (approximately age 19) through the beginning of middle age (approximately age 39). This is a rather broad age range, and 19-year-olds typically have greater physical capacity than 39-year-olds. However, as a group, young adults are relatively strong and capable of high-intensity cardiorespiratory and muscle resistance exercise. For

many young adults it is difficult to schedule long training sessions because the time pressures of work, family, recreation, and other commitments, so they might be best advised to perform exercise sessions of moderate duration.

- **Middle-aged adults.** Middle age means different things to different people, but most 40- to 55-year-olds fit into this category. This might be the most important time of life to perform regular exercise. During these years, men and women who do not engage in training rapidly lose muscle tissue. This results in a lower physical capacity, a reduced metabolic rate, and a premature onset of old age. A well-designed personal training program can maintain muscle mass, metabolic rate, and physical capacity at a high level throughout an adult's middle years. Because middle-aged adults typically have busy schedules, they often respond well to brief exercise sessions.

- **Older adults.** Although people in this category have attained a certain *quantity of life*, too many have sacrificed a desirable *quality of life*. Because many are sedentary, they function at a much lower level than they should, and they accept their lack of fitness as part of the aging process. We must address this problem by introducing older adults to a more active lifestyle. One step is developing individualized exercise that will increase their muscle strength and physical capacity. Personal training sessions should be of moderate effort and reasonable duration and in the company of other older adults whenever possible.

BEING THE BEST

Good YMCA personal training instructors know their stuff. They understand the basic principles of cardiorespiratory and muscular fitness, incorporate safe movements and exercises into individual programs, try to prevent injuries by teaching correct exercise technique, and motivate participants at all skill and fitness levels. They effectively apply their knowledge and communicate it to participants and implement the YMCA's philosophy of helping each person achieve his or her personal best through sensible training and educational programs. Let's look at each of these areas.

Knowing Your Stuff

As a personal training instructor you must do much more than demonstrate exercises. You are also expected to provide accurate fitness information, plan effective programs, and address participants' questions. Knowledge you gain from the exercise sciences will strengthen your preparation to lead. For example, understanding basic principles of fitness will help you better plan each warm-up, workout, and cool-down, and insights from sport psychology can provide useful ways to motivate your participants. Throughout this book you'll become familiar with information from the exercise sciences to apply to training programs. The more you learn about all dimensions of effectively planning and leading personal training, the more you will inspire and benefit your participants.

Reaching Your Participants

You might be the most knowledgeable personal training instructor at your YMCA, but if you can't motivate and communicate with participants, they're not likely to stay with your program very long. Only highly self-motivated people will stick with an instructor who does a poor job of motivating or communicating with them before, during, and after the workouts. You must be aware of individual members' different interests and abilities in order to provide a relevant and engaging exercise experience that keeps them motivated and active.

Some instructors are naturally talented at motivating and communicating with participants; others must do more conscious planning to make sure encouragement comes across. Reading this book will give you ideas for motivating and communicating with your participants. But reading suggestions is only one way to improve your skills. Probably the best way to learn successful motivation and communication techniques is to watch effective instructors in action. Pay close attention to these instructors at your YMCA. Note what they say, verbally and nonverbally, as they work with individual members. Exchanging ideas with other YMCA instructors is a rewarding way to learn.

Implementing the YMCA's Philosophy

The YMCA has been a recognized leader in health and fitness for the spirit, mind, and body since 1891. YMCAs view personal training as a means to develop, grow personally, and have fun. YMCAs address all aspects of a participant's good health through comprehensive programs. Preparticipation health screening, fitness testing, exercise plans, and education programs all meet tough standards set by physicians, exercise physiologists, and health educators.

Programs should be open to all individuals, no matter what their current level of fitness or their economic status. YMCAs pride themselves on offering equal opportunities for people of any sex, age, shape, or size to participate in fitness programs. Many YMCAs offer classes for a variety of groups: multilevel, multiage, seniors, visually impaired, hearing impaired, prenatal and postpartum women, people with physical disabilities, and people who use wheelchairs. YMCA programs are taught in inner cities as well as in smaller urban and suburban communities; they're held in schools, churches, hospitals, and recreation facilities as well as in YMCA buildings.

PERSONAL TRAINING AS A YMCA PROGRAM

As with all YMCA programs and services, personal training should be offered at your YMCA in a way that is consistent with the mission, goals, and values of the YMCA movement.

Mission and Values

The YMCA's mission statement was adopted in the 1980s by the YMCA of the USA and is considered a contemporary expression of the purpose statement published in the YMCA's national constitution. **The YMCA mission is to put Christian principles into practice through programs that build healthy spirit, mind, and body for all.** Local Ys may have the same statement or one that is different, but for the most part, the essence is the same.

Local YMCAs help people develop values and behavior that are consistent with Christian principles. They focus on fostering four core values adopted by the YMCA of the USA in the 1990s as part of a recommitment to character development:

- *Caring*: to love others; to be sensitive to the well-being of others; to help others (related values are compassion, forgiveness, generosity, and kindness)
- *Honesty*: to tell the truth; to act in such a way that you are worthy of trust; to have integrity, making sure your choices match your values (related values are integrity and fairness)
- *Respect*: to treat others as you would have them treat you; to value the worth of every person, including yourself (related values are acceptance, empathy, self-respect, and tolerance)
- *Responsibility*: to do what is right, what you ought to do; to be accountable for your behavior (related values are commitment, courage, health, service, and citizenship)

Goals

In the 1970s, a set of eight goals was adopted by the National Council of YMCAs (to which all Ys in the United States belong) and was published in the preamble to its constitution and by-laws. The preamble states that the goals are for "our members and their constituents," i.e., local YMCAs and the children, teens, and adults they serve and involve. All YMCA programs, activities, and endeavors should help people develop and enhance each of these characteristics and behaviors. (Note: the words in bold are contemporary summaries of each goal; they are not published in the constitution).

YMCAs build healthy spirit, mind, and body by helping people develop . . .

Self-Worth: To develop self-confidence and self-respect and an appreciation of their own worth as individuals.

Christian Principles: To develop a faith for daily living based upon the teachings of Jesus Christ, that they may thereby be helped in achieving their highest potential as children of God.

Positive Relationships: To grow as responsible members of their families and citizens of their communities.

Holistic Health: To appreciate that health of mind and body is a sacred gift and that physical fitness and mental well-being are conditions to be achieved and maintained.

Appreciation of Diversity: To recognize the worth of all persons and to work for interracial and intergroup understanding (Note: intergroup understanding represents a variety of dimensions including background, style, perspectives, beliefs, and competencies beyond race including gender, age, ethnicity, ability, sexual orientation, religious beliefs, and more).

International Awareness: To develop a sense of world-mindedness and to work for worldwide understanding.

Leadership and Service: To develop their capacities for leadership and use them responsibly in their own groups and in community life.

Environmental Stewardship: To appreciate the beauty, diversity, and independence of all forms of life and all resources that God has provided in this world, and to develop an ethical basis for guiding the relationships of mankind with the rest of God's natural community.

YMCAs prize instructors who genuinely care about and encourage the development of program participants. Caring about your members can be shown in many ways. Learning participants' names and their goals is a simple way to show that you care. Extending courtesy to all at all times is another characteristic of caring instructors. Good teaching practices, such as patience when you must explain the same movement several times, also show that you care. Many member-service educational materials are available from the YMCA Program Store.

FOLLOWING THE YMCA INSTRUCTOR CODE OF ETHICS

Like most professionals, YMCA exercise instructors have ethical standards that are broad based and serve as guidelines for behavior. Ethical behavior for any group of professionals begins with each person making decisions based on standards of morality, fairness, and honesty. Although most health and fitness professionals work diligently to be recognized for their role in helping people live healthy and balanced lives, their effectiveness may be undermined by negative interactions with members and among peers. YMCA exercise instructors are guided by the following code of conduct as they interact with members, the general public, and their colleagues in health and fitness:

- I understand the purpose and mission of the YMCA and its programs, which goes beyond skills and involves the spiritual, mental, and physical well-being of participants.
- I will teach the YMCA's values of caring, honesty, respect, and responsibility to participants by modeling those values, celebrating them, and holding them up as what is right. I will ask participants to practice those values. I will consistently reinforce participants for behaviors that support the values, and I will consistently confront participants whose actions are inconsistent with the values without devaluing those participants.
- I will set a good example in appearance, speech, and attitude.
- I will be reliable, prompt, and prepared.
- I will be a good role model for my participants, and I will not abuse alcohol, tobacco, or illegal drugs.
- I will speak clearly and use words whose meaning is clear to my participants. I will not use profanity.
- I will create a good learning atmosphere.
- I will strive to build positive and supportive relationships with all members and staff.
- I will be encouraging, respectful, and considerate to participants and instructors regard-

less of their race, physical ability or health status, religion, gender, or culture.

- I will always be conscious that the safety of my participants comes first.
- I am committed to keeping my certification and training up to date, and I will take part in learning opportunities to remain an effective instructor.
- I believe I am free of psychological or physical conditions that might adversely affect others' health, including significant fever and contagious conditions.
- I will report any suspected child abuse or molestation according to the proper procedures.
- I will refrain from socializing or associating with program participants and members under the age of 18 outside of YMCA activities.

KNOWING WHAT YOUR YMCA EXPECTS OF YOU

Ideally, YMCAs prefer to hire personal training instructors who are already well trained in exercise physiology or who have past experience training others. Although not everyone chosen to train has these extensive credentials, YMCAs do expect certain qualities of all instructors. These characteristics include physical fitness, high motivation, the ability to communicate well, a personable nature, the ability and willingness to work with people, and reasonable maturity. The YMCA has found that, although the professional backgrounds of instructors are diverse, these common traits exist in all effective instructors.

Regardless of your background in or knowledge of physical fitness, you will receive additional training upon joining the YMCA staff. In many YMCAs, a new instructor is teamed with an experienced instructor and serves an apprenticeship. This 20- to 30-day internship helps to acquaint you with the YMCA's way of leading personal training and helps ease you into working with your first member. If you aren't currently certified in CPR, you must become certified or renew your expired card. Classes to prepare you to pass the CPR exam are held frequently at the YMCA and in many other community programs. You might be required to attend a YMCA of the USA Personal Training Instructor certification course that covers such topics as exercise physiology, ways to give good instruction, safe exercises, and how to motivate participants.

ATTENDING ADDITIONAL TRAININGS

As a YMCA instructor, you should take pride in improving the quality of your program's content. Making improvements depends heavily on your commitment to continue learning. Many instructors attend additional YMCA of the USA Health and Fitness certification training and continually search for new ideas. The following are selected YMCA of the USA Health and Fitness courses that are useful for personal trainers:

- **YMCA Fitness Testing and Assessment Specialist.** This course certifies staff members and volunteers to conduct the YMCA Fitness Testing and Assessment protocol and develop individualized exercise plans with members. Course content includes applied anatomy and physiology, cardiorespiratory and neuromuscular exercise science, interpretation of test results and exercise prescription, and laboratory sessions on fitness testing protocol practice and examination.
- **YMCA Personal Fitness Program Director.** This course teaches the YMCA's innovative program of introducing inactive people to regular exercise. The program is based on the science of exercise behavior change and teaches staff how to manage staff, facilities, equipment, and activity issues by better understanding the needs and motivations of the ready-to-be-fit. Course content also includes effective goal setting and strategies for helping new exercisers identify and overcome barriers to exercise. Participants will be presented a staff training outline for use with instructors at their Ys. This training course is designed for the health and fitness director who will oversee the implementation of the YMCA Personal Fitness Program at his or her facility.
- **YMCA Pilates Instructor**. This course teaches exercise instructors the basic biomechanics and philosophical principles of Pilates exercise.

Participants will learn a series of Pilates mat exercises that are designed to improve muscle strength and flexibility, balance, posture, and overall well-being. Also included is information on how to incorporate Pilates exercises into effective group exercise and personal training programs. Practical sessions are included.

- **YMCA Group Cycling Instructor**. This course was developed in collaboration with Reebok University, originators of the Cycle Reebok program. It is designed to teach YMCA exercise instructors how to develop new and exciting indoor group cycle classes. The emphasis of this training is on providing instructors with the practical and theoretical skills needed to create a variety of safe and effective cycle exercise programs.
- **YMCA Martial Arts Exercise Instructor**. This course was developed in collaboration with Promise Enterprises, originators of The Box-Aerobic Exercise program. It is designed to teach YMCA exercise instructors how to develop new and exciting group exercise classes based on athletic movements adapted from martial arts such as boxing, kickboxing, taekwondo, and kung fu. The emphasis of this training is on providing instructors with the basic skills needed to create a variety of safe and effective martial arts–based exercise programs.
- **YMCA Walk Reebok Premier Instructor**. This is a course developed through a collaboration with Reebok University. Participants learn options for developing walking programs, clubs, clinics, and the exclusive "Walk Reebok" techniques for three different levels of walkers. Course content also includes the benefits of fitness walking, the YMCA Walk Reebok Walking Test, and safety and injury-prevention information. Now expanded to include a second-level training, the course also teaches techniques for distance and interval fitness training, effective goal setting and strategies for increasing walking mileage, and ways to increase conditioning intensity through the use of intervals.
- **Active Older Adult Exercise Instructor (Land).** This course is designed for people who lead or assist in teaching land exercise classes for active older adults. It focuses on adaptations for older adult participants and includes sample exercise classes. Related health and fitness programs for active older adults are introduced, including strength training and fitness walking.
- **YMCA/IDEA Get Real Weight Management Instructor**. This is a course developed in collaboration with IDEA Health and Fitness Association, based on the book *Get Real: A Personal Guide to Real-Life Weight Management* (Kosich 1996). This course teaches the techniques and strategies for conducting weight management group classes and individual sessions. It also shows how to incorporate this information into exercise and fitness programs. Content covers sensible nutrition, self-empowerment and body image, and the role of physical activity in successful lifelong weight management.
- **YMCA Water Fitness Instructor**. This course, based on the latest research, provides participants with the necessary knowledge and skills needed to lead YMCA Water Fitness classes. The course includes all components of fitness principles, information about designing purposeful exercises, and methods for targeting specific training objectives.
- **YMCA Active Older Adult Water Fitness Instructor**. This course provides participants with the necessary knowledge and skills needed to lead YMCA Water Fitness classes specifically for active older adults. The focus is on targeting functional fitness for activities of daily living.
- **Enhanced Qualification Courses.** These specialty courses for certified YMCA group exercise or personal training instructors are four hours in length and are on topics of specific interest to exercise instructors. Descriptions of enhanced qualification courses currently available can be found in the YMCA of the USA Training Course catalog.

These and many other YMCA programs are excellent opportunities to expand your fitness knowledge. You can continue your quest for information by becoming familiar with the materials available through the YMCA Program Store. These materials can keep you up to date on the latest techniques and program ideas.

Most instructors subscribe to reliable fitness-oriented magazines and journals to stay informed of the latest trends. A list of these resources can be found in the book *YMCA Healthy Lifestyle Principles* (YMCA of the USA, 2004). Taking courses, using available materials, and regularly reading fitness magazines help instructors make their programs more complete and more sound.

BEING A HEALTH AND FITNESS EDUCATOR

Although education programs are often offered as separate entities at the YMCA, education should be an integral and ongoing part of every fitness program. You can help participants learn by encouraging them to attend educational programs in addition to their fitness programs and by providing information as part of your personal training sessions. Appendix A includes outlines for health and fitness topics that you can share with participants. Select reliable information and apply that information to your participants.

Selecting Reliable Information

With the abundance of health and fitness materials available, trying to determine whether information is reliable can be frustrating and confusing. Add to this the need to include information about sports medicine and leadership abilities, and the task appears overwhelming. Fitness materials are plentiful and competitive, but be careful—not all information is accurate or reliable. So how exactly do you choose reliable sources or references to answer questions about exercise-related topics?

Competent authority is the main concern in evaluating fitness information. Whether the information comes from books or magazines, or even television, you should know the credentials of the person or people presenting it. Become familiar with reputable authorities in the areas in which you need information; otherwise you might get caught in the celebrity name game when you seek fitness information.

What's in a name? Apparently a lot. Books written by celebrities sell quite well, much better than those written by noted exercise physiologists. But don't let the popularity of a celebrity influence your search for accurate information. Your job is to sort out reliable information from all that is available. Subscribe to professional journals and magazines that strive to educate as well as to entertain. *YMCA Healthy Lifestyle Principles* lists some resources from which you can begin to compile fitness reference materials for you and your participants and to share with other YMCA staff.

Applying Exercise Science to Your Program

As important as finding reliable sources of information on exercise science is being able to read and understand them. Although you seek knowledge from exercise scientists, it might be difficult to sift through the scientific jargon to understand the practical implications. Exercise scientists, like other scientists, seem to speak a language all their own. This language is necessary for communicating precisely among fellow scientists, but the specialized terms that enhance scientific communication make it more difficult for lay readers to understand and apply what is said.

You must work at bridging the "technical-term gap" between personal training instructors and exercise scientists. Terms from exercise science appear frequently in popular as well as academic journals. But beyond merely recognizing these terms, you must understand what they mean and how they fit into the overall fitness scheme. Each of the following chapters uses the appropriate technical terms to discuss each topic. Once you understand the terms and general principles from each chapter, you can begin to apply them to your program. Having a good understanding of fitness information and how to apply it vastly improves the quality of your program.

BEING AN EFFECTIVE PERSONAL TRAINER

Establishing an exercise prescription and program for a member and then supporting the process over the long term is not a simple task. Not only must you be knowledgeable and skillful in exercise science and technique, you must also have the communication skills and personality traits required of a good consultant.

Provide your members the proper environment for growth by motivating and challenging them, giving them responsibility, and providing encouragement along the way. An effective personal trainer develops warm, personal relationships with each member he or she works with and regards everyone as worthy of respect, concern, and personal attention. Traits of a good instructor include the following:

- **Empathy.** Having the ability to put yourself in the member's position and communicate that you understand her or his concerns and feelings.
- **Respect.** Possessing genuine appreciation of the worth of each individual.
- **Genuineness.** Freely being yourself, not just playing a role.
- **Honesty.** Being truthful in all of your dealings and relationships with each member.
- **Concern.** Exhibiting a warmth that communicates your concern for each member.

In many respects, developing a personal, caring relationship with each member will go further in helping them become successful at exercise and maintain a program than possessing all of the technical knowledge available about exercise.

LOOKING AHEAD

The continued success of personal training programs at the YMCA depends on you. Programs will stay fresh and alive as long as instructors are creative, innovative, and hardworking. Although this might sound like a formidable task, if you are willing to assess your current abilities and learn how to develop new skills one step at a time, you will become a top-notch YMCA personal training instructor in no time at all. You are to be commended for taking on the challenge of teaching at the YMCA. As you read the next few chapters, take a close look at yourself—the skills you have, what you might lack, and what you can gain from your YMCA experience. You will find information to help you make quick, long strides in becoming the best instructor you can be.

CHAPTER 2

Cardiorespiratory Fitness

Rosemary Schaffner-Lindle, PhD

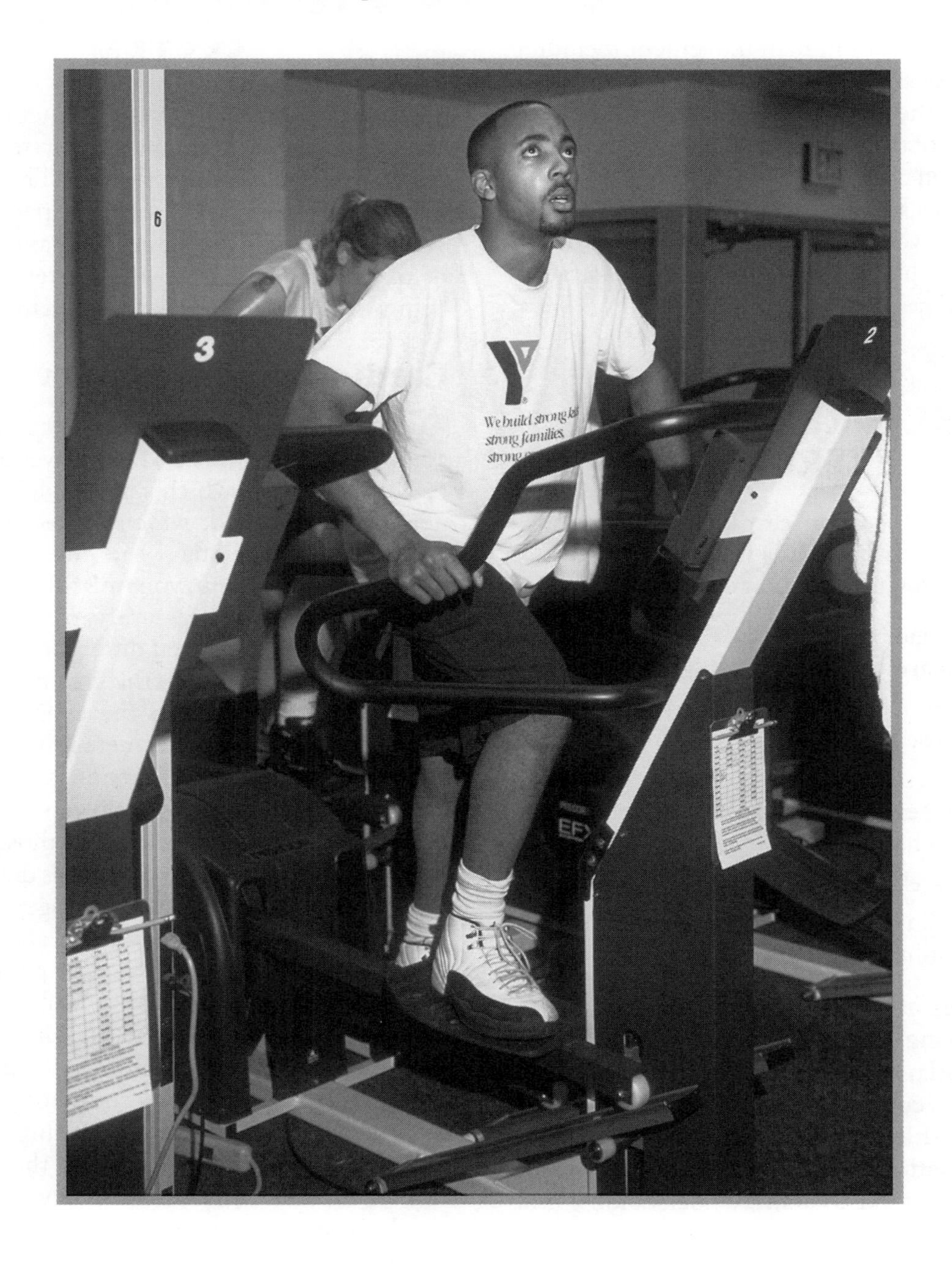

Individual exercise, primarily using cardio exercise machines, is a popular training method for helping members achieve aerobic fitness. To design safe and effective exercise programs for YMCA members, personal training instructors must understand how the body functions during exercise and how it adapts to training. Exercise science is a broad field that encompasses all of the different aspects of human movement including anatomy, the study of the structure of the body; physiology, the study of the function of the various systems of the body such as the cardiovascular, muscular, and nervous systems; and kinesiology or biomechanics, the study of the mechanical aspects of human movement. This chapter focuses on the anatomy and physiology of the cardiorespiratory and energy systems.

WHAT IS CARDIORESPIRATORY EXERCISE?

The various forms of cardiorespiratory (also referred to as cardiovascular or aerobic) exercises have the following common elements:

- They place a demand on the cardiorespiratory (cardio = heart; respiratory = lungs) system.
- They use large muscle groups.
- They predominantly use the aerobic (with oxygen) energy system (to be explained later in this chapter).
- They are rhythmic in nature.
- They can be safely performed at a moderate level of intensity.

Examples of aerobic activities include swimming, walking, jogging, running, cycling, stair climbing, step aerobics, and high–low aerobics. If performed consistently for 20 minutes or more, aerobic activities prompt adaptations, or training responses, within the cardiorespiratory, muscular, energy, and nervous systems. Understanding how these systems adapt can help you

- realize the importance of individualized fitness programs,
- plan safe and beneficial workouts,
- understand the training benefits gained from aerobic exercise,
- answer questions concerning exercise, and
- respond appropriately to injuries or emergencies.

CARDIORESPIRATORY SYSTEM

The cardiorespiratory system is composed of the cardiovascular (circulatory) system and the respiratory (ventilation) system. The following discussion describes specific aspects of each system, how they are integrated, and the basics of oxygen consumption and its recovery. Let's begin with the cardiovascular system.

Cardiovascular System

The cardiovascular system of circulation is composed of the heart, which serves as a pump; the blood vessels, which serve as delivery channels; and the blood, which serves as the fluid medium. To understand the physiology of the cardiovascular system, you must also understand the physics of blood pressure, cardiac output, and the arteriovenous oxygen difference.

The major function of the system is to deliver oxygen and nutrients to the cells throughout the body and to remove metabolic waste such as carbon dioxide. This function is critical. Cells need a continuous supply of oxygen. If blood flow is cut off to any part of the body, those cells will die quickly. For example, brain cells die after only three to four minutes without oxygen.

The heart is a muscular organ, about the size of a fist, weighing less than one pound. It has four chambers: two atria, which act as receiving chambers, and two ventricles, which circulate the blood. The right side of the heart receives the deoxygenated blood returning from the body through the veins and pumps it to the lungs (pulmonary circulation). In the lungs, the carbon dioxide is unloaded and oxygen is picked up. This process is referred to as gas exchange. The oxygen-rich blood then flows to the left side of heart for distribution to the entire body (systemic circulation). Let's take a closer look at the flow of the blood through the heart (figure 2.1).

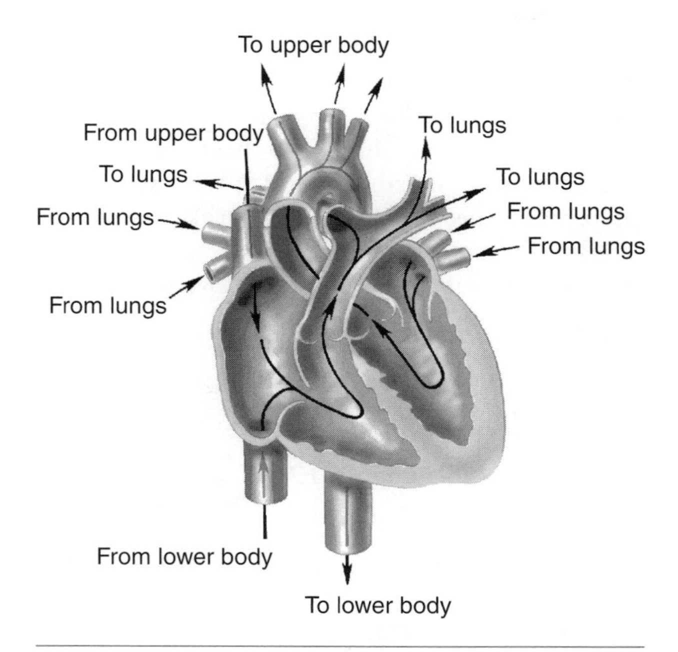

Figure 2.1 Path of blood flow through the heart.

The deoxygenated blood is returned through the superior and inferior vena cava to the right atrium (RA). Atrial contraction forces blood through the tricuspid valve into the right ventricle (RV). Contraction of the right ventricle forces blood through the pulmonary valve into the pulmonary artery and to the lungs. (Note that the pulmonary artery is the only artery in the body that transports deoxygenated blood.) After oxygen and carbon dioxide have been exchanged, the blood returns through the pulmonary vein to the left atrium (LA). Left atrial contraction forces blood through the bicuspid (mitral) valve into the left ventricle. Finally, from the left ventricle the blood is pumped through the aortic valve and on through the body.

Blood serves several vital functions, including the delivery of oxygen to all the cells of the body. Blood is composed of plasma, which is mainly water and formed elements that include the following:

- Platelets play a major role in clot formation.
- Red blood cells contain hemoglobin, an iron compound that binds and carries oxygen from the lungs to the cells of the body.
- White blood cells play a part in the body's immune system, which is responsible for protecting the body against foreign invaders including bacteria, viruses, parasites, and tumor cells.

The vascular system functions as the delivery channels for the cardiovascular system. The vascular system branches from larger to smaller vessels, much like a tree. The three primary components of the vascular system are the arteries, the capillaries, and the veins.

- Arteries are the vessels that distribute the oxygen-rich blood to all the cells of the body. The trunk of the arterial tree is the aorta, which is connected to the left ventricle. The oxygen-rich blood flows through the aorta into the arteries, then through arterioles, and finally to the capillaries.
- Capillaries, which are embedded in the muscles, are thin-walled vessels that allow the easy diffusion of oxygen and carbon dioxide. In the muscle, the hemoglobin releases the oxygen, and the oxygen diffuses into the muscle fibers. Mitochondria are specialized cells in the muscle fibers for aerobic metabolism. Capillaries and mitochondria facilitate the use of oxygen. The number of capillaries and mitochondria increases in response to aerobic training, thus increasing the aerobic capacity.
- Veins carry the deoxygenated blood that is high in carbon dioxide from the cells back to the heart. This is referred to as venous return and is facilitated by the squeezing action of contracting muscles against the veins, the "muscle pump." A system of one-way valves in the veins assists with this flow. Without muscle action, blood will pool in the extremities, causing a decrease in venous return and an insufficient supply of blood to the heart.

Blood Pressure

Blood pressure is the force exerted on the artery walls. Contraction of the heart forces blood into the arteries, creating pressure. This pressure exerted on the walls of the arteries can be measured using a sphygmomanometer. Blood pressure is measured in two phases: Systolic pressure occurs during heart contraction, and diastolic pressure occurs during the relaxation of the heart.

During aerobic activity, systolic pressure increases, but diastolic pressure stays the same or decreases slightly. However, during a resistance exercise bout, both systolic and diastolic blood pressure increase. The extent of the increase in blood pressure depends on the length of time the contraction is held, the intensity of the contraction, and the amount of muscle mass involved in the contraction.

Normal resting blood pressure values are 120/80 millimeters of mercury (mmHg). High blood pressure (hypertension) is defined as a resting blood pressure of 140/90 mmHg and higher. Chronically elevated blood pressure can damage the lining of the arterial walls leading to atherosclerosis. Hypertension also stresses the heart, which can result in a heart attack or a stroke.

Regular aerobic training can lower resting blood pressure in people with moderate hypertension. Results from strength training studies vary depending on the specific type of program, with some showing a decrease in resting blood pressure and others showing no change.

Cardiac Output

The function of the cardiovascular system is to circulate blood, which contains oxygen and nutrients, to all the cells of the body. Functional capacity is defined as the volume of blood that can be circulated per minute, or the *cardiac output.* This volume is expressed in liters (L) or milliliters (ml) of blood pumped per minute (min). The symbol Q is commonly used to represent cardiac output in scientific literature. Cardiac output is the product of stroke volume, the amount of blood in milliliters ejected during each beat of the heart, times the heart rate in beats per minute (BPM).

Cardiac output (Q) =
heart rate (HR) × stroke volume (SV)

Q (L/min) = HR (BPM) × SV(L)

Cardiac output changes proportionally with the intensity of the activity. The average resting cardiac output is approximately 5 liters of blood per minute. Interestingly, this represents the total blood volume. The average quantity of blood in the body is approximately 5 liters. Therefore, the total blood volume is circulated every minute at rest. Walking increases the cardiac output to about 7.5 liters per minute. Strenuous exercise can raise it to 25 liters per minute or as high as 35 liters per minute in a highly trained athlete. Aerobic training strengthens the heart muscle, thus increasing the stroke volume even at rest. Because of the larger stroke volume, the heart rate at rest and during submaximal workloads decreases. At maximal levels of exercise, the stroke volume in the trained state is larger than the untrained state, so the maximal cardiac output is larger.

Resting Values

Sedentary: 5 L/min =
70 BPM × .070 L = 4.9 L/min

Trained: 5 L/min =
50 BPM × .100 L = 5.0 L/min

Resting cardiac output is about the same for trained as for untrained people. Although the stroke volume increases with training due to the increased contractility of the heart, the heart rate decreases with training.

Maximal Values

Sedentary: 22 L/min =
195 BPM × .113 L = 22.035 L/min

Trained: 35 L/min =
195 BPM × .179 L = 34.905 L/min

Maximal heart rate does not change with training (it is related to age), but training does increase maximal stroke volume. Thus, maximal cardiac output increases, which contributes to increased delivery of oxygen to the working muscles (greater $\dot{V}O_2max$, discussed in the next section).

Arteriovenous Oxygen Difference

Arteriovenous oxygen difference ($a\text{-}\bar{v}O_2diff$) is the difference in blood oxygen content between the arteries and the veins, which reflects the amount of oxygen extracted and used by the muscles. As exercise intensity increases, the $a\text{-}\bar{v}O_2diff$ increases. Cardiac output is the delivery of the oxygen to the muscles. The $a\text{-}\bar{v}O_2diff$ reflects how much of that oxygen the muscles extract and use.

Respiratory System

The respiratory system is responsible for pulmonary ventilation, which refers to the intake of oxygen and removal of carbon dioxide. During exercise, as well as at rest, carbon dioxide and oxygen are continually exchanged between the tiny sacs (alveoli) of the lungs and the capillaries of the cardiovascular system. Air is inhaled through the nose or the mouth and flows through an elaborate system of elastic tubing (see figure 2.2). The trachea divides into the right and left bronchi. In the lungs, the bronchi branch into smaller tubes called bronchioles and finally terminate in microscopic air sacs called the alveoli. The alveoli interface with the pulmonary capillaries of the cardiovascular system. The alveoli are extremely thin-walled structures that facilitate a rapid exchange of oxygen (O_2) and carbon dioxide (CO_2) (see figure 2.3). Oxygen diffuses across the alveolar membrane into the pulmonary capillaries and binds to the iron component (hemoglobin) in the red blood cells.

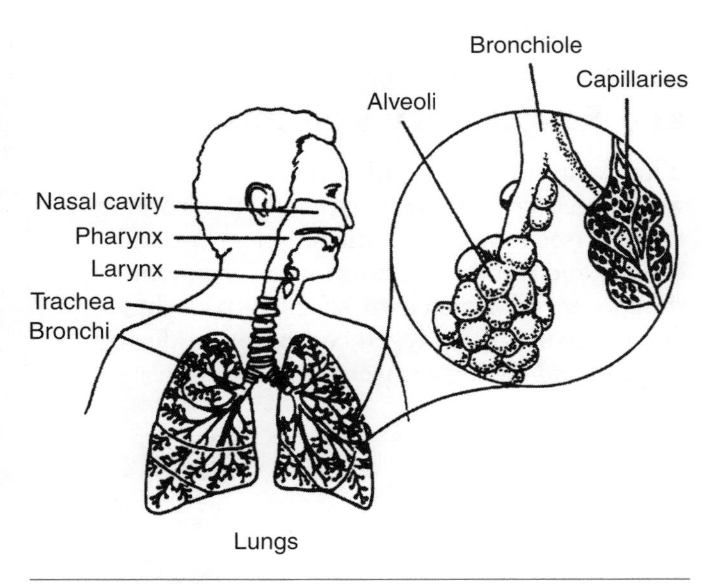

Figure 2.2 The tubular structure of the lungs.

Exercisers sometimes experience difficulties in breathing such as the following:

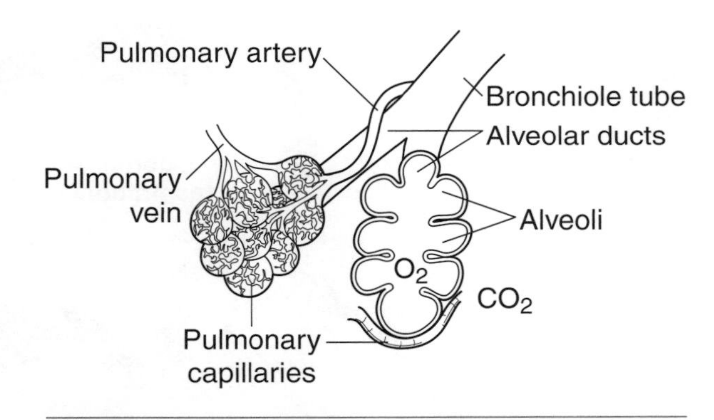

Figure 2.3 Exchange of carbon dioxide and oxygen between the alveoli and capillaries.

- **Shortness of breath (dyspnea).** Beginning exercisers often experience this when exercising. It is caused by a buildup of carbon dioxide in the blood. In fit people, ventilation increases in response to exercise in order to rid the body of the excess carbon dioxide. However, in untrained people, the respiratory muscles (the diaphragm and the intercostal muscles between the ribs) fatigue rapidly and are unable to sustain exercise. To counteract dyspnea, the exerciser simply needs to lower the exercise intensity. With continued training, the respiratory muscles, like the other muscles of the body, will adapt and get stronger, allowing greater ventilation.

- **Hyperventilation.** Anxiety or certain respiratory disorders (asthma and exercise bronchitis) can cause an individual to hyperventilate or "overbreathe." This causes a decrease in the carbon dioxide level in the blood, and as a result decreases the stimulus to breathe. Swimmers sometimes hyperventilate on purpose in order to increase the amount of time that they can hold their breath. The problem is that hyperventilation can result in light-headedness or even loss of consciousness. The immediate remedy for hyperventilation is to breathe into a paper bag. This increases the carbon dioxide levels and triggers the stimulus to breathe.

- **Valsalva maneuver.** The Valsalva maneuver, holding the breath while contracting the abdominal or chest muscles or both, can increase the pressure in the abdominal and thoracic (chest) cavities. The elevated pressure compresses the veins, decreasing the flow of blood back to the heart (venous return). This diminishes cardiac output and can result in light-headedness and loss of consciousness. Although the Valsalva maneuver can be helpful in certain circumstances such as powerlifting, most people should avoid it, particularly those who have hypertension or known cardiovascular disease.

Integration of the Cardiovascular and Respiratory Systems

The cardiovascular and respiratory systems work together to delivery oxygen to the working muscles (see figure 2.4). The muscles extract the oxygen and use it to perform work. To monitor the amount of oxygen used, scientists have developed measures for oxygen consumption during exercise and during recovery from exercise.

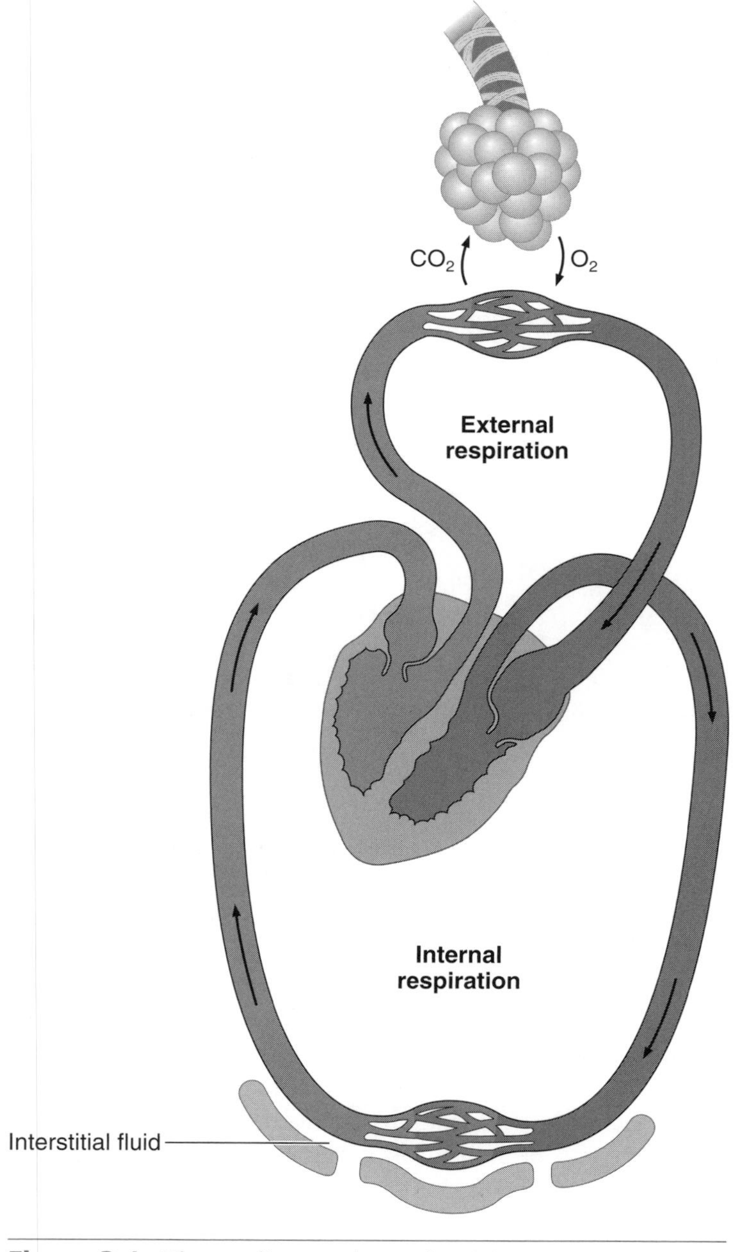

Figure 2.4 The cardiovascular and respiratory systems.

Oxygen Consumption

The amount of oxygen that the body uses is called oxygen consumption. Oxygen consumption, or VO_2, is commonly measured in liters of oxygen consumed per minute (L/min). To obtain a relative value that allows comparison between people of different sizes, this measure can be divided by the body weight and expressed as milliliters of oxygen used per kilogram of body weight (1 kg = 2.2 lb) per minute (ml/kg/min).

The amount of oxygen consumed at rest (for example, sitting and reading this book) is approximately 3.5 ml/kg/min. As the intensity of activity increases, oxygen consumption increases up to maximal levels of approximately 40 ml/kg/min in untrained people to as high as 70 to 90 ml/kg/min in world-class endurance athletes. Maximal oxygen consumption ($\dot{V}O_2$max) varies considerably depending on age, gender, and fitness level. In response to a six-month aerobic training program, $\dot{V}O_2$max will increase approximately 10 to 30 percent depending on initial fitness level, genetic endowment, and training regimen.

Increases in $\dot{V}O_2$max in response to aerobic training are due to several factors. The Fick equation states that $\dot{V}O_2$max is the product of the delivery of oxygen to the body (the cardiac output) and oxygen utilization by the muscles (the arteriovenous oxygen difference).

$$\dot{V}O_2\text{max} = \text{cardiac output (maximal)} \times \text{a-}\bar{v}O_2\text{diff (maximal)}$$

Both of these factors increase in response to aerobic training. Maximal cardiac output, which is the product of maximal stroke volume and maximal heart rate, increases because of increased maximal stroke volume. However, maximal heart rate is related to age and doesn't change with training (MHR = 220 – age). Various adaptations in the muscles contribute to the increase in a-$\bar{v}O_2$diff. These adaptations include an increase in the capillary network within the muscles, which facilitates the distribution of oxygen, as well as an increase in the number of mitochondria, the site of aerobic metabolism within the muscle, and in aerobic enzymes.

Recovery Oxygen Consumption or Excess Post-Oxygen Consumption (EPOC)

At the beginning of exercise, the supply of oxygen cannot meet the demand. This creates an oxygen deficit. During this period, anaerobic (without oxygen) energy sources supply the energy. In aerobic exercise, the body's ability to supply oxygen catches up with the demand. The point at which this happens is called *steady state* and is characterized by a stabilized heart rate. At this level, the body is able to carry on the activity for an extended time. At the end of exercise, the body must "pay back" the earlier deficit, so oxygen consumption remains elevated temporarily until the anaerobic sources used initially are replenished. This elevation in oxygen consumption is referred to as the recovery oxygen consumption or excess post-oxygen consumption (EPOC). See figure 2.5.

METABOLISM

Metabolism is the process by which the body generates the energy it needs for maintenance, repair, and growth of tissues and for muscle contraction and movement. The energy that we need is obtained from the food that we eat. We rely primarily on carbohydrate and fat, but protein can be used as a reserve fuel source during periods of starvation or carbohydrate depletion. When used to generate energy, both carbohydrate and protein yield approximately four calories per gram, whereas fat yields approximately nine calories per gram. A calorie, sometimes referred to as a kilocalorie, is a unit by which the energy in food is measured.

The chemical energy stored in the food that we eat is not directly used to fuel the body, but rather, it is used to generate adenosine triphosphate (ATP), the cell's energy currency. Only a small amount of ATP is stored in the muscle cells. When it is used up, the body regenerates it through the process of metabolism.

When we talk about metabolism, we distinguish two distinct types: aerobic and anaerobic. Aerobic metabolism literally means "with oxygen"; the oxygen supply is equal to the demand. The anaerobic system functions without oxygen and serves as a short-term reserve system.

Most of the time our activities are aerobic. Sitting and reading a book is aerobic, walking is aerobic, jogging for some people is aerobic. However, as the intensity of the activity increases, a point comes when the oxygen delivery to the muscles cannot keep up with the demand. To

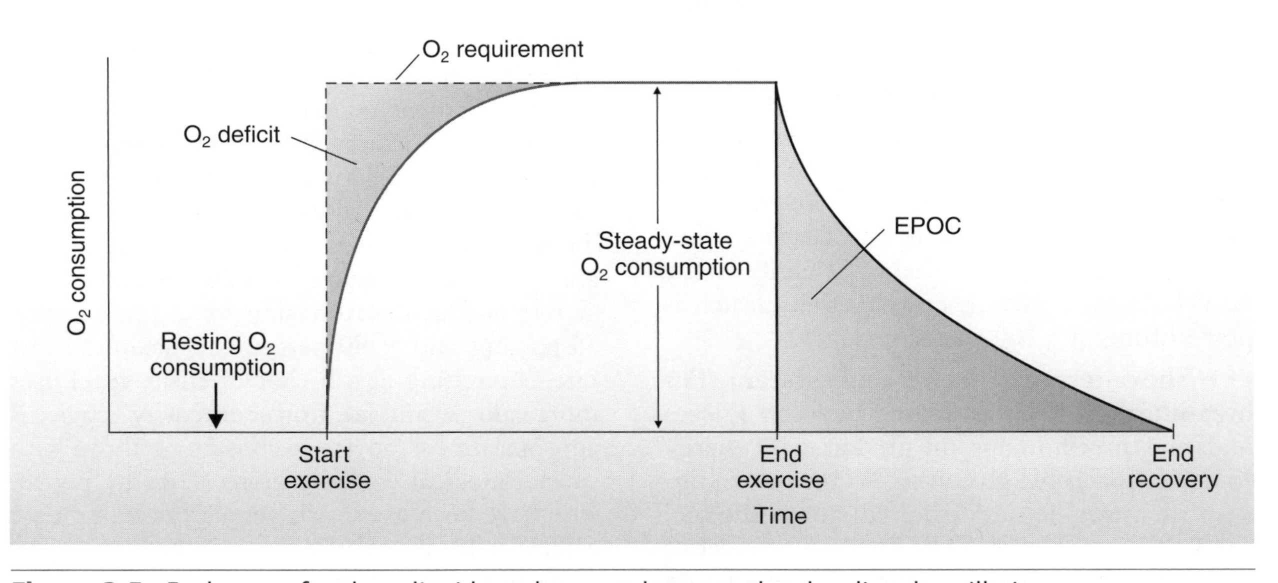

Figure 2.5 Exchange of carbon dioxide and oxygen between the alveoli and capillaries.

compensate, more energy is derived from the anaerobic system, which leads to a buildup of lactic acid. This elevated intensity level can only be maintained for a short time before the buildup of lactic acid forces the individual to slow down and recover.

Let's look at the energy systems our bodies use and how our bodies store unused energy.

Energy Systems

The three main sources of energy in the body are the energy stored in the muscles in the ATP-CP system for immediate use, the lactic-acid system for short-term use, and the aerobic system for long-term use. These three energy systems are integrated and work concurrently. Our bodies shift among them depending upon the intensity and duration of the activity.

Anaerobic Energy Systems

The anaerobic systems serve as short-term reserves; the energy for the first two to three minutes of an aerobic workout is predominantly supplied by anaerobic systems. During this period, an oxygen deficit occurs because the oxygen supply hasn't "caught up" to the demand. After two to three minutes, the oxygen supply catches up and reaches steady state. The oxygen supply is equal to the demand. The two anaerobic systems are these:

- **Immediate, or ATP-CP, system.** As stated earlier, a small amount of ATP and another high-energy compound, creatine phosphate (CP), are stored in the muscles. ATP and CP supply energy initially and for approximately 15 seconds of all-out maximal effort. The stored ATP-CP is used up quickly, and then the body relies on the metabolism of carbohydrate and fat to synthesize more ATP. Activities that rely mainly on the ATP-CP system include power activities such as powerlifting or a 100-meter sprint.
- **Short-term, or lactic-acid, system.** For high-intensity activities lasting between 15 seconds and three minutes, the predominant energy source is anaerobic glycolysis. As the name suggests, it uses glucose (carbohydrate) as the fuel source for generating ATP. The end product of anaerobic glycolysis is lactic acid. Accumulation of lactic acid in the muscle leads to momentary muscle fatigue, "the burn." Stopping the activity or lowering the intensity facilitates the removal and recycling of lactic acid. With training, the body becomes better equipped to handle lactic acid. Depending on the specific type of training, adaptations occur that decrease the production of lactic acid, increase its removal from the blood stream, and increase the tolerance (the buffering capacity) of the muscle.

Aerobic Energy System

The aerobic energy system is also called the oxidative system. This is the long-term energy system that takes over energy production after approximately three minutes of activity. It is fueled by a mixture of carbohydrate (glucose) and fat, which varies depending on the intensity and duration of the activity. Activities using the aerobic energy system, such as a three-mile walk or jog, are characterized by submaximal exertion. In aerobic metabolism, oxygen is necessary. When you generate energy aerobically from carbohydrate and fat, you end up with carbon and hydrogen molecules. These must be removed from the body. Oxygen acts as the terminal receptor of these molecules, binding with carbon to form carbon dioxide and with hydrogen to form water. These byproducts are then transported through the blood stream to the lungs, where they are removed.

One common fallacy is that low-intensity aerobic exercise more effectively burns calories, particularly those from fat, than higher-intensity aerobic exercise. Although it is true that the percent contribution of fat decreases with increasing intensities of exercise, higher-intensity aerobic activity uses more total calories and, therefore, uses more total fat calories. Table 2.1 shows the comparison of fat utilization and caloric expenditure for a 200-pound person at rest and while exercising for 30 minutes at 55 percent and at 80 percent of maximal heart rate. Exercising at a higher intensity level uses more calories and fat. Lower-intensity activity is appropriate for novice exercisers or those with special medical considerations. Healthy people who have been exercising regularly can increase caloric expenditure by increasing the intensity or using interval training.

Energy Storage

The food we eat is digested and broken into its basic components: carbohydrate to glucose, fat to fatty acids, and protein to amino acids. These are absorbed and circulated throughout the body. If needed, they are used immediately to generate energy; if not, they are stored for later use as follows:

- **Glucose** can be stored as glycogen in the liver and the muscles, but these storage compartments are very limited. When they are completely filled, excess glucose is converted to triglyceride (fat) and stored in the adipose tissue.
- **Fat** is stored in small amounts in the muscle as intramuscular triglyceride, but most of the excess is stored in the adipose tissue.
- **Protein** that isn't needed for growth and repair of cells and tissues is converted to triglyceride and stored in the adipose tissue.

Table 2.2 shows an example of where the body stores fuel and energy. The body runs most efficiently on a mixture of carbohydrate and fat. Because carbohydrate stores are limited, they can be depleted by endurance or strength training workouts lasting more than an hour. Glycogen depletion, referred to by athletes as "hitting the wall" or "bonking," is a major cause of fatigue and exhaustion. Thus, before events, many athletes will practice carbohydrate loading by consuming larger-than-usual amounts of carbohydrates in an attempt to temporarily maximize their glycogen stores.

Table 2.1 Comparison of Fat Utilization and Caloric Expenditure for a 200-lb Person

% of HRmax	% fat	% carbohydrate	Total cal/30 min	Fat cal/30 min
Rest	60	40	50 cal	30 cal
55	50	50	225 cal	112 cal
80	40	60	315 cal	126 cal

Table 2.2 Body Stores of Fuel and Energy

Carbohydrate stores	Cal	Fat stores	Cal
Liver glycogen	451	Adipose tissue	70,980
Muscle glycogen	1,025	Intramuscular	1,465
Total glycogen	1,476	Total fat	72,445

These estimates are based on body weight of 65 kg (143 lb) with 12% body fat.

CHAPTER 3

Cardiorespiratory Fitness and Exercise

Ralph La Forge, M.S.

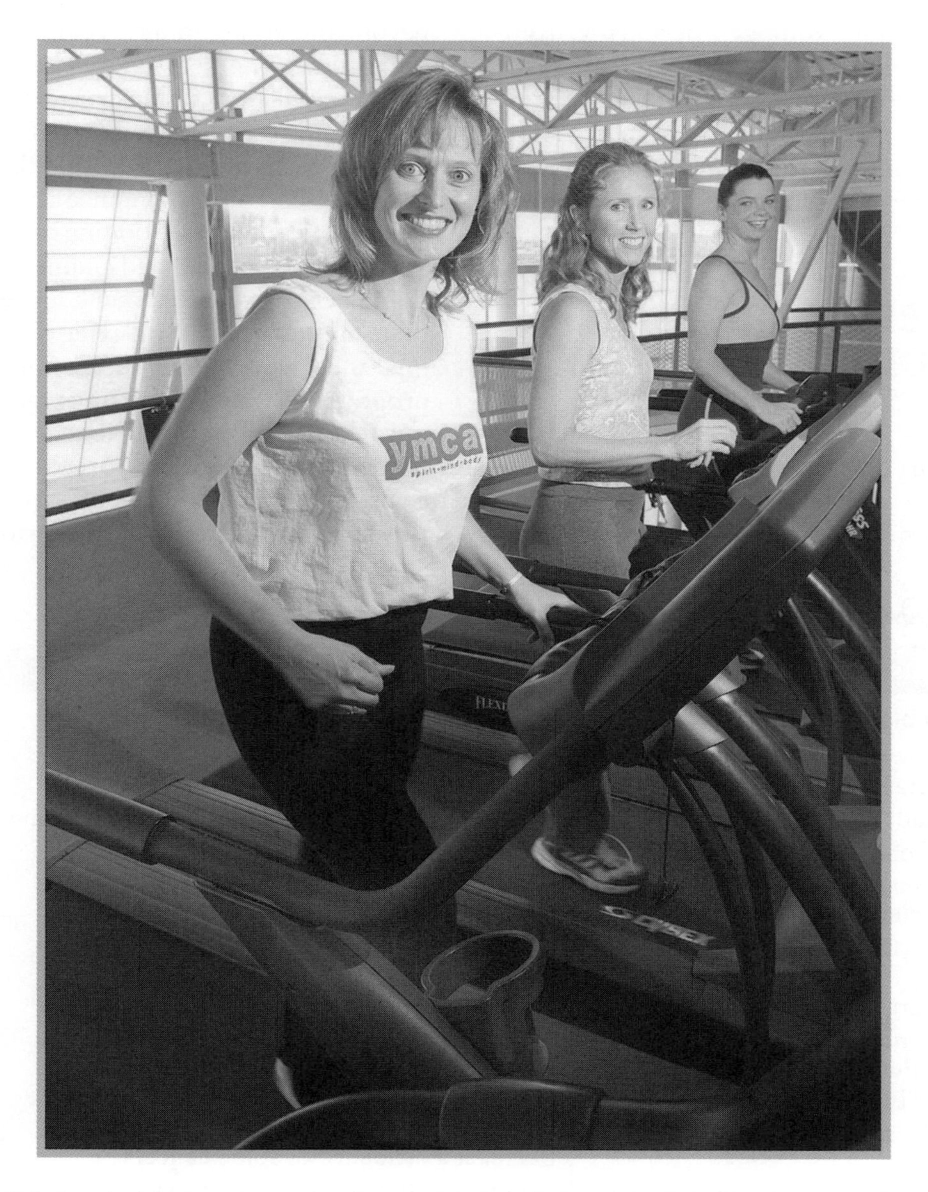

Ralph La Forge, M.S., is a physiologist and managing director of the Duke Lipid and Metabolic Disorder Training Program, Duke University Medical Center, Endocrine Division, Durham, NC. He has worked for 25 years in clinical cardiology/endocrinology and as an instructor of exercise physiology at the University of California, San Diego. La Forge has authored more than 300 consumer and professional publications on cardiovascular disease management, applied exercise science, and preventive cardiology and is the exercise science research editor for IDEA Health & Fitness Source. He has helped organize and inaugurate cardiovascular disease risk reduction and preventive endocrinology programs for more than 450 healthcare institutions and medical groups throughout the United States, including the Department of Defense.

Cardiorespiratory fitness is an essential component of physical fitness and has grown to receive equal acclaim for improving cardiovascular health in both primary and secondary prevention. For health and fitness applications, the terms cardiorespiratory fitness, cardiovascular fitness, and aerobic endurance fitness are synonymous. Cardiorespiratory fitness best describes the health and function of the heart, lungs, and circulatory system and is related to cardiorespiratory endurance, which is the ability to persist or sustain activity for prolonged periods. Cardiorespiratory fitness also describes the capacity of the lungs to exchange oxygen and carbon dioxide with the blood and the circulatory system's ability to transport blood and nutrients to metabolically active tissues for sustained periods without undue fatigue.

BENEFITS OF CARDIORESPIRATORY FITNESS

The numerous benefits of cardiorespiratory fitness (table 3.1) are related to a variety of adaptive physiologic responses to aerobic exercise. Physiologic responses to training—such as an increase in body-fat utilization, a decrease in **peripheral vascular resistance,** and an increase in **maximal oxygen consumption**—help decrease the risk of cardiovascular disease and diabetes by favorably modifying **risk factors** like **obesity, hypertension,** insulin resistance, and elevated **triglycerides** and **LDL cholesterol.** When such risk factors are removed from clients' health profiles, the clients can attain an acceptable level of cardiovascular health. Cardiovascular health goes beyond merely attaining aerobic fitness. It defines the status of the heart muscle, its blood vessels, and the circulatory system it serves. Acquiring and maintaining cardiorespiratory fitness is one of the primary pathways to cardiovascular health.

Likewise, aerobic endurance activities have been effective in other conditioning and clinical therapies, such as cardiac and pulmonary rehabilitation, sleep disorder treatment, diabetic treatment, prenatal/post-partum and renal dialysis conditioning, and anxiety- and depression-management programs. In clinical settings, aerobic exercise must be prescribed and managed carefully by trained exercise specialists or other qualified clinicians. Experienced and qualified personal trainers may form adjunct relationships with clinicians to

Table 3.1 Reported Benefits of Cardiorespiratory Exercise Training

Health benefits	Adaptive physiologic responses
Reduction in blood pressure	Increased lactate threshold
Increased HDL cholesterol	Decreased resting heart rate
Decreased total cholesterol	Increased heart volume
Decreased body fat stores	Increased resting and maximum stroke volume
Increased aerobic work capacity	Increased maximum cardiac output
Decreased clinical symptoms of anxiety, tension, and depression	Increased maximum oxygen consumption
Reduction in glucose-stimulated insulin secretion	Increased capillary density and blood flow to active muscles
Increased heart function	Increased total blood volume
Reduction in mortality in post-myocardial infarction patients	Increased maximal ventilation
Prevention of type 2 diabetes	Increased lung diffusion capacity
Adaptive physiologic responses	Increased mobilization and utilization of fat
	Reduced all-cause mortality
	Decreased anxiety and depression
	Decreased incidence of some cancers
	Improved arterial endothelial function
	Increased insulin sensitivity

Adapted, by permission, from American College of Sports Medicine, 2000, *ACSM's guidelines for exercise testing and prescription*, 6th ed. (Philadelphia, PA: Lippincott, Williams & Wilkins).

effectively manage the patient. Referrals from such programs depend on your relationship and knowledge of local clinical rehabilitation programs or affiliated healthcare institutions.

Cardiorespiratory fitness also serves as a foundation for other fitness programs. The conditioning and health of the heart, lungs, and blood vessels are prime ingredients in the safety and performance of nearly all sports and recreational programs. Activities such as tennis, golf, skiing, dancing, skating, basketball, volleyball, boxing, and nearly all muscular strength-training programs will benefit from attaining acceptable levels of cardiorespiratory fitness. Clients with adequate cardiorespiratory fitness generally have more stamina, which translates to less fatigue and fewer risks for certain types of injuries.

COMPONENTS OF AN AEROBIC EXERCISE PROGRAM

It is imperative for you to understand the physiologic rationale and application of each component of the cardiorespiratory exercise program.

The essential components of the written plan are:

1. Warm-up and cool-down
2. Primary cardiorespiratory activity criteria:
   a. Mode of exercise
   b. Frequency of exercise session
   c. Duration of exercise session
   d. Intensity of exercise session
3. Supportive conditioning exercise (e.g., strength and flexibility)
4. Progression plan
5. Safety and cautions

Each of these components must be discussed with the client and presented in a legible and succinct written form.

Warm-up and Cool-down

Although most fitness professionals teach a variety of warm-up and cool-down techniques, few fully understand their physiological and psychological rationales (table 3.2). Graduated low-level aerobic exercise is essential for maximizing safety and economy of movement during the cardiorespiratory conditioning phase of an exercise session. The warm-up should gradually increase the heart rate, blood pressure, oxygen consumption, dilation of the blood vessels, elasticity of the active muscles, and the heat produced by the active muscle groups. The warm-up should consist of two distinct components:

1. Graduated aerobic warm-up activity (e.g., walking or slow-tempo rhythmic calisthenic movements)
2. Flexibility exercise specific to the biomechanical nature of the primary conditioning activity (e.g., calf, quadriceps, and Achilles stretching prior to running or hiking).

Because a warm muscle is more easily stretched than a cold muscle, the flexibility component should be preceded by five to eight minutes of low-level aerobic activity using the same muscle groups. For instance, a 10-minute walk will increase muscle temperature and circulation of the legs, thereby promoting easier and safer stretching of the same muscle groups.

Table 3.3 on page 25 lists sample warm-up and cool-down activities for a variety of aerobic exercises. The intensity of the warm-up should be well below that of the primary conditioning activity. The warm-up duration depends on the level and intensity of the primary conditioning activity, as well as the fitness level of the client.

The cool-down is an integral part of the exercise program. The purpose of the cool-down is to slowly decrease the heart rate and overall metabolism, both of which have been elevated during the conditioning phase. Low-level aerobic exercise, similar to that of the conditioning exercise, is recommended (see table 3.3). Walking, slow jogging, cycling with little or no resistance, and slow aquatic activity or swimming are good examples. Cool-down helps prevent the sudden pooling of blood in the veins and ensures adequate circulation to the skeletal muscles, heart, and brain. Cool-down may aid in preventing delayed muscle stiffness and reduces

Table 3.2 Physiological and Psychological Rationale for Warm-up and Cool-down

Warm-up
1. Permits a gradual metabolic adaptation (e.g., oxygen consumption), which enhances cardiorespiratory performance (e.g., a higher maximum cardiac output and oxygen uptake)
2. Prevents the premature onset of blood lactic acid accumulation and fatigue during higher level aerobic exercise
3. Causes a gradual increase in muscle temperature, which decreases the work of contraction and reduces the likelihood of muscle injury
4. Facilitates neural transmission for motor unit recruitment
5. Improves coronary blood flow in early stages of the conditioning exercise, lessening the potential for myocardial ischemia
6. Allows a gradual redistribution of blood flow to active muscles
7. Increases the elasticity of connective tissue and other muscle components
8. Provides a screening mechanism for potential musculoskeletal or metabolic problems that may increase at higher intensities
9. Provides a psychological warm-up to higher levels of work (i.e., increases arousal and focus on exercise)
Cool-down
1. Prevents postexercise venous blood pooling and too rapid a drop in blood pressure, thereby reducing the likelihood of postexercise lightheadedness or fainting
2. Reduces the immediate postexercise tendency for muscle spasm or cramping
3. Reduces the concentration of exercise hormones (e.g., norepinephrine) that are at relatively high levels immediately after vigorous aerobic exercise. This reduction will lower the probability of postexercise disturbances in cardiac rhythm

Adapted, by permission, from American College of Sports Medicine, 2000, *ACSM's guidelines for exercise testing and prescription*, 6th ed. (Philadelphia, PA: Lippincott, Williams & Wilkins).

any tendency toward postexercise fainting and dizziness. For high cardiovascular risk clients, a gradual decrease in the intensity of exercise is crucial. Sudden cessation of exercise without cool-down may adversely affect cardiac function because a relatively high concentration of adrenaline remains in the blood from the conditioning exercise. Sudden exercise cessation also may adversely affect filling pressures of the heart, putting a weak heart at risk. The length of the cool-down phase is proportional to the intensity and length of the conditioning phase. A typical 30- to 40-minute conditioning phase at 70% of maximum heart rate would warrant a 5- to 10-minute cool-down. The aerobic component of the cool-down phase should be followed by several minutes of stretching those muscle groups active in the conditioning phase.

Primary Cardiorespiratory Exercise Criteria

For maximum effectiveness and safety, the cardiorespiratory exercise program must include specific instructions on the mode, frequency, duration, and intensity of exercise. Most of these criteria originate from the American College of Sports Medicine (ACSM) exercise guidelines and position statements to ensure standardization and validity in the broad field of exercise science (American College of Sports Medicine 2000).

To avoid confusion, the exercise criteria listed in this section are those needed for measurable improvements in cardiorespiratory fitness (e.g., increase in **$\dot{V}O_2$max**). This is an important clarification because the exercise threshold criteria for health enhancement are generally lower (Ameri-

Table 3.3 Sample Warm-Up and Cool-Down Activities (Including Stretching Exercise)

Primary conditioning exercise	Warm-up/cool-down activity
Aerobics (group exercise)	Graduated low-level aerobic activity utilizing same muscle groups
Circuit weight training	Low-level aerobic activity (e.g., walking or cycling, and/or beginning the circuit training session with a set of relatively high-repetition, low-resistance exercises)
Hiking	Graduate from relatively flat terrain at minimal altitudes to steeper terrain and higher altitudes
Jogging and running	Walking, walk-jogging, or jogging at a slower pace
Outdoor cycling	Begin with relatively flat terrain in lower gears; gradually shift to higher gears and steeper terrain
Racquetball, handball, or squash	Walk-jog and/or graduated tempo volleying
Rope skipping	Graduated walking or walk-jogging pace and/or slow tempo rope-skipping pace
Sprinting	Jogging and graduated pace in running intervals
Stationary cycling	Start with cycling against little or no resistance at 2/3 of the pedal crank rpm used in the conditioning phase
Stationary exercise devices	Begin with 50 to 60% of intended conditioning workload or speed; the duration of submaximal graduated warm-up should be proportional to the peak intensity of the conditioning work load
Stepping/standing exercise (e.g., stair climber, elliptical crosstrainer)	Low-level aerobic activity (e.g., walking or cycling and/or relatively low-tempo step exercise)
Swimming	Begin with slow crawl and gradually increase arm stroke and pace, and/or begin with short one- or two-lap slow intervals
Tennis (competitive)	Walk-jog and/or graduated tempo volleying proportional to the level of the game

can College of Sports Medicine 2000; Haskell 1994). For instance, the minimum duration and intensity of physical activity required for health enhancement is 15 minutes at 40% of $\dot{V}O_2$max. Here, health enhancement refers to reduced risk of degenerative disease, such as cardiovascular disease and diabetes.

Exercise Mode

Selection of the exercise mode is made on the basis of the client's **functional capacity,** interests, time availability, equipment and facilities, and personal goals. Any activity that uses large muscle groups, is rhythmical and cardiorespiratory in nature, and is maintained continuously can be used. The American College of Sports Medicine classifies **cardiorespiratory endurance** activities into three groups:

GROUP 1: Physical activities in which exercise intensity is easily maintained at a constant level, and interindividual variation in energy expenditure is relatively low. Examples are walking and cycling, especially treadmill and cycle ergometry.

GROUP 2: Physical activities in which energy expenditure is related to skill, but for a given individual can provide a constant intensity: aerobic dance, aerobic step exercise, slide exercise, swimming, skating, and cross-country skiing.

GROUP 3: Physical activities that are quite variable in both skill and intensity: soccer, basketball, and racquet sports.

Group 1 activities are recommended when precise control of the exercise intensity is necessary, as in the beginning stages of a conditioning program. These activities can be performed in a continuous or discontinuous (interval) format, depending upon the client's fitness level and personal preference, and are useful during all stages of conditioning. Group 2 activities are useful because of the enjoyment provided by group exercise and settings other than an exercise gym. Adding Group 2 exercise to a training program helps foster compliance and reduce boredom. Because of the skill and variable intensity nature of Group 3 activities, they require a base level of conditioning using Group 1 activities. Group 3 activities tend to be group- or team-sport oriented and, therefore, provide greater interest and compliance for many individuals. Group 3 activities should be cautiously considered for high-risk, deconditioned, or symptomatic individuals.

Exercise Frequency

Frequency refers to the number of exercise sessions per week included in the program. The frequency of exercise depends on the duration and intensity of the exercise session. Lower-intensity exercise performed for shorter periods can warrant more sessions per week. To improve both cardiorespiratory fitness and maintain body fat at near-optimum levels, a client should exercise at least three days per week with no more than two days between sessions. The American College of Sports Medicine recommends three to five days per week for most aerobic programs. When a client starts an aerobic exercise program, exercising every other day for at least the first eight weeks is appropriate. For those with a poor functional capacity, one to two daily sessions may be recommended. Those with an average functional capacity should exercise at least three times per week on alternate days. In general, clients who are just beginning weightbearing exercise, such as traditional aerobics, step training, and jogging, should have at least 36 to 48 hours of rest between workouts to prevent **overuse injuries** and promote adequate bone/joint stress recovery. This is especially true with those who are overweight.

Exercise Duration

Duration refers to the number of minutes of exercise during the conditioning period. The conditioning period, exclusive of the warm-up and cool-down, may vary from as little as 5 to 60 or more minutes. The duration required for cardiorespiratory benefits is dependent upon the exercise intensity. Take a given intensity of exercise, for example 75% of functional capacity, and compare it to an exercise duration of 5 minutes versus 20 minutes at this intensity. Obviously, more total energy is expended during the 20-minute exercise session.

The conditioning response to an exercise session is the result of the product of the intensity and duration of exercise (total energy expenditure). Beginners who are in the lower cardiorespiratory fitness classifications should begin with 10 to 20 minutes of aerobic conditioning. Very deconditioned individuals may be more suited for multiple sessions of short duration, such as 5 to 10 minutes. Those in the average classification should go for 15 to 45 minutes, and those in the high fitness classification can go for 30 to 60 minutes.

Intensity of Exercise

Intensity refers to the speed or exercise workload. The American College of Sports Medicine (2000) recommends an intensity range of 55 to 90% of **maximum heart rate**, or between 40 and 85% of **heart-rate reserve** or **oxygen uptake reserve ($\dot{V}O_2R$).** The $\dot{V}O_2R$ is the difference between $\dot{V}O_2max$ and resting $\dot{V}O_2$. It is important to see that the 55 to 90% of maximum heartrate range approximates 40 to 85% of what was formerly referred to as $\dot{V}O_2max$ but now is oxygen uptake reserve ($\dot{V}O_2R$). It is important for you to understand that for any given percentage of maximum oxygen uptake, except for maximum exercise intensities, the percentage of maximum heart rate will be somewhat higher (table 3.4).

From a physiologic point of view, this 50 to 85% of maximum oxygen uptake range is the goal for cardiorespiratory training benefits. Lower intensities, such as 50 to 60% of maximal oxygen consumption and **heart-rate maximum reserve,** are advised for beginners in the lower cardiorespiratory fitness levels. Persons with very low fitness levels, however, can benefit from training intensities as low as 40 to 50% of maximal oxygen uptake. Exercise intensities as high as 75 to 85% of maximal oxygen uptake and heart-rate reserve may be more appropriate for those who are apparently healthy and in the higher fitness classifications. Overall, the average

Table 3.4 **Classification of Physical Activity Intensity**

	Relative intensity			Absolute intensity in healthy adults, METs*			
				Age			
Intensity	O_2max, %	Maximum heart rate, %	RPE†	(20–39)	(40–64)	(65–79)	(80+)
Very light	<20	<35	<10	<2.4	<2.0	<1.6	<1.0
Light	20–39	35–54	10–11	2.4–4.7	2.0–3.9	1.6–3.1	1.1–1.9
Moderate	40–59	55–69	12–13	4.8–7.1	4.0–5.9	3.2–4.7	2.0–2.9
Hard	60–84	70–89	14–16	7.2–10.1	6.0–8.4	4.8–6.7	3.0–4.25
Very hard	>85	>90	17–19	>10.2	>8.5	>6.8	>4.25
Maximum	100	100	20	12.0‡	10.0‡	8.0‡	5.0‡

*Based on 8 to 12 repetitions for persons <50–60 years old and 10 to 15 repetitions for persons >50–60 years

†Borg rating of Relative Perceived Exertion (RPE), 6–20 scale.

‡Maximum values are mean values achieved during maximum exercise by healthy adults. Absolute intensity values are approximate mean values for men.

Mean values for women are 1 to 2 METs lower than those for men.

Adapted, by permission, from American Heart Association, 2001, "Exercise standards for testing and training," *Circulation*, 104: 1694.

exercise intensity for apparently healthy adults is usually between 60 and 70% of their maximum oxygen uptake.

Table 3.4 classifies and compares age-related relative exercise intensity (% of $\dot{V}O_2$max or heart-rate max) to absolute exercise intensity (actual or estimated MET cost). This classification system is important for the personal trainer to learn because it establishes a common exercise intensity language with other trainers and healthcare professionals.

Exercise Intensity and Health-Related Outcomes

Years of research on exercise and health has made it clear that such health-related outcomes as increased HDL cholesterol, decreased blood pressure, improved glucose tolerance, reduced blood clotting tendency (fibrinolysis), reduced anxiety, and decreased risk of cardiovascular disease, diabetes, and all-cause mortality can result from moderate intensities of exercise (i.e., 40 to 60% of maximum oxygen uptake). In some cases, even lower intensities are recommended (Blair et al. 1995). Employing exercise intensities as low as 30% of $\dot{V}O_2$max, the diabetes prevention program (DPP) demonstrated a 58% reduction in type 2 diabetes in glucose intolerant obese individuals (Diabetes Prevention Program Research Group 2002). The volume of exercise attained in this three-year study was just 700–900 kcal/week.

Monitoring Exercise Intensity

Of the numerous methods for monitoring exercise intensity, five have been somewhat standardized and are recommended for the personal trainer. The method you choose will depend on your client's exercise program and level of fitness, your access to exercise test data (e.g., treadmill stress test heart rates, work loads, functional capacity), and your experience. The following are the primary methods of monitoring exercise intensity:

1. Heart Rate
    a. Percentage of maximal heart rate
    b. Percentage of heart-rate reserve
2. Rating of perceived exertion
3. The "talk test" method
4. METs

Percentage of Maximal Heart Rate

This method of monitoring intensity of exercise calculates the exercise heart rate as a percentage of maximal heart rate. Maximal heart rate can be determined by a maximal functional capacity test, using a bicycle or treadmill ergometer, or by age-predicted maximal heart-rate tables, which frequently use the 220-minus-age formula. If this method of estimating maximal heart rate is used, the following formula applies:

Training Heart Rate = maximal measured or predicted heart rate × 60 to 90% (desired percent of maximal HR)

For example:
A 40-year-old man for whom an intensity of 70% of maximal heart rate is desired:

220 – 40 = 180 (predicted max HR)

180 (predicted max HR) × 0.70 (70% exercise intensity) =126 (exercise HR)

You should use caution when using age group average maximal heart-rate tables because these tables only estimate a "rule of thumb" maximal heart rate, usually from the "220-minus-age" formula. This method has a variability of plus or minus 10 to 12 beats per minute (Durstine & Pate 1993). In addition, women generally have a higher heart-rate response than men to the same absolute work output. Research has also demonstrated that older individuals (older than age 65) may have significantly higher maximal heart rates than predicted by the 220-minus-age formula (Whaley et al. 1992).

It is essential for you to understand the relationship between exercise heart rate and aerobic capacity (maximal oxygen consumption). An important point is often overlooked in aerobic exercise: For nearly all levels of submaximal exercise, the percentage of heart-rate maximum does not equal the same percentage of aerobic capacity unless the heart-rate maximum reserve method **(Karvonen formula)** is used. As described in table 3.4, for any given percentage of maximal heart rate, the corresponding percentage of maximal oxygen consumption (aerobic capacity) is 5 to 10% less.

Percentage of Heart-rate Reserve (Karvonen Formula)

The heart-rate reserve method is similar to the percentage of maximal heart-rate method, except resting heart rate is factored in:

Training Heart Rate = maximum heart rate – resting heart rate × desired intensity (50 to 85%) + resting heart rate

For example: What is the target heart rate for a 40-year-old client with a resting heart rate of 80 bpm at an intensity of 70%?

THR = (maximum HR – RHR) × intensity + RHR

220 – 40 = 180 (predicted maximum HR)

180 (predicted maximum HR) – 80 (RHR) = 100 (heart-rate reserve) × 0.70 (70% intensity) = 70

70 + 80 (RHR) = 150 (target HR at 70% of heart-rate reserve)

Maximum Heart Rate: How Useful Is the Prediction Equation?

Two methods exist for determining maximum heart rate (MHR). The most accurate way is to directly measure the MHR with an EKG monitoring device during a graded exercise test. The other way is to estimate MHR by using a simple prediction equation or formula. In 1970, the formula "220 – age" was introduced and was widely accepted by the health and fitness community. Recently, however, the validity of the formula has come under attack for several reasons. The subjects used in the study to determine the formula were not representative of the general population. In addition, even if the prediction equation did represent a reasonable average, a significant percentage of individuals will not fit the average. In fact, standard deviations of plus or minus 10 to 20 beats per minute have been observed. Consequently, basing a client's exercise intensity (i.e., training heart rate) on a potentially flawed estimation of MHR is somewhat dubious. When the training heart rate is based on an estimated MHR, it should be used in combination with the perceived exertion scale (see table 3.5). Modify the intensity of the workout if your client reports a high level of perceived exertion, even if his or her training heart rate has not been achieved.

Note that this exercise heart rate of 150 bpm is 24 bpm higher than the straight percentage of maximum heart-rate method illustrated previously. Therefore, you must be careful when recommending exercise intensity using only the heart-rate reserve (Karvonen) method.

The physiological basis for the heart-rate reserve method is that the difference between resting and maximal heart rates for a given client represents the reserve of the heart for increasing cardiac output. Like the percentage of maximal heart-rate method, the accuracy of the Karvonen formula is somewhat compromised when the predicted maximal heart rate is estimated from tables or 220-minus-age rather than determined from an actual functional capacity test. Still, this method is one of the most popular for determining exercise heart rates.

Rating of Perceived Exertion

Exercise intensity also can be measured by assigning a numerical value (6 to 20 or 0 to 10) to subjective feelings of exercise exertion. The popular name for this method is the **ratings of perceived exertion (RPE)**. Originally designed by Dr. Gunnar Borg, it is sometimes called the Borg Scale. RPE takes into account all that the exercising client is perceiving in terms of exercise fatigue, including psychological, musculoskeletal, and environmental factors. The RPE response also correlates very well with cardiorespiratory and metabolic factors such as heart rate, breathing rate, oxygen consumption, and overall fatigue. This level of perceived physical effort is assigned a rating from either of the two rating scales in table 3.5. For instance, using the Borg Scale, an RPE of 12 to 13 corresponds to approximately 55 to 69% of maximal heart rate, or 50 to 74% of maximal oxygen consumption or heart rate reserve (see table 3.4). An RPE of 16 would correspond to about 90% of maximal heart rate or 85% of maximal oxygen consumption or heart-rate reserve. Thus, as a rule, most clients would exercise between 12 and 16 on the Borg Scale. The Borg Scale begins at 6 because originally it was used to approximate exercise heart rate. For example, an RPE of 6 would approximate a heart rate of 60; an RPE of 15 would approximate a heart rate of 150.

In recent years, a revised Borg Scale (see the Category Ratio Scale in table 3.5) has made it easier to use because of its simpler 0 to 10 rating. On this revised RPE Scale, a client should exercise between an RPE of 4 (somewhat strong) and an RPE of 5 or 6 (strong) (Carlton & Rhodes, 1985). Perhaps the most appropriate use of RPE is as an adjunct to heart-rate monitoring. Ideally, the trainer or exercising client will monitor and record both intensities to ensure close observation of the cardiac and physiological exercise response.

Dishman and colleagues believe that the standard scales can be prone to error, and have been researching an alternative approach known as "preferred exertion" (Dishman, Farquhar, & Cureton 1994). In this method, the exercisers self-select exercise intensity (e.g., power output on a stationary cycle) according to their own volition, as long as the selected intensity is within an effective exercise intensity range. It has been

Table 3.5 Ratings of Perceived Exertion

RPE	Category ratio scale
6	0 Nothing at all
7 Very, very light	0.5 Very, very weak
8	1 Very weak
9 Very light	2 Weak
10	3 Moderate
11 Fairly light	4 Somewhat strong
12	5 Strong
13 Somewhat hard	6
14	7 Very strong
15 Hard	8
16	9
17 Very hard	10 Very, very strong
18	* Maximal
19 Very, very hard	
20	

Adapted, by permission, from American College of Sports Medicine, 2000, *ACSM's guidelines for exercise testing and prescription*, 6th ed. (Philadelphia, PA: Lippincott, Williams & Wilkins).

suggested that complementary use of "preferred intensities" may be safer and may better promote long-term exercise adherence than a strict exercise program based on more precise physiological criteria, especially if those criteria conflict with a person's intensity preference.

The Talk-Test Method

Another means of evaluating the intensity of exercise is the talk test. Like the RPE method, the talk test is subjective, but it is quite useful in determining a "comfort zone" of aerobic intensity. Clients should be able to breathe comfortably and rhythmically throughout all phases of a workout to ensure a safe and comfortable level of exercise, especially for those just beginning an exercise program. Those who progress to higher functional capacities and higher-level workouts may find this technique somewhat conservative, especially at intensities greater than 80% of functional capacity.

In summary, you can modify criteria such as the mode, frequency, duration, and intensity of exercise to suit the client's level of fitness, program goals, and schedule. As a rule, however, building a foundation of endurance at a relatively low-to-moderate intensity prior to performing higher-intensity workouts or competition is clearly justified for safety and comfort. This may mean moving the client, for the first few weeks, through gradual increases in duration, while holding intensity nearly constant until an acceptable level of endurance, such as 20 to 30 minutes, has been achieved. Within each of these criteria, you have an enormous range of choices, such as variations in modes and intensities, with which to vary the exercise stimulus and maximize the client's interest and adaptation to increasing levels of exercise.

Intensity Measured by METs

Exercise intensity can be assessed by a graded exercise test (bicycle or treadmill) (table 3.6). Based on the time the client stays on the treadmill or bicycle ergometer, the maximal oxygen consumption (i.e., aerobic or functional capacity) can be estimated and converted to a **MET** equivalent. A MET is a multiple of resting oxygen consumption. One MET equals a person's oxygen uptake at rest, which is equal to approximately 3.5 milliliters of oxygen per kilogram of body weight per minute (3.5 mL/kg/min). The intensity of exercise may be determined as a specified percentage of the client's maximal oxygen consumption or functional capacity (e.g., 50 to 85%), and then choosing activities that are known to require energy expenditure at the desired level (table 3.7). For example, if a client has a functional capacity of 10 METs and you recommend he or she begins at 60% of functional capacity, then 60% times 10 METs equals 6 METs beginning intensity.

10 METs (functional or aerobic capacity) × 0.60 (60% recommended exercise intensity) = 6 METs (beginning exercise intensity)

Table 3.6 Training Method Selection

Cardiorespiratory fitness level	Aerobic capacity (METs)	Training method
Poor	1–3.9	Low-level (2–3 METs) aerobic interval training
Low	4–6.9	Aerobic interval training at 3–5 METs
Average	7–10.9	Aerobic interval training at 6–8 METs; continuous training at 5–8 METs
Good	11–13.9	Aerobic interval training at 9–12 METs; continuous training at 8–12 METs; aerobic composite training at 8–12 METs; moderate anaerobic interval training
High	14+	Aerobic interval training at 10–13+ METs; continuous training at 9–13+ METs; aerobic composite training at 9–13+ METs; anaerobic or Fartlek training

Table 3.7 Leisure Activities in METs: Sports, Exercise Classes, Games, Dancing

	Mean	Range
Archery	3.9	3–4
Backpacking	—	5–11
Badminton	5.8	4–9+
Basketball		
Game play	8.3	7–12+
Nongame play	—	3–9
Billiards	2.5	—
Bowling	—	2–4
Boxing		
In-ring	13.3	—
Sparring	8.3	—
Canoeing, rowing, and kayaking	—	3–8
Conditioning exercise	—	3–8+
Climbing hills	7.2	5–10+
Cricket	5.2	4–8
Croquet	3.5	—
Cycling		
Pleasure or to work	—	3–8+
10 mph	7.0	—
Dancing (social, square, tap)	—	3–8
Dancing (aerobic)	—	6–9
Fencing	—	6–10+
Field hockey	8.0	—
Fishing		
From bank	3.7	2–4
Wading in stream	—	5–6
Football (touch)	7.9	6–10
Golf		
Power cart	—	2–3
Walking (carrying bag or pulling cart)	5.1	4–7
Handball	—	8–12+
Hiking (cross-country)	—	3–7
Horseback riding		
Galloping	8.2	—
Trotting	6.6	—
Walking	2.4	—
Horseshoe pitching	—	2–3
Hunting (bow or gun)		
Small game (walking, carrying light load)	—	3–7
Big game (dragging carcass, walking)	—	3–14
Judo	13.5	—
Mountain climbing	—	5–10+
Music playing	—	2–3
Paddleball, racquetball	9	8–12
Rope jumping	11	—
60–80 skips/min	9	—
120–140 skips/min	—	11–12
Running		
12 min per mile	8.7	—
11 min per mile	9.4	—
10 min per mile	10.2	—
9 min per mile	11.2	—
8 min per mile	12.5	—
7 min per mile	14.1	—
6 min per mile	16.3	—
Sailing	—	2–5
Scuba diving	—	5–10
Shuffleboard	—	2–3
Skating, ice and roller	—	5–8
Skiing, snow		
Downhill	—	5–8
Cross-country	—	6–12+
Skiing, water	—	5–7
Sledding, tobogganing	—	4–8
Snowshoeing	9.9	7–14
Squash	—	8–12+
Soccer	—	5–12+
Stair climbing	—	4–8
Swimming	—	4–8+
Table tennis	4.1	3–5
Tennis	6.5	4–9+
Volleyball	—	3–6

Reprinted, by permission, from American College of Sports Medicine, 2000, *ACSM's guidelines for exercise testing and prescription*, 6th ed. (Philadelphia, PA: Lippincott, Williams & Wilkins).

Exercise intensity determined by METs has some disadvantages. Environmental influences such as wind, hills, heat, humidity, altitude, air pollution, and a variety of mechanical factors, such as the mechanical efficiency of a bicycle, can alter the energy cost of the activity. In addition, as the client improves cardiorespiratory endurance, higher MET levels will be required to ensure an adequate training stimulus. As a rule, training by heart rate and perceived exertion may be an easier and more accurate method for determining effective aerobic exercise.

Exercise Program Relative Versus Absolute Intensity

Personal trainers may find it more appropriate to use a relative scale to gauge exercise intensity instead of an absolute scale. Recent research by Lee and others (2003) has demonstrated that the relative intensity of physical activity (e.g., perceived exertion) is a better predictor of health outcomes than recommending that someone exercise at an absolute intensity (e.g., a specific MET level). This research and recommendations made by the National Institutes of Health Consensus Development Panel (National Institutes of Health 1996) and the DC/ACSM guidelines (Pate et al. 1995) clearly de-emphasize recommending absolute exercise levels across age levels. Physical activity recommendations need to be tailored to the individual in contrast to a flat MET level for all.

Supportive Conditioning Exercise

All cardiorespiratory exercise programs must be supported by flexibility, strength, and even neuromuscular fitness exercise to enhance the efficiency of aerobic exercise (exercise economy) and minimize musculoskeletal injury. Although some of this supportive exercise, such as stretching, can be part of the warm-up and/or cool-down, it is prudent to add several separate sessions per week that improve the strength of the back, legs, and abdomen. Stretching and range-of-motion exercises are fundamental to a successful cardiorespiratory fitness program. Incorporating various neuromuscular relaxation activities into the cool-down phase of the program is appropriate for those coming from high-stress work environments who need more than just aerobic exercise. You can help your clients relax both mentally and physically by teaching them easy stretching and mental relaxation skills simultaneously. Chapters 9 and 10 describe strength and flexibility exercises in more detail.

Cardiorespiratory Fitness Goals

The goals of cardiorespiratory exercise must be clearly stated in the written exercise plan to reinforce compliance and motivation and for assessment during follow up. The client's implementation and progression plan must reflect these goals and depict means of achieving them safely and realistically. Chapter 10 contains an excellent discussion of goal formulation. The following are examples of areas that can be addressed in the formulation of cardiorespiratory exercise and activity goals:

1. Overall acquisition and maintenance of cardiorespiratory fitness (e.g., kcal/day energy expenditure, mastery of jogging, 20-pound weight loss)
2. Cardiovascular risk-factor modification
    a. Body composition
    b. Blood pressure reduction
    c. Cholesterol control
    d. Stress and anxiety reduction
3. Performance objectives
    a. Personal accomplishment (e.g., 10K run, 1-mile swim, or 6-mile hike)
    b. Increase physical stamina

Caloric Expenditure Goals

An alternative means of programming exercise is to recommend specific energy expenditure goals. Many health benefits are related to total session and weekly energy expenditure (e.g., weight loss and reduction in risk of chronic disease such as diabetes and obesity). The American College of Sports Medicine (2000) recommends 150 kcal energy expenditure in physical activity or exercise per day or 1,000 kcal per week as a *minimal* initial goal for previously sedentary individuals.

You must become skilled in estimating and/or calculating the energy costs of various activities. One practical method to approximate the caloric cost of exercise is to use the following equation based on the MET level of the activity:

$$(\text{METs} \times 3.5 \times \text{body weight in kg}) = \text{kcal/min } 200$$

It is important to understand that this energy expenditure method for setting exercise goals is less precise than assigning specific target heart-rate ranges. However, it still has much utility from a health risk–reduction perspective. For a more comprehensive list of physical activities and their approximate metabolic cost, refer to *Compendium of Physical Activities: Classification of Energy Costs of Human Physical Activities* (Ainsworth et al. 2001).

Calculating Energy Expenditure

Personal trainers should be able to calculate energy expenditure for any type of cardiorespiratory assessment or activity. To calculate energy expenditure, maximal oxygen consumption (or $\dot{V}O_2$) must first be assessed. Oxygen consumption is linearly related to energy expenditure, and this provides an indirect measurement of an individual's maximal capacity to do work aerobically.

All metabolic calculations are based on direct measurements of oxygen consumption, which are typically performed in a laboratory setting where a person performs a graded maximal exercise test on a treadmill, bike, or other apparatus wearing a specialized headgear that has a nonrebreathing valve attached to it. The person mouth-breathes through the valve and the amount of oxygen and carbon dioxide is computed by a metabolic measurement cart. Maximal oxygen consumption can be calculated from the final state of exercise where the workload increases but oxygen consumption does not increase. With most standardized exercise test protocols, a person of average fitness will complete a test in approximately 10 to 15 minutes. Since direct measurement of oxygen consumption requires specialized and expensive equipment, it is more practical to determine oxygen consumption by estimating it in a fitness setting. Numerous studies have quantified the average oxygen consumption required to maintain certain workloads on a treadmill or stationary cycle, and as a result, equations to estimate energy expenditure have been formulated.

Since oxygen consumption is expressed in mL/kg/min, you simply need to fill in the missing values to calculate energy expenditure:

1. Milliliters of oxygen ($\dot{V}O_2$max or percentage of $\dot{V}O_2$max)
2. Weight in kilograms
3. Total minutes of exercise

Conversion formulas:

Calories: 1 L of O_2 = 5 kilocalories

Power: 1 MET = 3.5 mL O_2/kg/min

Weight: 1 kg = 2.2 lbs

Volume: 1,000 mL = 1 L

Example 1

If a person weighs 175 lb, has a $\dot{V}O_2$max of 50 mL/kg/min, and is exercising at a steady intensity of 80% of $\dot{V}O_2$max [or heart-rate reserve (HRR)] for 30 minutes, how many calories are expended during exercise?

Step 1: conversion to SI units

kg: 175 lb ÷ 2.2 = 80 kg

mL: 0.80 × 50 mL/kg/min × 80 kg = 3,200 mL/min

min: 30 minutes

Step 2: calculation of oxygen consumption (Note: 1 L = 1,000 mL)

3,200 mL/min ÷ 1,000 = 3.2 L/min

Step 3: calculation of calories burned during the workout (Note: 1 L of O_2 = 5 kilocalories)

3.2 L/min × 5 kcal/L × 30 minutes = 480 calories

Note: the determination of energy expenditure is more accurate if the assessment used is a direct measurement, such as in a laboratory setting where a true maximal heart is obtained, and less accurate with an indirect measurement where the maximal heart rate is estimated. Also, energy expenditure may be underestimated or overestimated if the intensity at which the person exercises varies.

Progression Plan

A written progression plan with periodic reevaluation is crucial. This plan must provide details for a graduated progression in the frequency, duration, and intensity of exercise. There must be sufficient flexibility in the rate of progression so that the plan comfortably adjusts to the client's cardiorespiratory and musculoskeletal response. The rate of progression depends upon a number of factors:

- individual level of fitness (aerobic capacity)
- age
- health status
- cardiorespiratory response to exercise
- individual preferences and goals
- social and family support
- level of exercise initiative and motivation
- access to appropriate facilities and equipment

Three stages of progression for the cardiorespiratory endurance exercise plan are identified in the American College of Sports Medicine guidelines (2000): the initial conditioning stage, the improvement conditioning stage, and the maintenance conditioning stage.

Initial Conditioning Stage

This stage usually lasts four to six weeks or longer and includes low-level aerobic activities, stretching, and light calisthenics. Exercise frequency should begin with every other day. Depending upon initial level of fitness and functional capacity, duration should start with 10 to 20 minutes and gradually increase according to the client's cardiorespiratory and musculoskeletal response. For those with low functional capacity (4 to 7 METs or less), it may be appropriate to prescribe low-level aerobic interval exercise of two to five minutes at a time. The most important thing to remember during the initial conditioning stage is to be conservative with the exercise intensity. For example, if the individual has a 9 MET functional capacity (31.5 mL/kg/min $\dot{V}O_2max$), begin at a conservative 40 to 60% of this value, or at about 4 METs. Here, exercise heart rate should begin at approximately 40 to 60% of heart-rate reserve (Karvonen).

Improvement Conditioning Stage

This is the primary conditioning stage for most aerobic-training programs. It may last from 8 to 20 weeks, and the rate of progression in intensity is more rapid. The exercise intensity can be increased to the next highest level than that completed in the initial conditioning stage, and within the 60 to 90% of maximal heart rate (50 to 85% of $\dot{V}O_2max$ or heart-rate reserve) depending on fitness level and age. Exercise duration should be increased every two to three weeks according to the client's response and goals. It is important to periodically review progress at two- to four-week intervals during this stage, either by direct monitoring or by assessing selfreport data (RPE, heart rate, symptoms, caloric expenditure).

Maintenance Stage

When clients reach their target functional capacity or primary goals, the maintenance stage begins. This stage is usually reached after the first 6 months of training, but it may be delayed as long as 12 months, depending upon goals. In any case, it is important to reassess goals at the beginning of this stage. Maintenance of a particular level of cardiorespiratory fitness can be derived from an exercise program that has similar energy requirements to that of the conditioning program. Cardiorespiratory fitness can often be maintained by regularly engaging in a variety of endurance-related sports activities that are fun and enjoyable.

Safety and Cautions

The last component of an exercise plan involves using individual information to ensure each client's exercise safety with specific precautions. List any personal or environmental information that reduces the risk of exercise injury or that may compromise exercise safety. Individualized comments such as those describing hot, humid environments or avoiding musculoskeletal symptoms specific to the client should be included. Another useful format is to list several cautions that are standard for nearly all exercise programs:

- Do not exercise for at least 90 minutes after a meal.
- Avoid continuing exercise with chest discomfort, lightheadedness, or dizziness.

- Reduce exercise intensity in response to very hot or humid environments or to altitudes above 5,000 feet.
- Avoid exercise with tenderness in a joint (for example, a knee or ankle) that tends to worsen with activity.
- Avoid strenuous aerobic exercise during viral infections such as the flu or upper respiratory tract infection.
- If you are receiving care from a physician for a chronic medical condition (e.g., diabetes, cardiovascular disease, hypertension), you should obtain clearance from your doctor before proceeding with this exercise program.

TRAINING METHODS

Once the mode, frequency, duration, and intensity of exercise has been established, you must choose the appropriate training method. The choice provides the foundation for the exercise progression plan. Selection requires understanding the physiological response to various training methods and, preferably, personal experience with each of those methods. As with exercise intensity and progression, the training method depends on the functional fitness level and the goals of the participant. There are five major training methods (Heyward 1984; Wells & Pate 1988):

1. Continuous training
    a. Intermediate slow distance
    b. Long slow distance
2. Interval training
    a. Aerobic interval training
    b. Anaerobic interval training
3. Fartlek training
4. Circuit training
5. Aerobic cross training

Continuous Training

Continuous training involves conditioning stage exercise, such as walking, jogging, cycling, swimming, and aerobic dancing. The intensity is maintained continuously between 50 and 85% of functional capacity (maximal oxygen uptake). For those with initially low functional capacities, continuous training may be initiated at 40% of functional capacity and is usually preceded by four to six weeks of interval training in the initial conditioning stage. In practice, continuous training is divided into two types:

- Intermediate slow distance: Generally from 20 to 60 minutes of continuous aerobic exercise—the most common type of sustained aerobic exercise for fitness improvement. Body-fat reduction, improvement in cardiorespiratory fitness, and cardiovascular risk factor management—all are responsive to this type of continuous training.
- Long slow distance (LSD): 60 or more minutes of continuous aerobic exercise, usually employed for athletic training in such sports as cycling and long-distance running. Cardiorespiratory and metabolic demands are great for LSD training. At least six months of successful intermediate slow distance training should precede LSD training. Increased risk of musculoskeletal injury (e.g., Achilles tendinitis) accompanies this type of prolonged aerobic training.

Interval Training

Interval training involves alternating relatively more intense bouts of cardiovascular exercise with those that are relatively less intense. Interval training has useful applications for beginning exercisers, as well as experienced, conditioned clients who wish to improve aerobic power. You can use two types of interval training: aerobic and anaerobic. The following four variables should be considered when designing an aerobic or anaerobic interval training program:

- intensity of work interval (e.g., speed)
- duration of work interval (e.g., distance or time)
- duration of rest or recovery interval
- number of repetitions or repeat intervals

Aerobic Interval Training

Aerobic interval training is best suited for those beginning in the poor- or low-cardiorespiratory fitness classifications because it is less intense (table 3.8). Generally, aerobic interval training uses exercise bouts of 2 to 15 minutes at an intensity between 60 and 80% of functional capacity

Table 3.8 Percentile Values for Maximal Aerobic Power (mL/kg/min)

	Age				
Percentile	20-29	30-39	40-49	50-59	60+
Men					
90	51.4	50.4	48.2	45.3	42.5
80	48.2	46.8	44.1	41.0	38.1
70	46.8	44.6	41.8	38.5	35.3
60	44.2	42.4	39.9	36.7	33.6
50	42.5	41.0	38.1	35.2	31.8
40	41.0	38.9	36.7	33.8	30.2
30	39.5	37.4	35.1	32.3	28.7
20	37.1	35.4	33.0	30.2	26.5
10	34.5	32.5	30.9	28.0	23.1
Women					
90	44.2	41.0	39.5	35.2	35.2
80	41.0	38.6	36.3	32.3	31.2
70	38.1	36.7	33.8	30.9	29.4
60	36.7	34.6	32.3	29.4	27.2
50	35.2	33.8	30.9	28.2	25.8
40	33.8	32.3	29.5	26.9	24.5
30	32.3	30.5	28.3	25.5	23.8
20	30.6	28.7	26.5	24.3	22.8
10	28.4	26.5	25.1	22.3	20.8

Adapted, by permission, from the *Physical Fitness Certification Manual*, 2003, (Dallas, TX: The Cooper Institute); adapted, by permission, from American College of Sports Medicine, 2000, *ACSM's guidelines for exercise testing and prescription*, 6th ed. (Philadelphia, PA: Lippincott, Williams & Wilkins).

Study population for the data set was predominately white and college educated. A modified Balke treadmill test was used with $\dot{V}O_2max$ estimated from the last grade/speed achieved. The following may be used as descriptors for the percentile rankings: well above average (90), above average (70), average (50), below average (30), and well below average (10).

(modified from Wells & Pate 1988). Those with poor or low functional capacity should start with two- to three-minute exercise intervals at 60 to 70% of functional capacity. Rest intervals should take approximately the same time as a complete exercise interval. Intervals can be repeated 5 to 10 times depending on the client's response and program goals; for example, stationary bicycling for three minutes at a work load intensity of 60 to 70% of functional capacity with a two-minute "rest period" of cycling at zero resistance or load. Hypothetically, this would be repeated 5 to 10 times for a total workout of 25 to 50 minutes. Higher-intensity and longer-duration aerobic interval training (e.g., 5- to 15-minute bouts at 70 to 90% of functional capacity) should be reserved for those in higher cardiorespiratory fitness classifications seeking increased aerobic endurance and speed.

Anaerobic Interval Training

Anaerobic interval training is primarily reserved for those in the higher cardiorespiratory fitness classifications who desire to increase speed, lactate threshold, and overall aerobic power. Such training usually results in greater lactic acid concentrations in exercising muscles and is accompanied by greater muscular discomfort. Because of the relatively high metabolic and cardiorespiratory demands, beginners or those below a 10-MET aerobic capacity should refrain from anaerobic interval training. Although there are many derivations of anaerobic interval training, the training stimulus is usually between 30 seconds and four minutes at an intensity of 85% to greater than 100% of functional capacity (maximal oxygen uptake). The probability of musculoskeletal injury is greater because of high muscle contraction velocities and forces. The client, frequently an athlete, should engage in substantial low-level aerobic warm-up and stretching before vigorous activity.

Fartlek Training

Fartlek training is similar to interval training. However, the work-rest intervals are not systematically or accurately measured. Work-rest intervals and intensity are usually determined by how the participant feels. Over the years, Fartlek training has blossomed in many aerobic-training regimens, primarily to prevent boredom and to enhance aerobic endurance. One of its most useful applications is in running, where the warm-up consists of running for 10 to 20 minutes, then the pace is significantly varied every 5 to 10 minutes. Like long, slow distance aerobic training, this form should be reserved for those in the average or above-average cardiorespiratory fitness levels because of the relatively high demand on the cardiorespiratory system.

Circuit Training

Circuit training takes the client through a series of exercise stations, with relatively brief rest intervals between each station. The number of stations may range from 4 to 10. Historically, circuit training was designed to enhance muscular endurance and incorporated mostly low-weight, high-repetition exercises. A circuit of 4 to 10 stations with a low-level aerobic warm-up and cool-down station (for example, the stationary bicycle) could be followed by exercise stations using either free weights or single-station weight machines. A good example of circuit training in a more natural environment is par course exercise, which intersperses walking or jogging with a variety of stations that feature flexibility, muscular endurance, and strength exercises.

Aerobic circuit-training programs are also popular. Between four and eight aerobic exercise stations with one to five minutes per station and a 15-second rest break between stations constitute a circuit. Stations may include stationary cycling, treadmill exercise, elliptical training, moderate stair climbing, and rowing. Depending on the number of stations, the workout provides 20 to 50 minutes of aerobic exercise. One key to success is to avoid excessive workloads at each station. Each station should be set at 50 to 70% of the client's functional capacity.

Aerobic Cross Training

Aerobic **cross training** is an individualized combination or composite of all aerobic training methods and is characterized by a variety of intensities and modes. It is primarily for exercisers in the maintenance phase of conditioning who want variety and an intensity corresponding to how they feel during a given exercise workout. A good example is a 50-minute workout in which the client warms up by jogging 15 minutes to a nearby pool, swims for 20 minutes, and then jogs 15 minutes back home. Another example is bicycling 20 minutes to a track or running course and, after 20 minutes of running, cycling back home. Combining a group of aerobic activities into one workout at steady or various intensities is an excellent method of cross training to fight boredom from the same daily workout mode and intensity. This method can also be applied to circuit training in a gym by combining a continuous, relatively low-level aerobic session, such as 20 minutes of stationary cycling, with 10 to 20 minutes of a variety of higher intensity aerobic intervals on various aerobic ergometers, and concluding with a 5- to 10-minute cool-down of stationary cycling. The many obvious permutations of this method should begin and end with a continuous low-level cardiorespiratory exercise effort for effective physiological warm-up. This method instills variety and is a mini-version of a "training triathlon."

Domestic Forms of Physical Activity

Although not often thought of as a training method per se, continuous or intermittent physical movement during household chores has the capacity to generate small increases in cardiorespiratory fitness and more significant improvements in cardiovascular health. Domestic activities such as yard work, cleaning, scrubbing, gardening, and repair work generate energy costs of 3 to 6 METs and are important contributors to disease prevention. While these activities do not generate the same cardiorespiratory stimulus as running or cycling, they clearly should not be viewed as insignificant contributors to weekly activity energy expenditure and cardiovascular and metabolic health.

GUIDELINES FOR CARDIORESPIRATORY ACTIVITY

The best resources for detailed aerobic activities are those that adopt sensible progression guidelines with adequate instruction for each form of exercise (e.g., American Council on Exercise 2000; American College of Sports Medicine 2003; Neporent & Schlosberg 1999; Howley & Franks 1998; Nieman 1990). Following are guidelines for popular aerobic and sport activities.

Walking

Walking is the easiest aerobic-conditioning activity and is often preferred because of its low injury rate, relative simplicity, and adaptability to busy schedules. Although nearly anyone can incur significant health benefits from walking, several types of clients will respond particularly well to a graduated walking program:

- Those with low functional capacity (2 to 7 METs) who need an initial low-intensity workout
- Those over 60 years of age who have been sedentary and are just beginning an exercise program
- Those who are 20 or more pounds overweight

The energy cost of walking is relatively low compared to that of jogging because of slower speeds; however, at walking speeds of five miles per hour and faster, the oxygen and caloric cost per minute approaches that of jogging or running (table 3.9). There still exists an abundance of misinformation regarding the energy costs of walking versus running. Despite the longstanding claim that walking 1 mile is equivalent to running 1 mile, this is not the case, with the exception of very fast walking speeds of greater than 5 miles per hour (Howley & Franks 2003; Howley & Glover 1974). In general, the **net caloric cost** per mile* of walking is 50 to 60% of that for running. This is an important point if you intend to program and quantify walking mileage for weight-management purposes.

Table 3.9 Energy Costs of Walking (kcal/min)

Body Weight (lb)	Miles Per Hour						
	2.0	2.5	3.0	3.5	4.0	4.5	5.0
110	2.1	2.4	2.8	3.1	4.1	5.2	6.6
120	2.3	2.6	3.0	3.4	4.4	5.6	7.2
130	2.5	2.9	3.2	3.6	4.8	6.1	7.8
140	2.7	3.1	3.5	3.9	5.2	6.6	8.4
150	2.8	3.3	3.7	4.2	5.6	7.0	9.0
160	3.0	3.5	4.0	4.5	5.9	7.5	9.6
170	3.2	3.7	4.2	4.8	6.3	8.0	10.2
180	3.4	4.0	4.5	5.0	6.7	8.4	10.8
190	3.6	4.2	4.7	5.3	7.0	8.9	11.4
200	3.8	4.4	5.0	5.6	7.4	9.4	12.0
210	4.0	4.6	5.2	5.9	7.8	9.9	12.6
220	4.2	4.8	5.5	6.2	8.2	10.3	13.2

Adapted, by permission, from E. Howley and B.D. Franks, 2003, *Health fitness instructor's guide*, 4th ed. (Champaign, IL: Human Kinetics), 49.

**Note*: The net cost of exercise is the exercise energy expenditure minus resting energy expenditure. The net cost measures the energy expenditure used over that when at rest.

Walking is generally less intense than jogging or running, meaning that longer sessions can be maintained with less likelihood of musculoskeletal injury. When hilly terrain is gradually added to the walking program, there is greater energy expenditure. Perhaps the safest and most effective cardiorespiratory weight-control exercise for those who are 20 to 30 pounds (9 to 13.5 kg) overweight is progressive variable-terrain walking. This walking protocol graduates from walking approximately 2 miles on flat terrain to walking up to 5 or more miles over a variety of grades, such as those found on many urban and rural park and nature trails. It is not difficult to achieve and maintain the walking intensity and duration necessary for acceptable cardiorespiratory fitness. As a general rule, achieving acceptable fitness will require at least 20 minutes (preferably 30 minutes or more) of fast-paced, flat-ground walking or slightly slower variable-terrain walking. When walking, three things are important:

1. When walking is the primary activity, footwear is important. Specialized walking or hiking shoes are available from many stores, although many walkers will prefer a good pair of running shoes.

2. Always warm up and cool down. Begin each session by walking for about five minutes and then stretch the Achilles tendons, calves, and low-back muscles. After the primary conditioning phase, cool down by walking at a slower pace and stretching the muscles that were previously stretched.

3. Give special emphasis to gradually increasing the duration—for example, from 15 to 60 minutes—over the length of the program. Progression in intensity should follow successful duration progression. Emphasize duration first, then gradually add faster-paced walking. Keep in mind that adding hilly terrain increases the intensity, so be sure that the terrain is within the client's capacity.

Adhere to guidelines for proper walking and running form when using a motor-driven treadmill. These guidelines include:

- Safely mounting and dismounting the treadmill
- Maintaining a relatively upright posture
- Keeping the hips tucked directly under the torso
- Looking straight ahead
- Letting the arms swing naturally

Pedometer Walking

Wearing a pedometer or step-counter to quantify walking distance as well as other domestic and recreational activities has proven to be an effective means of motivating inactive clients. Numerous health plans and health-care institutions have adopted the 10,000-steps-a-day program, in part popularized by the diabetes prevention program study (Diabetes Prevention Program Research Group 2002). Although there is significant inter-individual variation in the number of steps per mile, most popular step-counters record approximately 2,000 steps per mile of walking. These devices can objectively score a client's daily and weekly physical activity, which can be of great value to both the participant and personal trainer.

Jogging and Running

Jogging and running are superb cardiorespiratory-endurance activities. The essential difference between the two is that jogging is "slower running," or as some authorities define it, jogging is running slower than eight minutes per mile. For beginners, a natural sequence of progression might be:

1. Walk/jog intervals: walk 50 yards, jog 50 yards, repeat 10 to 20 times; over time, gradually increase the jogging interval to 2 or more miles
2. Jogging: gradually increase jogging distance to desired distance or energy expenditure
3. Running: as jogging endurance improves, increase stride frequency and stride length to a comfortable running style

It is not necessary to graduate to running if desired goals can be achieved by jogging. However, running is a natural progression for those who orthopedically and psychologically respond well to jogging. Table 3.10 shows the energy cost in calories per minute for jogging and running. Note that the energy cost increases proportionately with increasing speed. These proportional increases in energy cost mean that a client who runs a mile at 9 miles per hour (6.6 minutes per mile) will finish the mile twice as fast as when jogging 4.5 miles per hour (13.3 minutes per mile), but energy cost per mile is about the same. Numerous benefits can be obtained from successful jogging and running programs that are adequately balanced with appropriate muscular-strength and flexibility exercises. Some of these benefits include increased maximum oxygen uptake, improved body composition (decrease in body-fat stores), coronary risk reduction, increased bone strength, and enhanced psychological well-being. Four things are important when jogging or running:

1. Wear appropriate footwear. A comfortable pair of running shoes designed for distance jogging/running should have adequate sole cushion, good heel support, and sufficient sole flexibility.
2. Always accompany jogging or running exercise with appropriate flexibility exercise. Stretching the Achilles tendons, calves, hamstrings, quadriceps, feet, and low-back muscles will help improve jogging and running efficiency.
3. For beginners, jog every other day (no more than four days per week) with a day of rest between workouts to allow for adequate recovery of the weightbearing joints, ligaments, and tendons. Limit the initial duration to no more than 25 to 30 minutes per workout for the first six to eight weeks.

Table 3.10 Energy Costs of Jogging and Running (kcal/min)

	Running/jogging speed (MPH)							
Body weight (lb)	3.0	4.0	5.0	6.0	7.0	8.0	9.0	10.0
110	4.7	5.9	7.2	8.5	9.8	11.1	12.3	13.6
120	5.1	6.4	7.9	9.3	10.6	12.1	13.4	14.8
130	5.5	7.0	8.6	10.0	11.5	13.1	14.6	16.1
140	5.9	7.5	9.2	10.8	12.4	14.1	15.7	17.3
150	6.4	8.1	9.9	11.6	13.3	15.1	16.8	18.5
160	6.8	8.6	10.5	12.4	14.2	16.1	17.9	19.8
170	7.2	9.1	11.2	13.1	15.1	17.1	19.1	21.0
180	7.6	9.7	11.8	13.9	15.9	18.1	20.2	22.2
190	8.1	10.2	12.5	14.7	16.8	19.1	21.3	23.5
200	8.5	10.8	13.2	15.4	17.7	20.1	22.4	24.7
210	8.9	11.3	13.8	16.2	18.6	21.1	23.5	25.9
220	9.3	11.8	14.5	17.0	19.5	22.2	24.7	27.2

Adapted, by permission, from E. Howley and B.D. Franks, 2003, *Health fitness instructor's guide*, 4th ed. (Champaign, IL: Human Kinetics), 52.

4. Increase jogging pace and add hills only gradually. Emphasize a gradual increase in distance at a relatively slow pace, and then slowly increase pace or speed. Aerobic interval training will facilitate a safe and gradual increase in distance.

Elliptical trainers are a relatively new form of aerobic exercise machine. With elliptical trainers, the lower-body motion is a relative combination of the cycling and stair climbing motions, except that the feet move in an elliptical (i.e., egg-shaped) pattern, as opposed to a circular movement path. Like stair climbers, elliptical motion trainers are low-impact (since the user's feet never leave the footpads) and weightbearing.

Cycling

Cycling is another excellent cardiorespiratory activity with benefits similar to jogging and running. It is a good alternative for those who do not like to jog or run or who have orthopedic limitations to weightbearing exercise. Two types are outdoor cycling and indoor stationary cycling. Both have advantages and disadvantages; however, with sufficient frequency, duration, and intensity, both can be an excellent stimulus to cardiorespiratory fitness.

Outdoor Cycling

The benefits of outdoor cycling are sunlight, fresh air, adequate cooling, and variety of terrain and scenery. And it can be a good source of inexpensive transportation. Most clients find that cycling outdoors makes it easier to prolong duration of exercise because of distances between destinations and more interesting environments. Disadvantages include inclement weather, nightfall, and some unsafe city environments. However, convenient outdoor cycling, combined with indoor stationary cycling, can be a stimulating year-round program.

Guidelines for outdoor bicycling include the following:

1. Use a bicycle with at least 10 speeds so that the cyclist can easily adapt to nearly any change in grade or wind.

2. For beginners, keep a relatively constant pedal crank speed by adjusting the gears to variable grades and headwinds. This pedal crank speed can vary depending on fitness and comfort, but will usually be between 70 and 90 rpm per leg. This will help minimize fatigue and maximize blood flow and nutrients to the legs.

3. Bicycle seat height should be high enough so that the leg that is on the downstroke is not quite completely extended when the ball of the foot is on the pedal.

4. Use toe clips, especially with significant hill climbing. Toe clips improve pedaling efficiency by delivering more muscular power to the pedal crank axis throughout the entire revolution.

5. Wear bicycling apparel. Always wear a cycling helmet. Padded shorts and gloves will increase comfort for cycling lasting longer than 45 minutes.

Indoor Stationary Cycling

The advantages of indoor stationary cycling include its convenience and relative safety. Most health clubs and fitness centers have two types of stationary cycles: those with mechanically braked flywheels and those that are electronically braked. Either type will provide a good aerobic or anaerobic workout; however, the electronically controlled cycles generally display digital workload information that may be helpful to motivate clients. On electronically controlled cycles, some beginners do not always get an adequate warm-up when selecting certain exercise programs on the display monitor. Regardless of the type of cycle, always warm up by cycling against low pedal crank resistance for at least 5 to 10 minutes. Many stationary cycles are not accurately calibrated, so there may be noticeable differences in pedal crank resistances for similarly indicated workloads between cycles.

For a thorough review of group indoor cycling refer to ACE's *Group Indoor Cycling* (Shechtman 2000).

The following guidelines apply to stationary cycling machines:

1. Ensure proper ventilation. If necessary, a fan gives adequate cross ventilation to enable good evaporative heat loss. Cooling the body by the evaporation of sweat is necessary to prevent a rapid rise in body temperature. Unlike outdoor bicycling, indoor cycling requires adequate ventilation for prolonged exercise.

2. As in outdoor bicycling, adjust seat height for a slight bend in the knee at the downstroke position.

3. Adjust the handlebars so that the client is relaxed and leaning slightly forward.

4. Hold pedal crank speed relatively constant for beginners in the range of 70 to 90 rpm per leg.

5. Always warm up and cool down with 5 to 10 minutes of low-resistance cycling.

6. Because of the relatively intense nature of group indoor cycling, it is paramount to incorporate a more graduated warm-up and cool-down and to ensure that adequate convective cooling (i.e., crosscurrent ventilation) is made available.

Swimming and Vertical Water Exercise

Swimming activities are another excellent form of cardiorespiratory endurance exercise. Swimming is a good alternative for those with chronic orthopedic problems or a recent musculoskeletal injury. Relatively experienced swimmers generate a lower heart-rate response for any level of effort compared to cyclists and runners. The diminished cardiac work is due to the prone position and the effect of immersion in a relatively cool environment. This is important when determining a target heart-rate range, which may be as much as 10 beats per minute lower with lap swimming than with cycling or running. This does not mean that swimming is not a significant cardiorespiratory stimulus. However, swimming generally requires a higher level of motor skill that may take significantly longer to learn than that of cycling or running. Several factors determine swimming efficiency and early success with any swimming program, including body buoyancy, swimming skill and style, and body dimensions. Women are generally more efficient swimmers than men, partly because of greater body fat stores and a more even distribution of body fat, which improves buoyancy. For an efficient swimmer, the energy cost of swimming 1 mile has been estimated to be more than 400 kcal. Unskilled swimmers may require twice the energy expenditure for a given velocity compared to skilled swimmers and often fatigue early.

Vertical water exercise (upright in the water) is an excellent way to develop cardiorespiratory and overall fitness without requiring swimming skills. Many clients may benefit greatly from training in the water, especially those who have problems with balance or coordination, or who need to begin exercising at a very low intensity. In addition, clients who want to achieve a relatively high-intensity workout with reduced impact can use the surrounding resistance of water as an effective exercise environment. Essentially, there are two types of vertical water exercise: shallow water exercise, which is conducted in water navel- to nipple-deep (standing position), and deep-water exercise, which is conducted in a depth where the lungs are fully submerged and the feet may be touching the bottom of the pool slightly or not at all. Flotation devices are generally used for support. Equipment that increases surface area (paddles for the feet in deep water or shoes for better traction in shallow water) may be added to progress intensity.

For additional information on water exercise, refer to *YMCA Water Fitness for Health* (YMCA of the USA, 2000), available from the YMCA Program Store.

The following guidelines should be followed for swimming:

1. Assess swimming or aquatic exercise skill by evaluating exercise history or by observation. If skill level (i.e., stroke efficiency and style) is low, supervision and swimming lessons should precede swimming as a cardiorespiratory-conditioning exercise.

2. Keep pool temperature for lap swimming at 76 to 84°F (24 to 29°C).

3. Ideally, use a lap pool with, at the most, 80 lengths per mile to enable the swimmer to attain a reasonable stroke rhythm before turning.

4. Use interval training for the beginning swimmer. For example, swimming either the width or length of the pool one to two times may be appropriate. Each of these would constitute a set with a rest interval of walking one or two widths in waist-high water. This could be repeated 4 to 10 times, depending on skill and cardiorespiratory fitness.

5. For the beginner, include a good warm-up and cool-down exercise, such as walking the width of the pool in waist- or chest-high water for 5 to 10 minutes.

6. For those who are not comfortable in the pool and perhaps cannot swim, flotation devices can help (e.g., small life-vests, kick-boards, pull-buoys).

Rowing

Rowing machines are sometimes used in gyms and fitness centers for cardiorespiratory exercise, as well as for attaining a reasonable degree of arm, back, and thigh muscular endurance. As with any stationary aerobic exercise device, a fan should provide air circulation to facilitate sweat evaporation and prevent overheating. There are numerous manufacturers of rowing machines, some very basic and some quite sophisticated with hydraulic action of the arm movement and workload display monitors. However, most operate on the principle of coordinated effort of lower-extremity muscular work with arm rowing action. Rowing intensity (rowing motion resistance) can be varied in most machines by changing the force angle of the rowing arm of the machine, by changing the hydraulic pressure in the pressure cylinder, or via electronic programming. Intensity also can be varied by increasing the rowing rate, or number of rows per minute. Those just learning should note that several sessions are required to learn how to perform repetitive, efficient rowing motions that require synchronizing the arms, back, and legs. Several guidelines may be helpful:

1. Secure feet in the anchors on the front part of the machine.
2. Use a smooth rowing action (coordinate arm and back rowing movements with leg extensions).
3. Begin with a relatively low intensity (low resistance) with approximately 8 to 10 rows per minute for hydraulic rowers, for 5 to 10 minutes.
4. Graduate the speed to approximately 15 to 30 rows per minute and gradually increase duration to 15 to 30 minutes.
5. Gradually increase intensity according to heart rate and perceived exertion.

Stair Climbing

Stair climbing can be an effective means of attaining cardiorespiratory fitness. The client may use either a staircase or one of the electronically braked stair-climbing machines that are found in most fitness centers. The advent of computer-interactive, electrically braked stair-climbing machines brought effective and well-controlled stair climbing to the health club and fitness center. They allow for a more effective warm-up and cool-down as well as a variety of training intensities because most of these devices regulate the intensity of climbing based on step rate, depth of step, or exercise resistance. It should be noted that many people incorrectly support their weight by leaning onto guard rails, so the actual work performed is less than that indicated on the monitor. Many people find these machines challenging and fun, and they can provide an interesting addition to circuit training programs or be a primary means of attaining cardiorespiratory fitness.

Safety precaution: A fan or other means of convective cooling should always be used because of the tendency to overheat on stationary exercise machines.

Because the energy cost of actual stair climbing is largely dependent upon body weight, a large anaerobic component is possible for those who are overweight or unaccustomed to regular stair climbing. Adequate warm-up and cool-down periods must be incorporated due to the potentially large energy costs. Walking for 5 to 10 minutes on relatively flat terrain, either on a track or treadmill, usually provides adequate warm-up or cool-down. Interval-training methods are best when beginning a program with regular stairs or steps in a stadium. After warming up, repeating a sequence of walking four flights of stairs and taking a 60-second walk on flat ground 4 to 10 times is one example of an interval approach. To provide protection to your client's knee joints, instruct stair climber users to keep their knees aligned with their toes. If the knees are allowed to move far past the toes, significant stress may be placed on the anterior aspect of the knee.

Traditional Aerobics

Studies on the effects of traditional aerobics show it to be an excellent form of cardiorespiratory endurance exercise. To gain significant benefits, the client must maintain the aerobic phase for at least 20 to 30 minutes, three to four times per week. The tempo (speed or pace) should be adjusted to fit the desired intensity or heart-rate range. Like swimming, traditional aerobics requires a degree of motor skill and coordination, and may take more time to learn than walking, jogging, or cycling. For those who are significantly overweight or have a history of orthopedic injuries, this type of exercise may create undue demands on the cardiorespiratory and musculoskeletal systems.

For a thorough review of traditional aerobics refer to ACE's *Traditional Aerobics* (Bricker 2000).

For traditional aerobics, the following guidelines apply:

1. Wear appropriate footwear that adheres to four standards: cushion, support, flexibility, and traction compatibility.
2. For beginners, recommend low-impact aerobics—a form of traditional aerobics that features one foot on the ground at all times, reducing the risk of musculoskeletal injury, and may include the use of light weights.
3. For beginners, recommend a class that will adapt appropriately to functional capacity and skill level.
4. Lower the target heart rate slightly, because traditional aerobics may elicit heart rates 10 to 15 beats per minute higher than running or cycling for the same percentage of aerobic capacity (Parker et al. 1989).

This disproportionate relationship between oxygen consumption and heart rate is generally true for most aerobic-exercise routines using upper-body muscle groups.

Step Training

In the 1990s, step training gained wide popularity in fitness centers and health clubs across the United States and many parts of Asia and Europe. Available research indicates that the energy cost of step training (7 to 11 METs) is commensurate with that of traditional aerobic exercise, such as running and cycling, and is an adequate stimulus of aerobic endurance. Choices of step bench height generally range from 4 to 10 inches, with a standard stepping rate of 120 to 130 steps per minute. Advise beginners to use smaller step heights of 4 to 6 inches with a goal of 8 inches after four to eight weeks of successful training. Discourage the addition of hand-held weights for beginners and those who are coronary-prone, because of the increased blood pressure response for any given step rate and step height.

For a thorough review of step training refer to ACE's *Step Training* (Bonelli 2000).

Tennis, Racquetball, and Handball

Tennis, racquetball, and handball are all popular sports and deserve special attention for their ability to increase cardiorespiratory fitness. Each requires various motor skills and neuromuscular coordination and the level and duration of play depend on these skills. For the beginner, racquet sports demand more from anaerobic energy systems than aerobic. However, as one becomes more skilled and efficient with movement and play, it is easier to prolong the activity and obtain more cardiorespiratory benefits. Improvements in cardiorespiratory fitness are dependent upon several factors:

- skill level and style of the player
- level of competition (intensity)
- total duration of each point played
- time interval between points and games
- total duration of entire exercise session

As the intensity and duration of these sports meet the criteria for cardiorespiratory endurance fitness (that is, 50 to 85% of maximal oxygen uptake for 20 to 60 minutes), they become more of a cardiorespiratory stimulus.

Racquetball and handball often are played in hot, unventilated environments, and require more attention to regular fluid intake and signs of dehydration. Generally, these racquet sports require at least average cardiorespiratory fitness and are excellent activities for developing and maintaining fitness.

Hiking and Backpacking

Hiking and backpacking activities can require high levels of cardiorespiratory endurance. Although most clients do not engage in these activities more than once a week, they are an excellent adjunct to a cardiorespiratory fitness program using fundamental aerobic activities such as jogging, cycling, or step training. The energy cost (oxygen uptake and calories expended) per minute is lower for hiking and backpacking, depending on grade, packloads, and altitude. The duration of such activity is usually prolonged (two to eight hours) and, therefore, the total energy cost is well above most routine aerobic workouts. It is important to be in at least average cardiorespiratory fitness, preferably the "above average" classification (see table 3.8), before attempting prolonged variable-terrain hiking. One of the most important concerns with prolonged hiking is dehydration. Be sure to carry adequate water and glucose replacement on trips lasting longer than 60 minutes.

Many factors govern the cardiorespiratory and metabolic cost of hiking and backpacking. The following are among the most important:

- body weight of hiker
- duration of the hike
- number and size of the grades
- altitude at which the hike occurs
- speed of movement
- pack load
- air temperature

Tai Chi and Other Mind-Body Exercise Practices With an Aerobic Component

Tai chi (shorthand for tai chi chuan or taijiquan) is just one form of the more ancient practice of qigong (Chinese health exercise). Tai chi is a "moving meditation" that has been shown to clearly increase cardiorespiratory endurance when sufficient pace and movement sequences are learned. This aerobic benefit has been particularly demonstrated in seniors (Lan et al. 1998). Tai chi characteristically consists of more than 100 movements (Yang style). There are numerous styles of Tai chi (e.g., Chen, Yang, and Wu styles), all of which may require years of training before one becomes adequately proficient. Other mind-body exercise programs that have the capacity to increase cardiorespiratory fitness include NIA (Neuromuscular Integrative Action), Yogarobics, E-motion among others.

MONITORING CARDIORESPIRATORY EXERCISE

Monitoring cardiorespiratory exercise performance is necessary for assessing exercise response, regulating exercise intensity, documenting progress, and assuring safety. Essentially, three techniques are used to monitor cardiorespiratory exercise: heart rate, ratings of perceived exertion, and laboratory monitoring techniques.

Monitoring Heart Rates

As mentioned earlier, heart rate is a good guide for exercise intensity and cardiorespiratory responsiveness. The heart rate can be obtained by palpating (feeling) the pulse or by using a cardiotachometer or electrocardiogram. From a practical standpoint, palpation is the easiest method to assess heart rate. The pulse may be palpated in the neck (carotid artery), the head (temporal artery), the wrist (radial artery), or the chest (apical artery). For example, the carotid pulse may be felt by gently placing the index and middle finger over a carotid artery in the neck on either side of the larynx. It is important not to apply too much pressure, as there are carotid sensors in these arteries that are sensitive to pressure and may induce a sudden drop in heart rate. Assess the radial pulse in the wrist by placing the first two fingers (index and middle) on the underside and thumb side of the wrist.

Heart-Rate Response to Training

There are two trends to look for when monitoring the heart-rate response to cardiorespiratory exercise training. First is the tendency of the heart rate, for any given level of exercise, to decrease with training. This tendency primarily applies to submaximal exercise, such as that between 60 and 80% of maximum functional capacity. For example, expect a decrease in heart rate for the same submaximal workload on a stationary cycle after several weeks of training. The actual decrease in exercise heart rate and the length of time required to elicit this change is variable between clients, but is primarily dependent upon age, initial level of fitness, length of the training program, and the exercise program intensity. Resting heart rate also tends to decrease with training along with the decrease in submaximal exercise heart rate. You must understand that there are other physiological reasons why resting heart rate may be low beyond that induced by endurance exercise training. A low resting pulse rate by itself is not by any means a perfect predictor of fitness.

Required Time for Expected Increases in Aerobic Capacity

For young and middle-aged adults, the usual improvement in aerobic capacity will be 15 to 20% over 10 to 20 weeks of training (Pollock, 1973). However, aerobic capacity may increase up to 45 to 50% depending upon the following factors:

- initial level of fitness
- age
- frequency of training
- intensity of training
- duration of exercise and total training programs
- genetics (e.g., oxidative processes, muscle fiber type ratio)

Those who begin a moderately intense cardiorespiratory conditioning program with a relatively high aerobic capacity can expect little improvement in aerobic capacity compared to those with initially low capacities. Age is not a detriment to increasing aerobic capacity by itself; however, training generally shows smaller improvements in aerobic capacity because of lower exercise intensities.

Overall, you can expect greater improvements with greater intensity or duration of exercise up to a point. This range for aerobic improvement is reflected in the mode, frequency, duration, and intensity standards previously mentioned. For most clients, cardiorespiratory changes, including aerobic capacity, continue to take place over many months, perhaps up to 24, as depicted in figure 3.1. This figure illustrates the relationship between initial functional capacity represented by three cardiorespiratory fitness levels and the relative difference in time required to achieve maximal or near-maximal aerobic capacity (Pollock 1973; Saltin et al. 1977; McArdle, Katch, & Katch 2001). This will provide you with a general estimate of expected aerobic capacity changes compared to program duration. Note that early stages of training in those with low cardiorespiratory fitness levels improve CRF relatively quickly in contrast to those who have already achieved either by training or by nature a higher aerobic capacity. Endurance performance (increasing exercise duration) may increase with little or no further increase in aerobic capacity. This is more likely to occur during the latter stages of training, such as the maintenance stage. The time required for other changes to occur, such as body-fat reduction and coronary risk modification, will vary considerably.

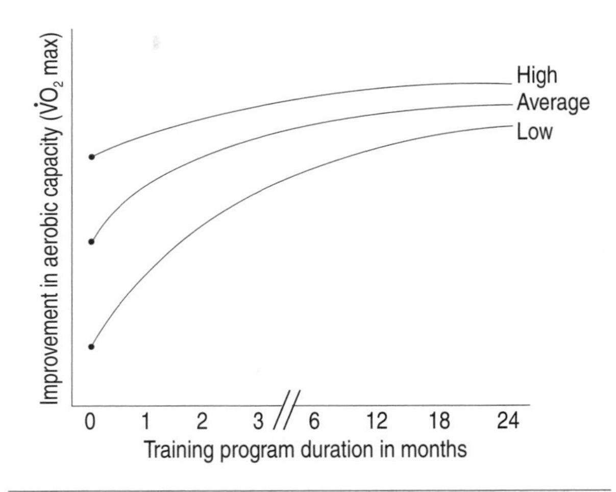

Figure 3.1 Hypothetical relationship between training program duration and improvements in aerobic capacity for three cardiorespiratory fitness levels (in healthy individuals).

SPECIAL CONSIDERATIONS AND SAFETY

You are responsible for determining current health status, developing an exercise program, and following up on a variety of clients. Two areas of special importance are understanding and differentiating the various sources of cardiorespiratory exercise fatigue and maximizing exercise safety.

The ability to recognize and differentiate exercise fatigue is especially helpful when evaluating self-report progress and teaching exertion limitation and safety precautions. Chapter 2 covers the physiology of aerobic and anaerobic capacity.

This section will discuss only basic sources of endurance exercise fatigue and list their basic characteristics. These sources often overlap. For example, during longer exercise bouts, there may be heat fatigue, glycogen depletion, and lactic acid accumulation. Becoming cognizant of each source of fatigue will better enable you to understand the spectrum of exercise responses. Following are six basic sources and manifestations of fatigue observed in cardiorespiratory exercise programs:

1. Exercise fuel depletion. Liver and muscle glycogen (storage forms of carbohydrate) are at relatively low levels after 60 to 80 minutes of intense cardiorespiratory exercise, depending on the level of endurance fitness. This form of fatigue is focused in the exercising muscle groups and, if exercise continues, leads to increasing anaerobic work.

2. Large increases in lactate production and/or accumulation in working muscle is a principal cause of exercise fatigue. This usually is caused by a decreased oxygen supply and/or a substantial increase in glycolysis. This form of fatigue usually comes with overpacing at too high an intensity, usually at levels greater than 80% of maximal oxygen consumption, or as a result of inadequate warm-up. An increase in the production or accumulation of lactic acid may also occur with exercise in hot weather or exercise at relatively high altitudes (more than 5,000 feet, or 1,524 meters). This fatigue has a relatively fast onset. It is characterized by the inability to sustain a pace or intensity, shortness of breath, and transient muscular weakness.

3. Hyperthermia-dehydration. This is a gradual increase in body temperature from prolonged aerobic exercise in hot, humid conditions and/or inadequate water replenishment during prolonged exercise. Elevated body temperatures, high heart rates, inability to sustain usual aerobic exercise intensities, and mental confusion can characterize this form of exercise fatigue.

4. Musculoskeletal (orthopedic). Musculoskeletal discomfort exhibits "fatigue-like" qualities. This discomfort is often the result of overuse, with prolonged repetitive movements or unusual stress on a joint or bone from weightbearing exercise such as jogging. This form of fatigue is nearly always focused on the muscle, ligament, tendon, or joint that is stressed, and is characterized by increasing joint or muscular tenderness that tends to worsen with repeated activity.

5. General overtraining syndrome, or staleness. This syndrome refers to the final stage in a proposed continuum of increasingly severe chronic fatigue states that develop as a result of overtraining, especially high-volume endurance overtraining. Overtraining syndrome is characterized by persistent plateau or worsening in performance that is not improved by short-term rest periods or reduced training. It also is associated with disturbances in mood and sleep, loss of appetite and weight, muscle soreness, a propensity for overuse injuries, and increased resting heart rate. Chapter 12 of this manual addresses injury prevention in much greater depth. Refer to Raglin and Moger (1999) and Raglin and Wilson (1999) for a current and detailed review of overtraining and staleness syndrome monitoring.

6. Abnormal cardiac symptoms or chest discomfort (angina). Although uncommon, this form of "fatigue" would represent a contraindication to continued exercise and justify a physician referral. This symptom usually characterizes coronary artery disease and someone who is prone to heart attack. Symptoms include chest discomfort (aching, pressure, burning, or tightness), that tends to come with physical effort and is relieved by rest. Always ensure that the client understands the seriousness of the symptoms and discontinues exercise, and require the client to report these symptoms to a physician without delay.

Maximizing Exercise Safety

You should be aware of and understand the behavioral and environmental factors that can either alter the response to exercise or predispose the client to increased risk of injury or cardiovascular complications. These factors include post-meal exercise, thermal stress, air pollutants, drugs and other substances, and the presence of unusual symptoms.

Exercise Following Meals

Vigorous aerobic exercise soon after a full meal can cause the heart to work harder, compromise oxygen and nutrient delivery to the working muscles, and cause gastric discomfort. Consequently, you should advise waiting at least 90 minutes after a full meal before beginning to engage in moderate- and higher-level aerobic exercise. The level of exercise and the amount and type of food ingested both affect the amount of time required for digestion to be completed before beginning exercise. The higher the exercise level and/or the greater the number of calories of food ingested, the longer the individual should wait between eating and exercise.

Thermal Stress

Exercise in hot, humid environments can place the client at risk for heat injury, as well as affect the usual intensity of exercise. Heat injury treatment is discussed on page 215. Methods recommended by the American College of Sports Medicine (2001) can prevent thermal or heat stress.

1. Allow 10 to 14 days for acclimatization to a hot, humid environment.
2. Defer exercise if the heat index is in the "high risk" zone.
3. Avoid training during the hottest part of the day, usually between 10 A.M. and 2 P.M., during summer months.
4. Drink 8 ounces of cold water about 20 minutes before exercising, and 4 to 8 ounces every 10 to 15 minutes during activity. Before and during exercise, replace fluid with either water or an approximately 6% glucose solution.
5. Wear loose-fitting clothing that allows for the evaporation of sweat.
6. Adjust training intensity down by monitoring heart rate.
7. Incorporate compulsory rest periods of at least 10 minutes for every 45 to 50 minutes of physical activity.
8. Closely monitor daily body weight. If losses are greater than 3% of body weight

they should be replaced by drinking fluids before the next training session.

9. Give special consideration to, and use caution with, the following heat-susceptible persons: those unacclimatized to the heat, the obese, and unfit (low cardiorespiratory fitness classifications), the dehydrated, and those with a previous history of heat stroke.

Air Pollutants

The principal air pollutants that may concern those who exercise outdoors in or near big cities are ozone, carbon monoxide, and sulfur dioxide. The major factors in determining the dose are the concentration of the pollutant, the duration of the exposure, and the volume of air inhaled. Since ventilation increases with the level of exercise, the effects of the pollutant will also depend on the intensity of exercise. See the *ACSM Resource Manual for Guidelines for Exercise Testing and Prescription*, 4th edition (2001), for a more detailed description of air pollution hazards and exercise.

Perhaps the most problematic of these pollutants is ozone, or smog (not stratospheric ozone), that is formed by the reaction of a combination of ultraviolet light and emissions from internal combustion engines. The level of ozone we breathe is a function of weather patterns, traffic density, and industrial output. Ozone exposure may impair lung function during moderate aerobic exercise at concentrations as low as 0.08 parts per million, which is at or below most air quality standards.

Carbon monoxide is another common air pollutant that can substantially reduce aerobic capacity. A 10% increase in carbon monoxide in the blood results in an approximate 10% reduction in maximal oxygen consumption. Moderate submaximal exercise in healthy individuals does not appear to be significantly affected by a 10 to 15% increase in blood carbon monoxide. Cardiac and pulmonary patients are generally affected by as little as a 5% increase in this pollutant. It also is noteworthy that because of the relatively slow removal of carbon monoxide from the blood (the clearance half-time is two to four hours), exposures that occur hours before an exercise session, on crowded freeways or in smoke-filled rooms, could influence aerobic performance.

Sulfur dioxide is most frequently produced in smelters, refineries, and other stationary sources and is not a major irritant for most apparently healthy individuals. However, those persons with asthma or bronchospasm tendencies may be quite sensitive to sulfur dioxide.

Particulate matter (e.g., dust and smoke) are minute particles that are generally 3 to 10 microns in size that may arise from dust in windy conditions or smoke from burning firewood. Smaller particles of 3 to 5 microns can easily penetrate the upper respiratory track, whereas those less than 3 microns can settle in the alveoli. Such particulate inhalation can cause bronchoconstriction (asthma symptoms) and inflammation and congestion of the lower respiratory track.

Be aware of the environmental air quality in your area. An excellent resource for local trends and standards of air quality is the county Air Quality Board or local Environmental Protection Agency. In most cities, one of these agencies or the weather bureau will periodically measure these pollutants and combine them into a Pollution Standards Index (PSI) that ranges from 0 to 500. Generally, PSI levels above 100 will affect those who are very unfit or who have cardiovascular or pulmonary disease, while levels greater that 150 will impair cardiorespiratory performance in healthy normal clients. By understanding environmental air quality standards and being knowledgeable of resources for more information, you can minimize unnecessary fatigue and respiratory distress in clients.

Drugs and Other Substances

There are a number of substances that, when combined with moderate- to high-level aerobic exercise, can increase the risk of cardiovascular complications or affect the response to exercise. These substances are certain prescription medications, alcohol, tobacco, strong stimulants, and over-the-counter medications. Although each is briefly discussed here, refer to a comprehensive review of drugs and substances and their effects on exercise performance in the *ACSM Resource Manual for Guidelines for Exercise Testing and Prescription, 4th edition* (2001).

Virtually all beta-blocking drugs and some of the calcium-channel blocking medications prescribed for a variety of hypertensive and cardiac disorders lower the heart-rate response to exercise. Although these medications may, in fact, increase the client's ability to perform safe exercise, it is important to understand that the heart-rate response to both submaximal and maximal exercise will be blunted. Psychological medications can have side effects that could make exercise more difficult. Some antianxiety medications, such as phenothiazines, can reduce blood pressure and cardiac output, each of which can reduce exercise capacity.

One of the most prevalent categories of drugs employed in medicine, and one that you are likely to at least occasionally observe in your clients, is antihypertensive drugs (i.e., blood pressure–lowering drugs). The major categories of antihypertensive drugs include diuretics, beta- and alpha-blockers, calcium channel blockers, and ACE inhibitors. Within limitations, all of these antihypertensive agents can make exercise safer for the patient with high blood pressure. Diuretic drugs (e.g., thiazides) can induce a relative depletion of blood volume, which can increase the vulnerability of a patient to hypotension in the postexercise period. This side effect of diuretics is of greater concern after prolonged exercise when dehydration may compound the problem.

Alcohol consumption before, during, or after exercise can impair normal exercise heat exchange during prolonged exercise in hot weather. Smoking tobacco in any form increases blood carbon monoxide levels, which will decrease the oxygen consumption of the heart and skeletal muscles.

Stimulants such as nicotine, amphetamines, and especially cocaine all have the potential to induce abnormal cardiac rhythms and decrease coronary blood flow. These substances also may mask important signs of exercise fatigue that are important for the client to discern to adjust exercise intensity. Mixing these or combining any of these substances with near-maximal or maximal aerobic exercise markedly increases the risk of cardiovascular complications, even sudden cardiac death.

Over-the-counter medications such as decongestants, antihistamines, and aspirin products are not contraindications to exercise by themselves but warrant attention because of the infections or ailments for which they are taken. You should caution clients who have viral infections to abstain from prolonged and/or intense aerobic exercise because of the potential for complications and cardiac rhythm disturbances.

Unusual Symptoms

Chest discomfort, musculoskeletal pain, dizziness, lightheadedness, or malaise are indications to discontinue exercise and, in some cases, consult a physician. Exceptional chest discomfort (not necessarily chest "pain") such as aching, pressure, tightness, or burning in the chest is always an indication to consult a physician. The client should never exceed the exercise threshold necessary to cause chest discomfort.

When a client experiences overall listlessness or recent onset lethargy (feelings of no energy) for no apparent reason, advise the client to either abort exercise or significantly decrease exercise intensity and duration. Such vague symptoms can precede viral infections and even be an indicator of future cardiovascular complications.

Musculoskeletal pain or tenderness in a muscle or joint that tends to increase with increasing exercise intensity or duration is an indication to discontinue that particular mode or intensity of exercise (see chapter 12). The beginner should be told to expect some minor muscle soreness and general postexercise fatigue. These minor symptoms usually resolve themselves in several weeks; however, those musculoskeletal symptoms that tend to reproduce themselves over the course of several weeks warrant special attention.

Exercise during viral infections, such as the flu and upper respiratory infections, may lead to complications including worsening of the infections, an increase in body temperature, and cardiac rhythm disturbances. Advise rest and the usual recuperative recommendations as long as malaise, congestion, or fever persist.

SUMMARY

Cardiorespiratory fitness, or the ability of the lungs to provide oxygen to the blood, and of the heart and circulatorysystem to transport blood and its nutrients to the tissues, is basic to all fitness programs. You must understand the physiology and application of each component of a cardiorespiratory exercise program: warm-up and cool-down; mode, frequency, duration, and intensity of an exercise session; importance of supporting cardiorespiratory exercise with flexibility and strength exercise; development of a written exercise progression plan that is updated on a regular basis; and information and guidance necessary to ensure each client's safety, including when to defer exercise.

You have a variety of training methods and cardiorespiratory activities with which to develop an exercise program that meets the needs of each client. You must be familiar with the application of, and the physiological response to, five basic training methods: continuous training, interval training, Fartlek training, circuit training, and aerobic composite training. You also must provide guidelines for such popular aerobic and sport activities as walking, jogging, indoor and outdoor cycling, swimming, rowing, traditional aerobics, stair-climbing, racquet sports, and hiking. These guidelines include teaching clients to monitor their exercise intensity using such self-monitoring techniques as heart rate or ratings of perceived exertion. Finally, you must understand the various sources of cardiorespiratory exercise fatigue, environmental considerations, and the effects of a variety of drugs and medications, and take proactive steps to maximize exercise safety for each client.

REFERENCES

Ainsworth, B.E. et al. (2001). Compendium of Physical Activities: Classification of Energy Costs of Human Physical Activities. In: *ACSM Resource Manual for Guidelines for Exercise Testing and Prescription* (4th ed.). Philadelphia: Lippincott Williams & Wilkins.

American College of Sports Medicine (2003). *ACSM Fitness Book* (3rd ed.). Champaign, Ill.: Human Kinetics.

American College of Sports Medicine (2000). *ACSM's Guidelines for Exercise Testing and Prescription* (6th ed.). Philadelphia: Lippincott Williams & Wilkins.

American College of Sports Medicine (2001). *ACSM Resource Manual for Guidelines for Exercise Testing and Prescription* (4th ed.). Philadelphia: Lippincott Williams & Wilkins.

American Council on Exercise (2000). *Group Fitness Instructor Manual.* San Diego: American Council on Exercise.

Blair, S.N. et al. (1995). Changes in physical fitness and all-cause mortality: a prospective study of healthy and unhealthy men. *Journal of the American Medical Association*, 273, 1093–1098.

Bonelli, S. (2000). *Step Training*. San Diego: American Council on Exercise.

Bonelli, S. (2001). *Aquatic Exercise*. San Diego: American Council on Exercise.

Bricker, K. (2000). *Traditional Aerobics*. San Diego: American Council on Exercise.

Carlton, R. & Rhodes, E. (1985). A critical review of the literature on the ratings scales of perceived exertion. *Sports Medicine*, 2, 198–222.

Diabetes Prevention Program Research Group (2002). Reduction in the incidence of type 2 diabetes with lifestyle intervention or Metformin. *New England Journal of Medicine*, 346, 6, 393–403.

Dishman, R., Farquhar, R., & Cureton, K. (1994). Responses to preferred intensities of exertion in men differing in activity levels. *Medicine and Science in Sports and Exercise*, 26, 783.

Durstine, L. & Pate, R. (1993). Cardiorespiratory responses to acute exercise. *ACSM's Resource Manual for Guidelines for Exercise Testing and Prescription* (2nd ed.). Philadelphia: Lea & Febiger.

Haskell, W.L. (1994). Health consequences of physical activity: understanding and challenges regarding dose response. *Medicine and Science in Sports and Exercise*, 26, 649–660.

Heyward, V.H. (1984). *Designs for Fitness.* Minneapolis, Minn.: Burgess Publishing.

Howley, E. & Franks, D. (2003). *Health Fitness Instructor's Handbook* (4th ed.). Champaign, Ill.: Human Kinetics.

Howley, E. & Glover, M. (1974). The caloric costs of running and walking 1 mile for men and women. *Medicine and Science in Sports and Exercise*, 6, 235–237.

Lan, C. et al. (1998). 12-month tai chi training in the elderly: its effect on health fitness. *Medicine and Science in Sports and Exercise*, 30, 345–351.

Lee, I-M. et al. (2003). Relative intensity of physicalactivity and risk of coronary heart disease. *Circulation*, 107, 1110–1116.

McArdle, W., Katch, F., & Katch, V. (2001). *Exercise Physiology: Energy, Nutrition, and Human Performance* (5th ed.). Philadelphia: Lippincott Williams & Wilkins.

National Institute of Health: Consensus Development Panel on Physical Activity and Cardiovascular Health (1996). Physical activity and cardiovascular health. *Journal of the American Medical Association*, 276, 241–246.

Neporent, L. & Schlosberg, S. (1999). *Fitness for Dummies* (2nd ed.). Hoboken, N.J.: John Wiley & Sons.

Nieman, D. (1990). *Fitness and Sports Medicine: An Introduction*. Palo Alto, Calif.: Bull Publishing.

Parker, S. et al. (1989). Failure of target heart rate to accurately monitor intensity during aerobic dance. *Medicine and Science in Sports and Exercise*, 21, 230.

Pate, R.R. et al. (1995). Physical activity and public health: a recommendation from the Centers for Disease Control and American College of Sports Medicine. *Journal of the American Medical Association*, 273, 402–407.

Pollock, M. (1973). The quantification of endurance training programs. *Exercise and Sport Science Reviews*, 1, 155–188.

Raglin, J. & Moger, L. (1999). Adverse psychological consequences of physical activity: when more is too much. In: *Lifestyles Medicine*, J.M. Rippe (Ed.). Worcester, Mass.: Blackwell Scientific.

Raglin, J.S. & Wilson, G.S. (1999). Overtraining in athletes. In: *Emotion in Sports*, Y.L. Hanin (Ed.). Champaign, Ill.: Human Kinetics.

Saltin, B. et al. (1977). Fiber types and metabolic potentials of skeletal muscles in sedentary men and endurance runners. *Annals of the New York Academy of Science*, 301, 3.

Shechtman, N. (2000). *Group Indoor Cycling*. San Diego: American Council on Exercise.

Whaley, M. et al. (1992). Questioning the routine use of 220 – AGE heart rate formula. *Medicine and Science in Sports and Exercise*, 24, 1173.

Wells, C. & Pate, R. (1988).Training for performance in prolonged exercise. In: *Prolonged Exercise* (Vol.1), 357–389, D. Lamb & R. Murray (Eds.) Carmel, Ind.: Benchmark Press.

SUGGESTED READING

American Heart Association (2001). Exercise standards for testing and training. *Circulation*, 104, 1694.

Astrand, P.O. & Rodahl, K. (1986). *Textbook of Work Physiology* (3rd ed.). New York: McGraw-Hill.

Borg, G. (1982). Psychological basis of perceived exertion. *Medicine and Science in Sports and Exercise*, 14, 377–381.

Borg, G. (1998). *Borg's Perceived Exertion and Pain Scales*. Champaign, Ill.: Human Kinetics.

Franks D. & Howley, E. (1990). *Fitness Facts*. Champaign, Ill.: Human Kinetics.

Greenberg, J. & Pargman, D. (1989). *Physical Fitness: A Wellness Approach* (2nd ed.). Englewood Cliffs, N.J.: Prentice-Hall.

Herbert, W. & Herbert, D. *The Exercise Standards and Malpractice Reporter*, 1987 to present.

Ketner, J.B. & Mekkion, M.B. (1995).The overtraining syndrome: a review of presentation, pathophysiology, and treatment. *Medicine, Exercise, Nutrition, & Health*, 4, 136–145.

Ockene, I. & Ockene, J. (1992). *Prevention of Coronary Heart Disease*. Boston: Little, Brown & Company.

Pollock, M. & Wilmore, J. (1990). *Exercise in Health and Disease* (2nd ed.). Philadelphia: W.B. Saunders.

Raglin, J.S. (1993). Overtraining and Staleness: Psychometric Monitoring of Endurance Athletes. In: *Handbook of Research on Sport Psychology*. R.B. Singer, M. Murphey, & L.Tennant (Eds.). New York: Macmillan.

Richie, D. (1989). Medical and legal implications of dance exercise leadership: the role of footwear. *Exercise Standards and Malpractice Reporter*, 3, 61.

Sanders, M. (Ed.) (2000). *YMCA Water Fitness for Health*. Champaign, Ill.: Human Kinetics.

Shapiro, U. & Seidman, D. (1990). Field and clinical observations of exertional heat stroke patients. *Medicine and Science in Sports and Exercise*, 22, 1.

Wilmore, J.H. & Costill, D. (1999). *Physiology of Sport and Exercise* (2nd ed.). Champaign, Ill.: Human Kinetics.

CHAPTER 4

Muscular Strength and Endurance

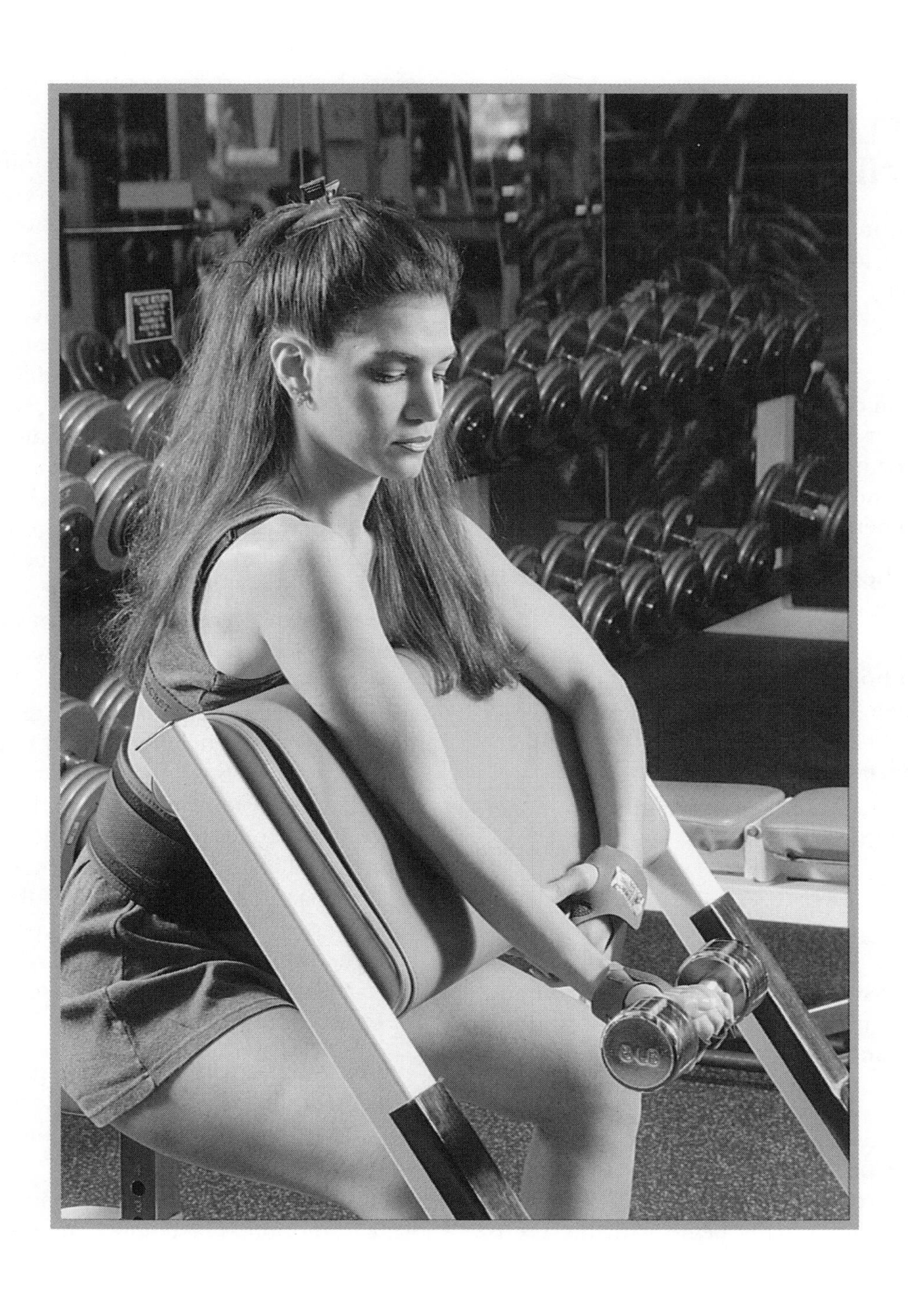

Every movement of the human body involves the muscular system. Muscles are unique in their ability to contract, relax, and produce force and movement. With appropriate exercise, muscles become larger and stronger. As a YMCA personal training instructor, you must be knowledgeable about the basic skeletal and muscle anatomy and physiology and the biomechanics of the musculoskeletal system. This chapter defines key terms and presents essential concepts from these areas of study and relates them to strength training exercise.

SKELETAL ANATOMY AND PHYSIOLOGY

In this section we look at the types of bones in the body, the joints, and the movements possible at the joints.

Bones

The skeleton consists of 206 bones that provide protection for the internal organs and a leverage structure for muscles. The skeleton also allows for growth and is the largest store of calcium in the body. There are four classes of bones:

- **Long bones.** These are found in the arms and legs, and they are associated with movement.
- **Short bones.** These are found in the hands and feet. Some short bones, such as the bones in the vertebral (spinal) column, are irregular in shape.
- **Flat bones.** These are found in the upper part of the skull.
- **Irregular bones.** These are found in vertebrae and in the pubic area.

Figure 4.1 (*a-b*) shows the front (anterior) and back (posterior) views of the skeleton and identifies the major bones, groups of bones, and anatomical landmarks.

Joints

A joint is the point where bones link or connect. Joints are also called *articulations*, and items associated with joints usually begin with the prefix *arthr-*, as in *arthroscope*, a device that is used to look into the joint spaces of a person with *arthritis*. Joints are classified on the basis of how much movement is permitted between the bones:

- **Synarthrodial joints.** These are immovable joints or those with limited movement, such as the joints between the bones in the skull.
- **Amphiarthrodial joints.** These are joints with slight movement, as seen in the connections between vertebrae in the spinal column.
- **Diarthrotic or synovial joints.** These are joints that have great potential for movement, as in the knee.

The diarthrotic or synovial joint is most important in physical activity. Movement occurs when the muscles move the bones through a range of motion within the limits of these joints. These joints are held together by connective tissue—*ligaments*, which cross over the joint, and *tendons*, which attach muscles to bones and also cross over joints to lend additional support. Because these joints move a great deal, the structure also contains slippery surfaces and a lubricant. The slippery surface in each movable joint is the *articular hyaline cartilage* that covers the ends of the bones. This cartilage also absorbs some of the shock of impact to reduce the chance that the bony surface will wear out. *Synovial fluid* is the lubricant secreted by the *synovial membrane* within the joint housing or capsule. In addition, *bursae*, or sacs containing synovial fluid outside the joint space, help to lubricate the movement of tendons, ligaments, and muscles over bony structures. Some of these joints (e.g., the knee) have additional cartilage in the joint space between the bones to take up some of the shock of impact. This is the type of cartilage that can be torn as a result of high-impact forces, and the smooth articular cartilage is the type that can be damaged by arthritis.

Diarthrodial (movable) joints are classified by the type of movement permitted:

- **Ball-and-socket joints.** These allow movement in all directions. An example is where the head of the humerus (the bone of the upper arm) fits into the shoulder.
- **Hinge joints.** These allow movement in one plane of motion. The elbow is an example.

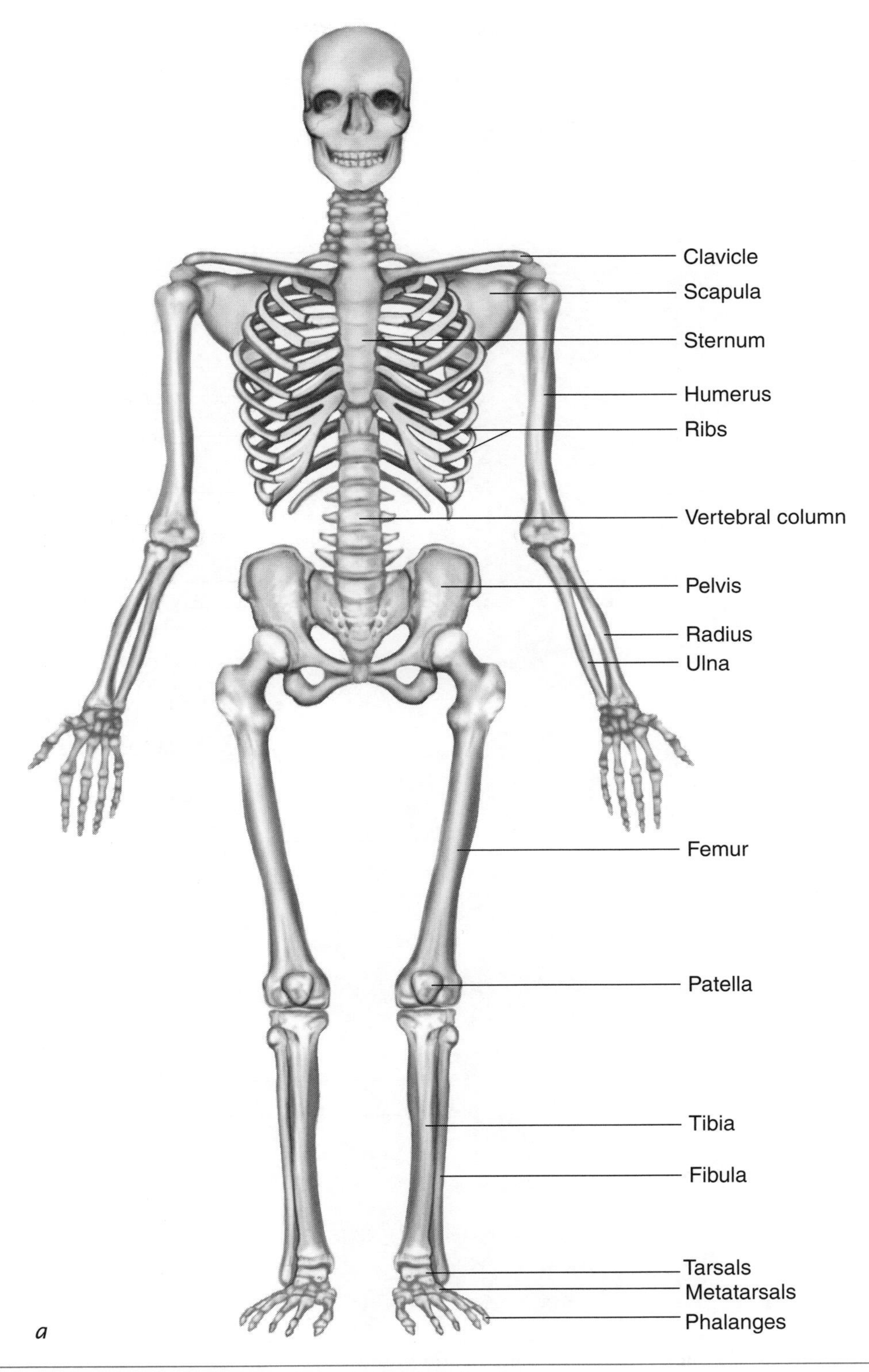

Figure 4.1 (*a*) Front (anterior) view of the human skeleton.

(continued)

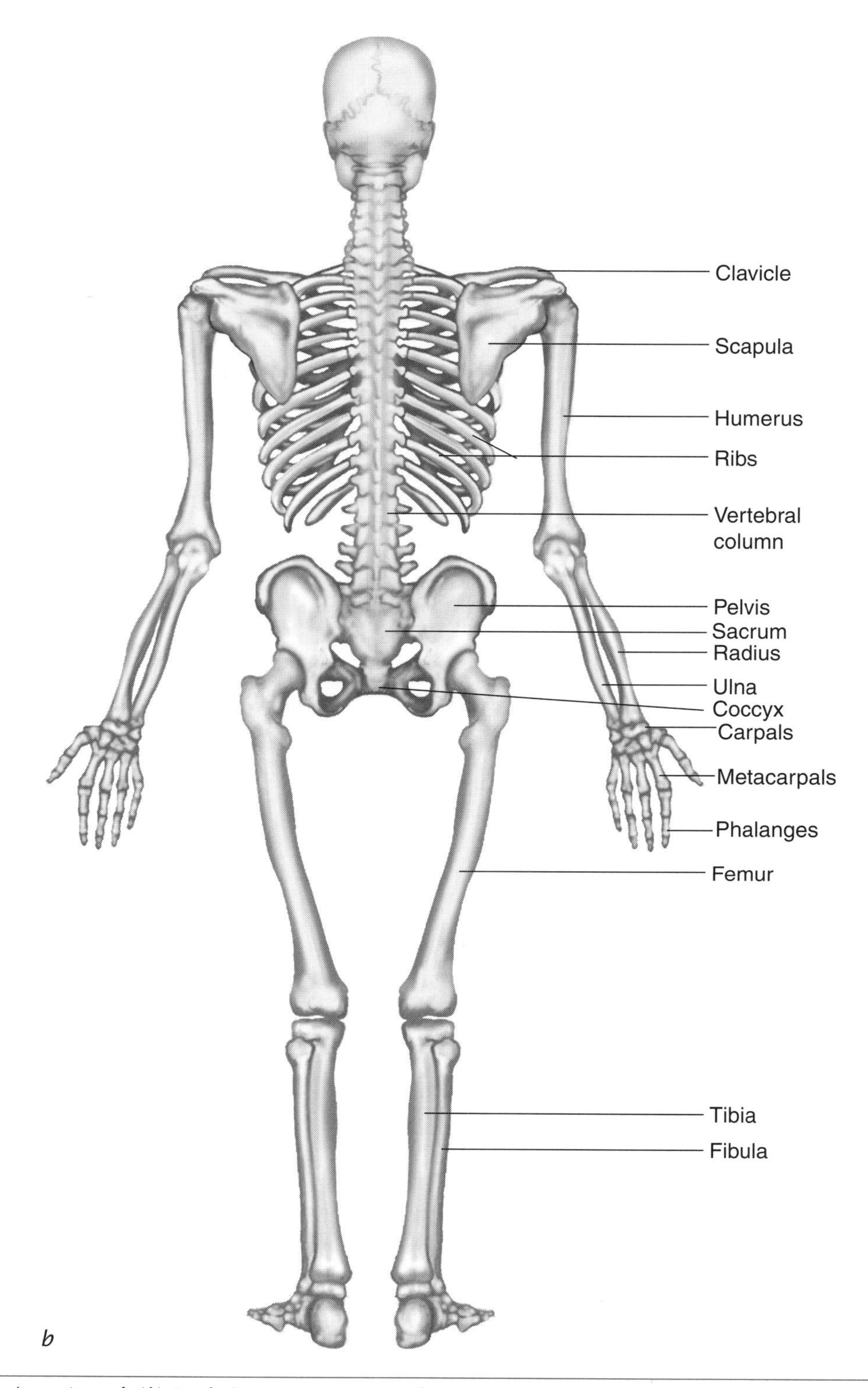

Figure 4.1 (*continued*) (*b*) Back (posterior) view of the human skeleton.

• **Saddle joints.** These allow movement in all directions. The metacarpal–carpal joint of the thumb is an example.

• **Pivot joints.** These allow rotation around the long portion of the bone. The radioulnar joint is an example because it allows rotation of the wrist to turn hand palm up (supinated position) or down (pronated position).

• **Gliding joints.** These allow only gliding or twisting. Examples are the joints between the wrist bones (carpals) or the ankle bones (tarsals).

Movements

The types of movements possible at each joint depend on the type of joint. It is important to know the terms that describe these movements before we present a summary of the muscles involved:

• **Flexion and extension.** Flexion describes a motion that decreases the angle of a joint, and extension is a movement that increases the joint angle. If your arm is hanging straight down, flexion is the movement of your hand toward your shoulder around the elbow joint; lowering the hand to its starting position is extension. The term *hyperextension* refers to a movement beyond a joint's ordinary resting position.

• **Abduction and adduction.** Abduction describes a movement away from the center line of the body; adduction is a return to the ordinary anatomical position. Moving the leg to the side, away from the body, is an example of abduction.

• **Rotation.** Rotation is movement around the long axis of a bone and describes a movement either toward (*inward* or *medial rotation*) or away from (*outward* or *lateral rotation*) the center of the body. With your forearm at a 90-degree angle relative to your upper arm and your hand in front of your body, movement of the wrist and lower arm toward the center line of the body is an example of medial rotation.

• **Pronation and supination.** If the forearm is held at a 90-degree angle relative to the upper arm, hand in front of the body with thumb up, pronation describes a movement of the forearm to turn the palm downward, and supination the reverse. These terms are also used to describe the manner in which the foot lands when walking or running. A person who lands with the inside, or medial aspect, of the foot striking first is said to be a "pronator." Because repeated steps on a pronated foot can cause pain or injury, many running shoes are designed to control this movement.

• **Dorsiflexion and plantarflexion.** These terms describe the movement of the foot from its normal position either toward the lower leg (dorsiflexion) or toward the bottom of the foot (plantarflexion).

See figure 4.2 for specific examples of these movements.

Ankle Extension (Plantarflexion)

Muscle Group

Gastrocnemius and soleus

Increasing the angle between the foot and the leg

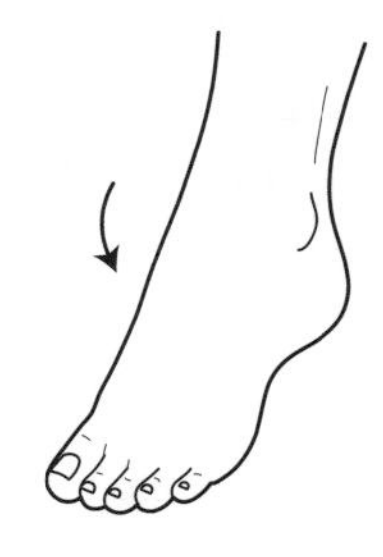

Ankle Flexion (Dorsiflexion)

Muscle Group

Tibialis anterior

Decreasing the angle between the foot and the leg

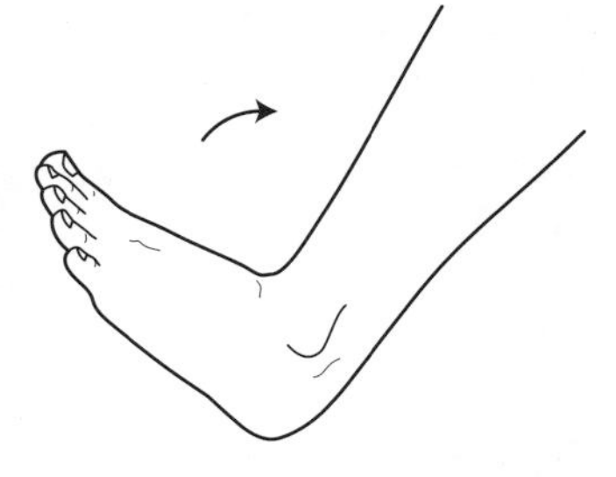

Figure 4.2 Movements in muscle groups.

(continued)

Knee Extension

Muscle Group

Quadriceps: rectus femoris, vastus lateralis, vastus medialis, and vastus intermedius

Increasing the angle between the thigh and the leg

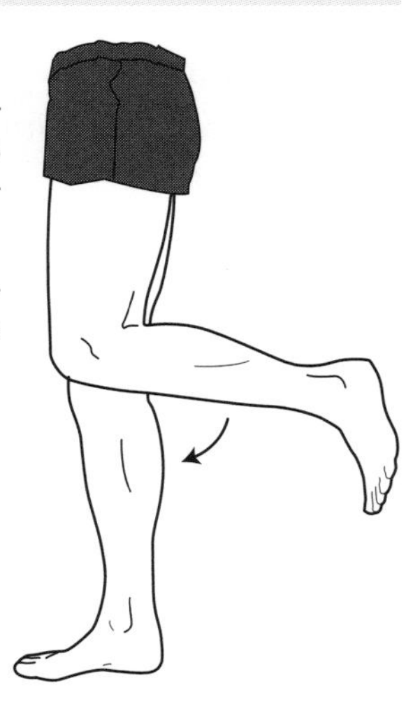

Knee Flexion

Muscle Group

Hamstrings: biceps femoris, semitendinosus, and semimembranosus

Decreasing the angle between the thigh and the leg

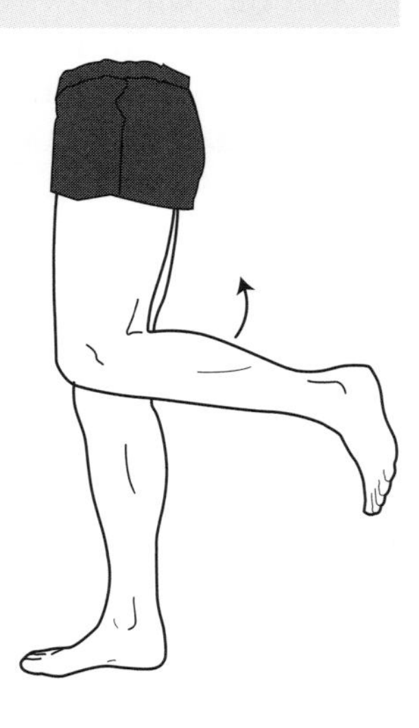

Hip Abduction

Muscle Group

Hip abductors: gluteus medius and tensor fasciae latae

Increasing the angle between the thigh and the mid-line of the body (outward–sideward movement)

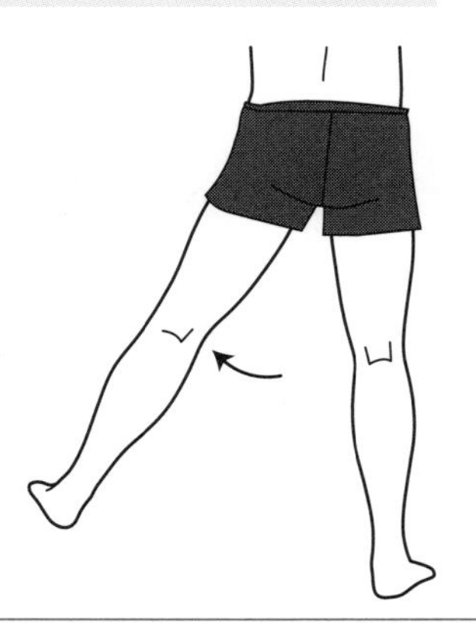

Hip Adduction

Muscle Group

Hip adductors: adductor magnus, adductor longus, adductor brevis, pectineus, and gracilis

Decreasing the angle between the thigh and the midline of the body (inward–sideward movement)

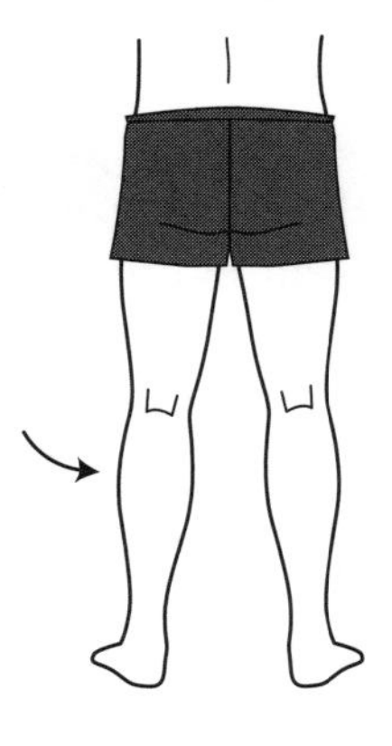

Hip Extension

Muscle Group

Gluteus maximus and hamstrings

Increasing the angle between the thigh and the torso

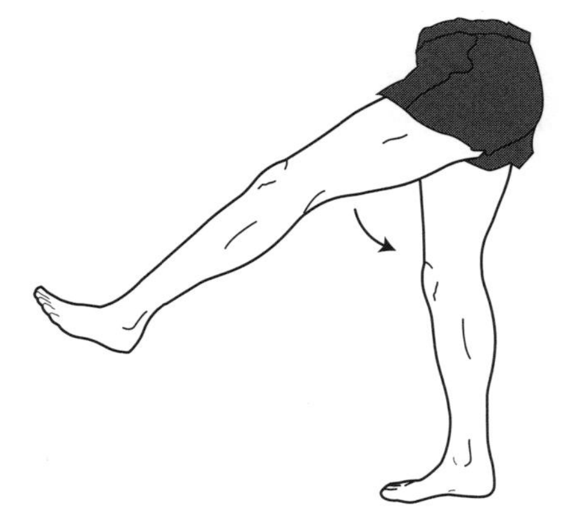

Hip Flexion

Muscle Group

Rectus femoris and iliopsoas

Decreasing the angle between the thigh and the torso

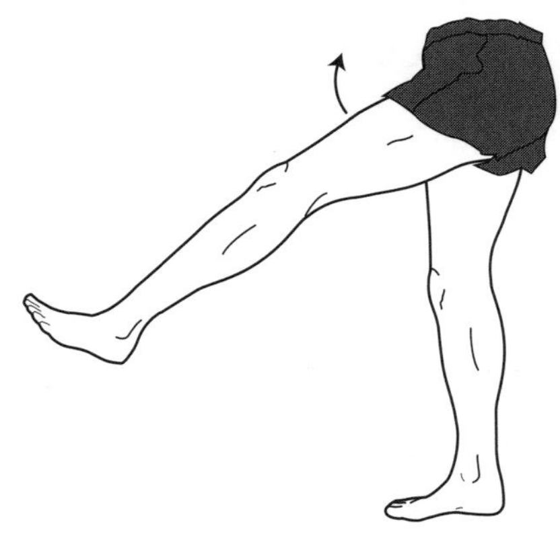

Figure 4.2 *(continued)*

Trunk Extension

Muscle Group

Erector spinae

Increasing the angle between the chest and the abdomen

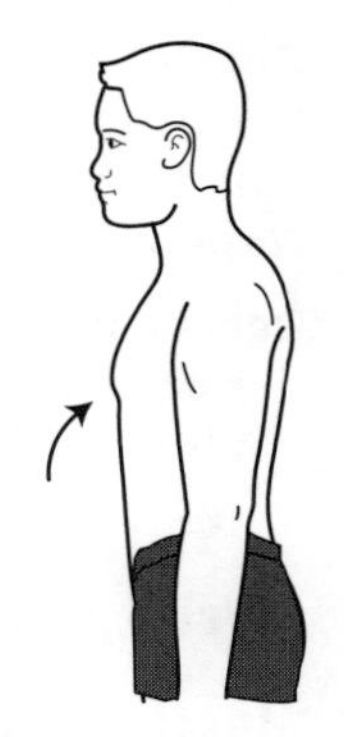

Trunk Flexion

Muscle Group

Rectus abdominis

Decreasing the angle between the chest and the abdomen

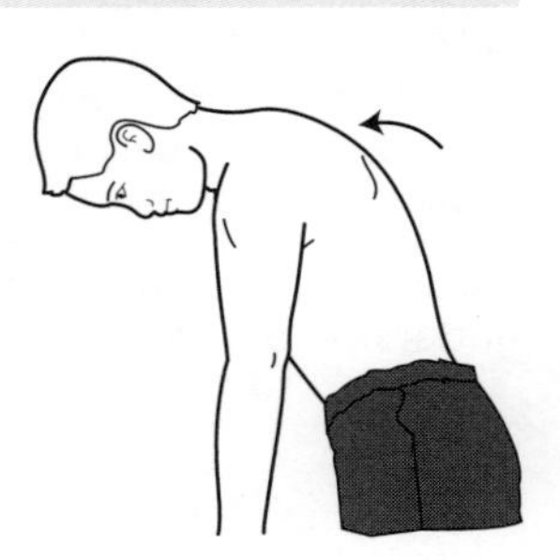

Shoulder Abduction

Muscle Group

Deltoids

Increasing the angle between the arm and the side (upward–sideward movement)

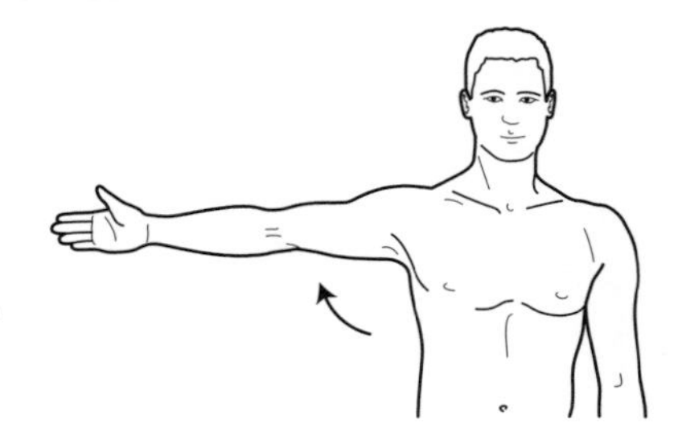

Shoulder Adduction

Muscle Group

Latissimus dorsi and pectoralis major

Decreasing the angle between the arm and the side (downward–sideward movement)

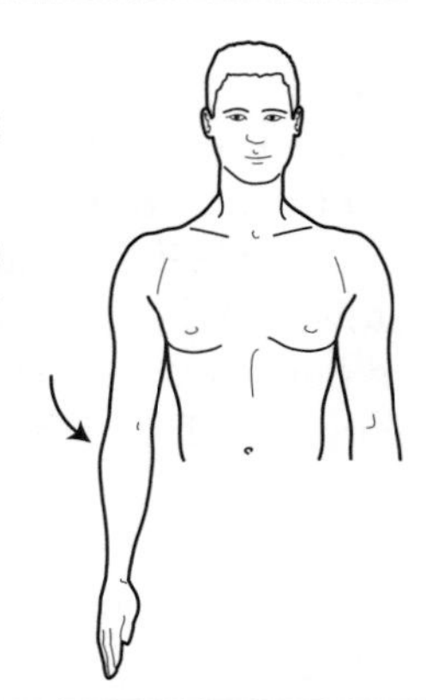

Shoulder Flexion

Muscle Group

Anterior deltoid

Increasing the angle between the arm and the chest (upward–forward movement)

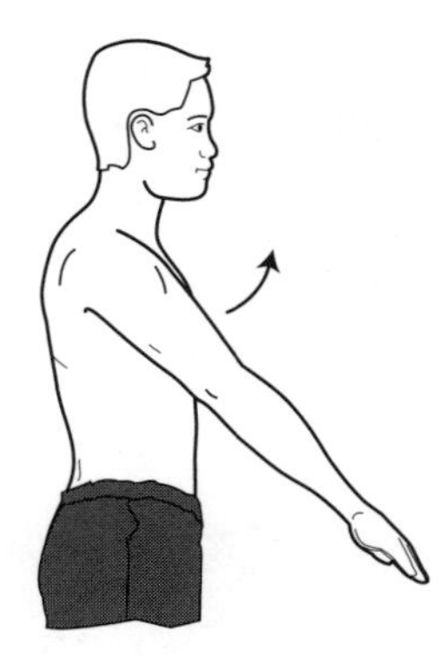

Shoulder Extension

Muscle Group

Posterior deltoid and latissimus dorsi

Decreasing the angle between the arms and the chest (downward–backward movement)

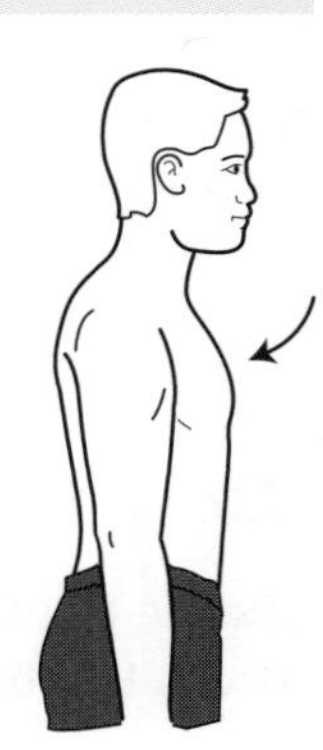

Shoulder Horizontal Flexion

Muscle Group

Pectoralis major and anterior deltoid

Decreasing the angle between the arms and the chest (forward movement with arms perpendicular to the chest)

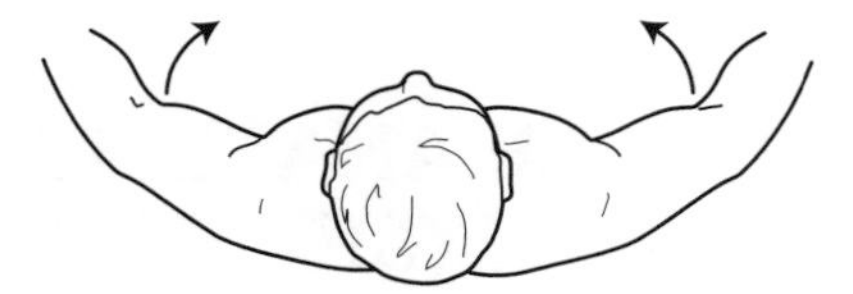

Figure 4.2 *(continued)*

(continued)

Shoulder Horizontal Extension

Muscle Group

Posterior deltoid and latissimus dorsi

Increasing the angle between the arms and the chest (backward movement with arms perpendicular to the chest)

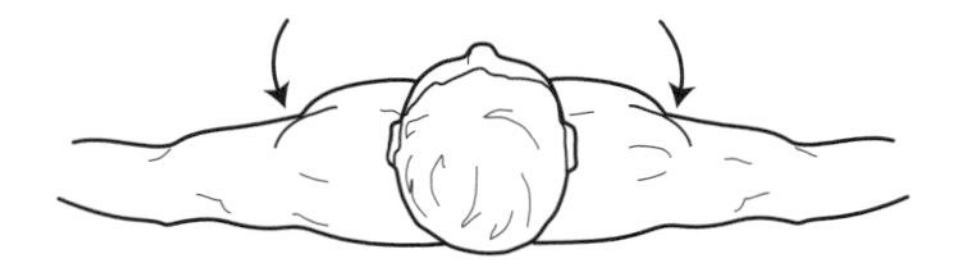

Elbow Flexion

Muscle Group

Biceps brachii

Decreasing the angle between the arm and the forearm

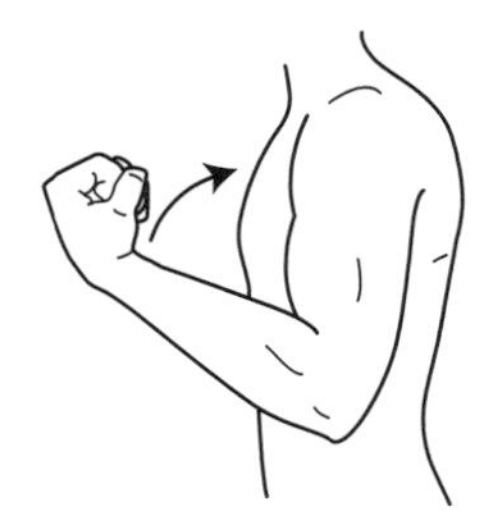

Elbow Extension

Muscle Group

Triceps brachii

Increasing the angle between the arm and the forearm

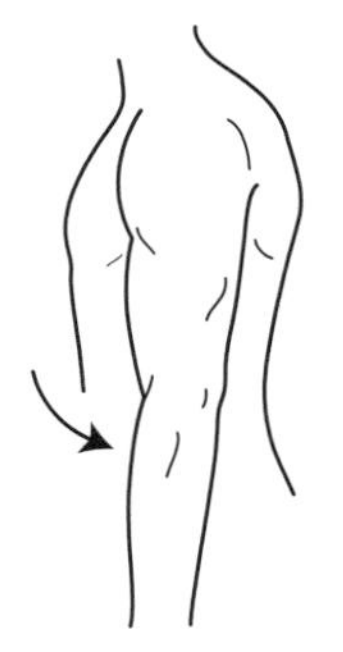

Wrist Flexion

Muscle Group

Forearm flexors: flexor carpi ulnaris, palmaris longus, flexor carpi radialis, and others

Decreasing the angle between the palm and the underside of the forearm

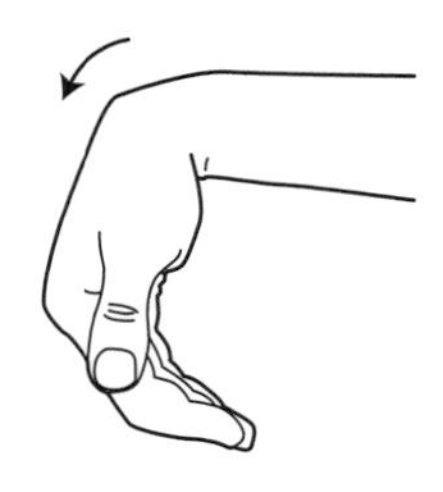

Wrist Extension

Muscle Group

Forearm extensors: extensor carpi ulnaris, extensor digitorum, extensor carpi radialis, and others

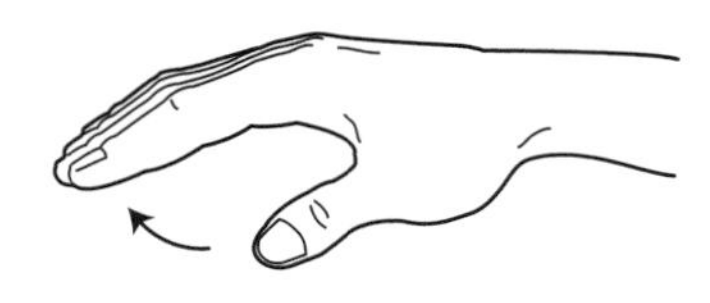

Increasing the angle between the palm and the underside of the forearm

Figure 4.2 *(continued)*

MUSCLE ANATOMY AND PHYSIOLOGY

Regardless of how well the cardiorespiratory system might function, no one could move without muscles and their phenomenal ability to contract. Muscles make up about 40 to 50 percent of total body weight. They are composed essentially of water (72 percent), lipids (8 percent), and proteins (20 percent). The muscle proteins are the keys to muscle contraction because they perform a unique function.

It is the anatomy of muscles that allows muscle contraction and relaxation to take place. This produces force, which takes the form of isometric, concentric, or eccentric contractions. Two types of muscle fibers are present—fast twitch and slow twitch, each best suited for a different type of performance. Muscles have both strength and endurance, which are different ways of exerting force.

The muscles can be overloaded using isometric, isotonic, or isokinetic exercises. How large muscles become or how quickly they develop as a result of overloading depends on the factors of muscle length, gender, and age. Each exercise movement uses three sets of muscles: the prime movers, the antagonists, and the stabilizers.

The following sections specifically discuss the anatomy, contraction and relaxation, force production, fiber types, strength and endurance, strength overload, and muscle size of the musculoskeletal system. We conclude with a brief summary of examples of common exercises and the muscles that are used in those activities.

Muscle Anatomy

Muscles are composed of muscle fibers, the individual muscle cells that are the functional components of muscles. As shown in figure 4.3, muscle fibers are cylindrical strands that contract as a unit when stimulated by an appropriate nerve impulse. *Myofibrils* are smaller cylindrical strands that run lengthwise within the muscle fiber. Each myofibril consists of numerous protein filaments that are sectioned into individual units called *sarcomeres* (see figure 4.3). Sarcomeres are the smallest units of contraction within muscles. As illustrated in figure 4.3, they form adjacent sections of each myofibril. Also shown is how sarcomeres are structured from two proteins that form a specific pattern and perform a specific function. Each sarcomere has thin actin proteins that surround thick myosin proteins. The thin actin proteins are coupled to the ends of the thick myosin proteins by means of small cross-bridges (see figure 4.3).

When properly stimulated, the thin actin proteins are pulled from both ends toward the center by the thick myosin proteins. As illustrated in figure 4.4, this results in a shortening of the activated muscle fibers and a bulging of the muscle.

Muscle Contraction and Relaxation

The pulling action between the actin and myosin proteins that produces the muscle contraction involves electrical, chemical, and mechanical interactions. The electrical stimulus arrives by means of a motor nerve, which is part of a motor unit. A *motor unit* consists of a single motor nerve and all of the individual muscle fibers that are

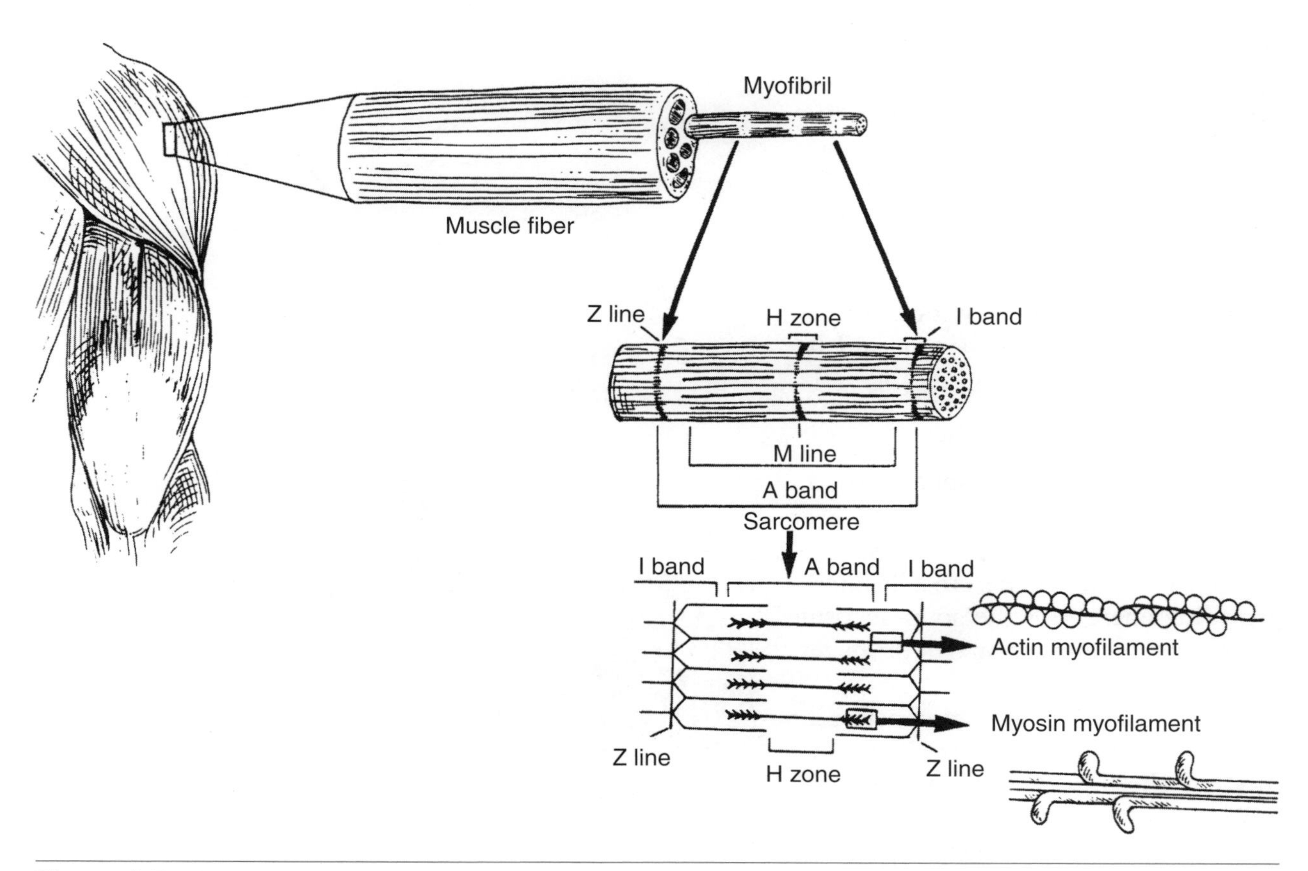

Figure 4.3 A sarcomere.

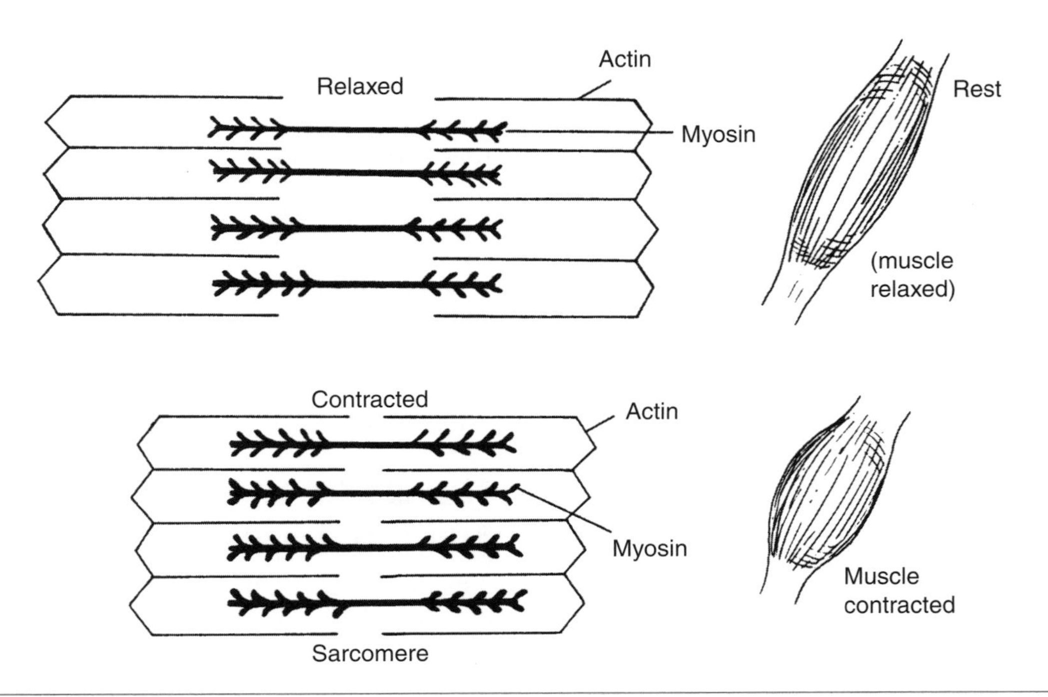

Figure 4.4 Shortening of muscle fibers.

activated by that nerve. As illustrated in figure 4.5, a typical motor unit involves several individual fibers throughout a muscle. Whenever a motor nerve sends a sufficient stimulus, all of the attached muscle fibers contract with maximum force. This is referred to as the *all-or-none principle of muscle contraction*. Consequently, to produce low force only a few motor units are activated, and to produce high force many motor units are activated.

The chemical process centers on splitting adenosine triphosphate (ATP), which produces the energy for muscle contraction. The ATP-splitting process appears to occur at the cross-bridges, providing energy for the actin–myosin linkage and pulling action that produces muscle contraction.

The mechanical interaction between the actin and myosin proteins is accomplished through the coupling and pulling movements of the connecting cross-bridges. During this process, the thin actin proteins are pulled toward

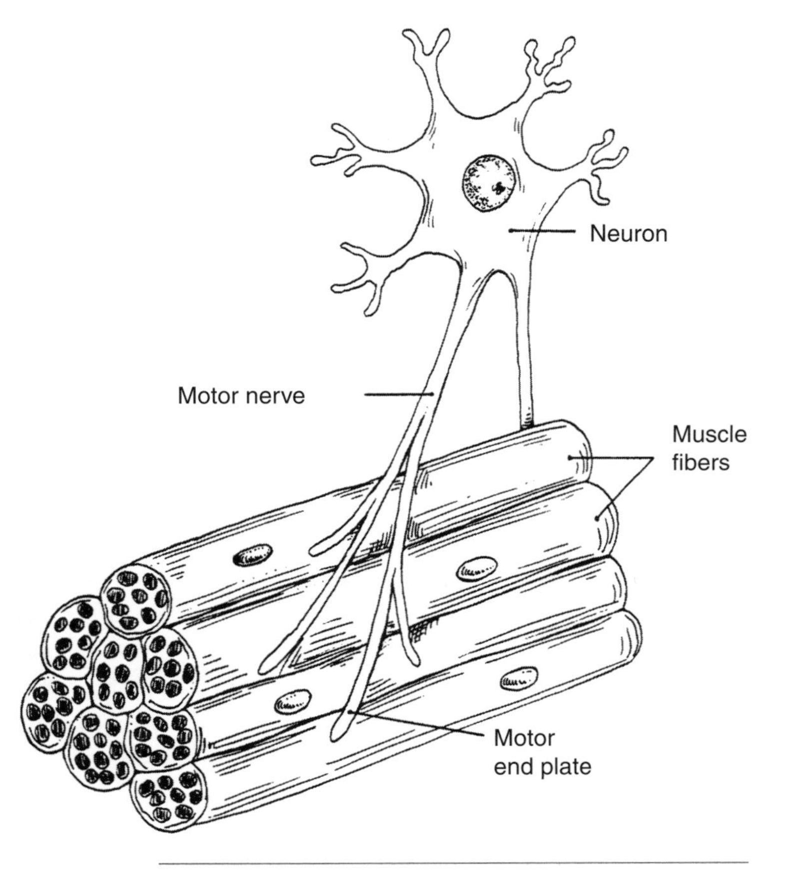

Figure 4.5 A motor unit.

the center by the thick myosin proteins, which shortens and bulges the muscle (see figure 4.4). The sliding action between the actin and myosin proteins produces muscle friction that alters the effective force output.

When the nervous stimulation that triggers muscle contraction ceases, the coupling and pulling movements between the actin and myosin proteins no longer occur and the muscle relaxes. Muscle relaxation is essential for every movement because as one muscle group contracts and shortens, the opposing muscle group must relax and lengthen. Fortunately, the nervous system precisely regulates concurrent muscle contraction and muscle relaxation to produce smooth movements with the desired degree of force and speed. Blocking nerve impulses to muscles that oppose a desired movement is termed *reciprocal inhibition.*

Force Production

A muscle possesses many motor units, and the tension that a muscle develops depends primarily on the number of motor units called into play. When little muscle force is required, the number of motor units activated is small and the frequency of nerve impulses is low. When a high level of muscle force is required, the number of motor units activated is large and the frequency of nerve impulses is high. When a muscle contracts, the ends of the muscle move toward each other. The following terms describe the different types of muscle contractions:

- **Isometric contraction.** An isometric contraction, also called a *static contraction*, occurs when a muscle exerts force and does not visibly change in length. The muscle force equals the resistance force, and the muscle neither shortens nor lengthens. Because there is no movement between the actin and myosin proteins, isometric contractions are not affected by frictional forces. Holding a 50-pound dumbbell at 90 degrees of elbow flexion (by producing 50 pounds of muscle force) is an example of isometric contraction (see figure 4.6*a*).
- **Concentric contraction.** A concentric contraction, often referred to as a *positive contraction*, occurs when a muscle exerts force as it shortens (generally a lifting movement). The muscle force is greater than the resistance force. The shortening process involves muscle friction that decreases the effective force output by about 20 percent. For example, if you can hold (isometric contraction) a 50-pound dumbbell at 90 degrees of elbow flexion, you should be able to slowly lift a 40-pound dumbbell (concentric contraction). Although you are still producing 50 pounds of biceps force, muscle friction subtracts about 20 percent for an effective force output of 40 pounds (see figure 4.6*b*).
- **Eccentric contraction.** An eccentric contraction, often referred to as a *negative contraction*, occurs when a muscle exerts force as it lengthens (generally a lowering movement). The muscle force is less than the resistance force. The lengthening process involves muscle friction, therefore increasing the effective force output by about 20 percent. For example, if you can hold (isometric contraction) a 50-pound dumbbell at 90 degrees of elbow flexion, you should be able to slowly lower a 60-pound dumbbell (eccentric contraction). Although you are still producing 50 pounds of biceps force, muscle friction adds about 20 percent for an effective force output of 60 pounds (see figure 4.6*c*).

Muscle Fiber Types

Two types of muscle fibers exist; each has different performance characteristics. *Slow-twitch (type I) muscle fibers* are better suited for low-force, long-duration activities because they possess more endurance enzymes, more blood capillaries, more mitochondria, and more intramuscular triglyceride stores for aerobic energy utilization. Marathon runners and triathletes typically have a high percentage of slow-twitch muscle fibers. *Fast-twitch (type II) muscle fibers* are better suited for high-force, short-duration activities because they possess more glycolytic enzyme activity, more myosin ATP activity, and more intramuscular phosphate stores for anaerobic energy utilization. Sprinters and jumpers typically have a high percentage of fast-twitch muscle fibers.

When maximum strength is required, both slow-twitch and fast-twitch muscle fibers are activated simultaneously. When submaximum strength is required, the slow-twitch muscle

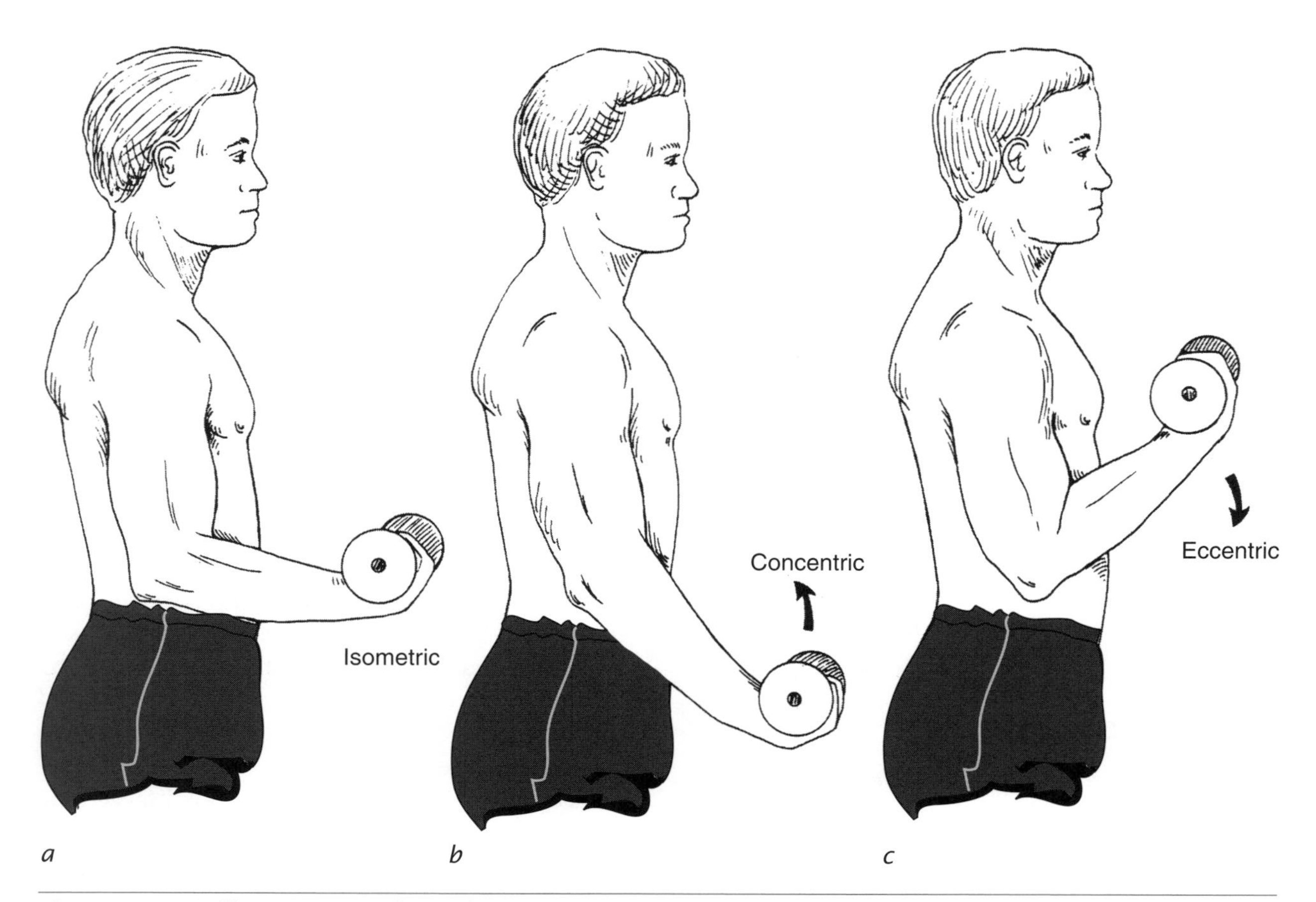

Figure 4.6 Different types of muscle contractions: *(a)* isometric, *(b)* concentric, and *(c)* eccentric.

fibers are recruited first, followed by the fast-twitch muscle fibers, if necessary. Although it is possible to increase both muscular strength and muscular endurance through proper training, it appears that the proportion of fast-twitch and slow-twitch muscle fibers is genetically determined and is not subject to change. However, fast-twitch fibers may take on more aerobic characteristics (type IIa) or more anaerobic characteristics (type IIb) depending on the type of training performed.

Muscle Strength and Endurance

Muscle strength is the ability to exert force against a resistance. It is usually assessed as the maximum resistance that can be performed one time in a given exercise, such as the heaviest weight you can bench press. *Muscle endurance* is the ability to repeatedly exert force against a resistance. It is usually assessed as the number of repetitions that can be performed with a submaximum resistance, such as the number of push-ups you can perform.

People with a high percentage of fast-twitch muscle fibers usually score higher on tests of muscle strength and lower on tests of muscle endurance. Conversely, people with a high percentage of slow-twitch muscle fibers typically score higher on tests of muscle endurance and lower on tests of muscle strength. In all cases, a rather consistent relationship exists between muscle strength and relative muscle endurance. For example, let's say that Ralph can perform one barbell curl with 50 pounds and six barbell curls with 40 pounds. If Ralph increases his strength to one barbell curl with 100 pounds, he will probably perform six barbell curls with 80 pounds. In other words, Ralph's relative muscle endurance (biceps) is six repetitions with 80 percent of his maximum resistance.

Types of Strength Overloads

For many years, strength training programs have been described based on the type of muscle contraction involved during the exercise. The three types of strength training programs are isometric, isotonic, and isokinetic.

- **Isometric exercise.** Isometric exercise is any activity in which the muscles exert force but do not visibly change in length. Pushing against a doorway, carrying a bag of groceries, and water skiing are examples of isometric exercise. Although isometric exercise is effective for increasing muscle strength, it has a few notable drawbacks. First, isometric strength gains are specific to the joint positions that were trained, with relatively little strength improvement in other joint positions. Second, isometric exercise occludes or restricts blood flow and often produces unacceptably high blood pressure responses. Third, it is difficult to assess the training effort and strength improvement associated with most types of isometric exercise.
- **Isotonic exercise.** Isotonic exercise refers to activity in which the muscles exert force and change in length as they lift and lower resistance. Strength exercises using a fixed amount of external resistance are now more accurately referred to as either *dynamic constant-* or *dynamic variable-*resistance exercises. As described in the next paragraphs, these names suggest how the resistance forces and muscle forces interact throughout the range of movement:
- **Dynamic constant-resistance exercise.** Dynamic constant-resistance exercise is characteristic of most muscular activities, such as lifting a baby or pressing a barbell. As the name implies, you lift and lower a constant resistance through a range of movement. Although the resistance does not vary (such as a 90-pound barbell), your muscle force capacity changes considerably throughout the movement range because of leverage factors. Consequently, the muscle force and the resistance force might be closely matched at only one point in the range of movement.
- **Dynamic variable-resistance exercise.** To better match muscle forces and resistance forces throughout the movement range, many types of strength training equipment incorporate dynamic variable-resistance exercise. Through the use of levers, cams, or linkage systems, this equipment automatically changes the resistance according to the muscle force capacity. The equipment provides less resistance in positions of lower muscle force capacity and more resistance in positions of higher muscle force capacity.

  Although dynamic variable-resistance exercise definitely better matches muscle forces and resistance forces throughout the movement range, it has not been shown to be more effective for strength development. In both dynamic constant-resistance exercise and dynamic variable-resistance exercise, the amount of resistance force you select determines the amount of muscle force you produce.
- **Isokinetic exercise.** Isokinetic exercise is an activity in which the resistance forces are closely matched to the muscle forces, thereby maintaining a constant movement speed. For this reason, isokinetic exercise is often referred to as *accommodating resistance*. Water activities are examples of isokinetic exercise because the water resistance accommodates your muscle force. If you push the water with low force, you encounter low resistance, but if you push the water with high force, you encounter high resistance. Isokinetic exercise can be performed on a variety of equipment using frictional resistance, hydraulic resistance, or electronic resistance. Although most isokinetic equipment uses only concentric contractions, some electronic machines provide accommodating resistance during both concentric and eccentric contractions. In isokinetic exercise, the amount of muscle force you produce determines the amount of resistance force you encounter.

Muscle Size Factors

Although many factors contribute to effective muscle strength, the most important one is the cross-sectional size of the muscle. Because most muscles produce approximately one to two kilograms of force per square centimeter of cross-sectional area, a larger muscle is usually a stronger muscle. Proper strength training can increase the cross-sectional size of a muscle by adding actin and myosin proteins. As a result, individual muscle fibers increase in size, which leads to a larger muscle circumference. An increase in muscle size is referred to as *hypertrophy*, and a decrease in muscle size is called *atrophy*.

Three factors that affect how large muscles can become and how quickly they can be developed are muscle length, gender, and age.

Muscle Length Factors

Although everyone can increase muscle strength and muscle size to some degree, one's potential muscle size is related to muscle length. A long muscle with short tendon attachments has more size potential than a short muscle with long tendon attachments. To see how long your muscles are, try this: Put your arm at a right angle and forcefully contract your biceps muscle. Place as many fingers as will comfortable fit between the end of your muscle bulge and your forearm (see figure 4.7).

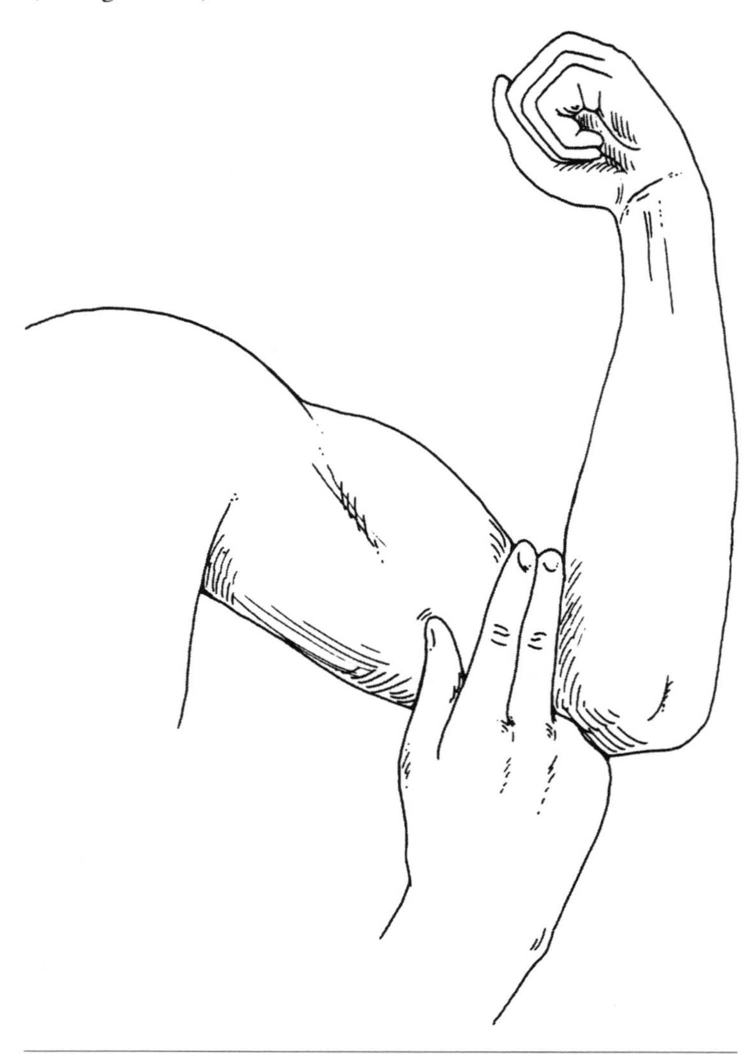

Figure 4.7 Measurement of biceps muscle length.

- If you can fit three fingers, you have a relatively short biceps muscle.
- If you can fit two fingers, you have a medium-length biceps muscle.
- If you can fit only one finger, you have a relatively long biceps muscle.

People who possess mostly long muscles are more likely to be successful in competitive bodybuilding and weightlifting activities.

Gender Factors

On a pound-for-pound basis, male muscle tissue and female muscle tissue are essentially the same. The average male is stronger than the average female not because he has better muscle tissue, but because he has more muscle tissue. Because of a larger frame size, the average man has more muscle mass than the average woman. Because of higher testosterone levels (the male sex hormone associated with muscle hypertrophy), the average man experiences larger increases in muscle size and strength as a result of progressive resistance exercise.

Age Factors

Age does not seem to affect strength development; a stimulus–response pattern associated with progressive resistance exercise produces similar strength results in 9-year-olds and 90-year-olds. However, age does appear to influence the rate of strength development. Research indicates that younger people gain muscle size and strength more quickly than older people. This is particularly true during the years of normal growth and maturation. Because a strong musculoskeletal system is desirable at every age, sensible strength training should begin in the preteen years and continue throughout life.

Muscles and Movements

In each movement we make, muscles are involved. Some provide most of the force for the desired movement, the prime mover muscles; others perform the movement opposite the desired movement, the antagonist muscles; and still others help maintain body posture while movement occurs, the stabilizer muscles.

• **Prime mover muscles.** The muscles primarily responsible for performing a particular movement are called the *prime mover* or *agonist* muscles. For example, in dumbbell curls the biceps muscles are primarily responsible for elbow flexion and serve as the prime mover muscles. More specifically, the biceps muscles contract concentrically to lift the dumbbell and contract eccentrically to lower the dumbbell.

• **Antagonist muscles.** The muscles primarily responsible for performing movement opposite that of the prime mover muscles are termed the *antagonist* muscles. For example, the triceps muscles are primarily responsible for elbow extension, and they function as the antagonist muscles to the biceps. For smooth elbow flexion, the triceps (antagonists) must lengthen as the biceps (prime movers) shorten. Conversely, for smooth elbow extension, the biceps (antagonists) must lengthen as the triceps (prime movers) shorten. Performance of these movements is regulated through the process of reciprocal inhibition (see figure 4.8, page 69).

• **Stabilizer muscles.** The muscles that stabilize certain joints to facilitate the desired movements in other joints are referred to as *stabilizer* or *synergist* muscles. For example, to properly perform barbell curls, the torso must remain erect and steady. This stabilizing function is performed by the low back and oblique muscles, which contract isometrically to maintain the torso in an erect posture.

The major muscle groups are described in figures 4.9 through 4.14, and the action of specific muscles at each joint are listed in table 4.1.

Table 4.1 Muscles That Are Prime Movers

Joint	Prime movers
Shoulder girdle	Abductors—serratus anterior, pectoralis minor
	Adductors—middle fibers of trapezius, rhomboids, upper and lower fibers of trapezius
	Upward rotators—upper and lower fibers of trapezius, serratus anterior
	Downward rotators—rhomboids, pectoralis minor
	Elevators—levator scapulae, upper fibers of trapezius, rhomboids
	Depressors—lower fibers of trapezius, pectoralis minor
Shoulder joint	Flexors—anterior deltoid, clavicular portion of pectoralis major
	Extensors—sternal portion of pectoralis major, latissimus dorsi, teres major
	Hyperextensors—latissimus dorsi, teres major
	Abductors—middle deltoid, supraspinatus
	Adductors—latissimus dorsi, teres major, sternal portion of pectoralis major
	External rotators—infraspinatus, teres minor
	Internal rotators—pectoralis major, subscapularis, latissimus dorsi, teres major
	Horizontal flexors—both portions of pectoralis major, anterior deltoid
	Horizontal extensors—latissimus dorsi, teres major, infraspinatus, teres minor, posterior deltoid

(continued)

Table 4.1 ***(continued)***

Joint	Prime movers
Elbow joint	Flexors—brachialis, biceps brachii, brachioradialis
	Extensors—triceps brachii
Radioulnar joint	Pronators—pronator quadratus, pronator teres, brachioradialis
	Supinators—supinator, biceps brachii, brachioradialis
Wrist joint	Flexors—flexor carpi ulnaris, flexor carpi radialis
	Extensors and hyperextensors—extensor carpi ulnaris, extensor carpi radialis longus and brevis
	Abductors (radial flexors)—flexor carpi radialis, extensor carpi radialis longus and brevis
	Adductors (ulnar flexors)—flexor carpi ulnaris, extensor carpi ulnaris
Lumbosacral joint	Forward pelvic tilters—iliopsoas
	Backward pelvic tilters—rectus abdominis, internal obliques
Spinal column	Flexors—rectus abdominis, external obliques, internal obliques (thoracic and lumbar areas)
	Extensors and hyperextensors—erector spinae group
	Rotators—internal obliques, external obliques, erector spinae, rotatores, multifidus
	Lateral flexors—internal obliques, external obliques, quadratus lumborum, multifidus, rotatores
Hip joint	Flexors—iliopsoas, pectineus, rectus femoris
	Extensors and hyperextensors—gluteus maximus, biceps femoris, semitendinosus, semimembranosus
	Abductors—gluteus medius
	Adductors—adductor brevis, adductor longus, gracilis, pectineus
	Lateral rotators—gluteus maximus, the six deep lateral rotator muscles
	Medial rotators—gluteus minimus, gluteus medius
Knee joint	Flexors—biceps femoris, semimembranosus, semitendinosus
	Extensors—rectus femoris, vastus medialis, vastus lateralis, vastus intermedius
Ankle joint	Plantar flexors—gastrocnemius, soleus
	Dorsiflexors—tibialis anterior, extensor digitorum longus, peroneus tertius
Intertarsal joint	Inverters—tibialis anterior, tibialis posterior
	Everters—extensor digitorum longus, peroneus brevis, peroneus longus, peroneus tertius

Adapted, by permission, from E. Howley and B.D. Franks, 1992, *Health fitness instructor's handbook*, 2nd ed. (Champaign, IL: Human Kinetics), 69.

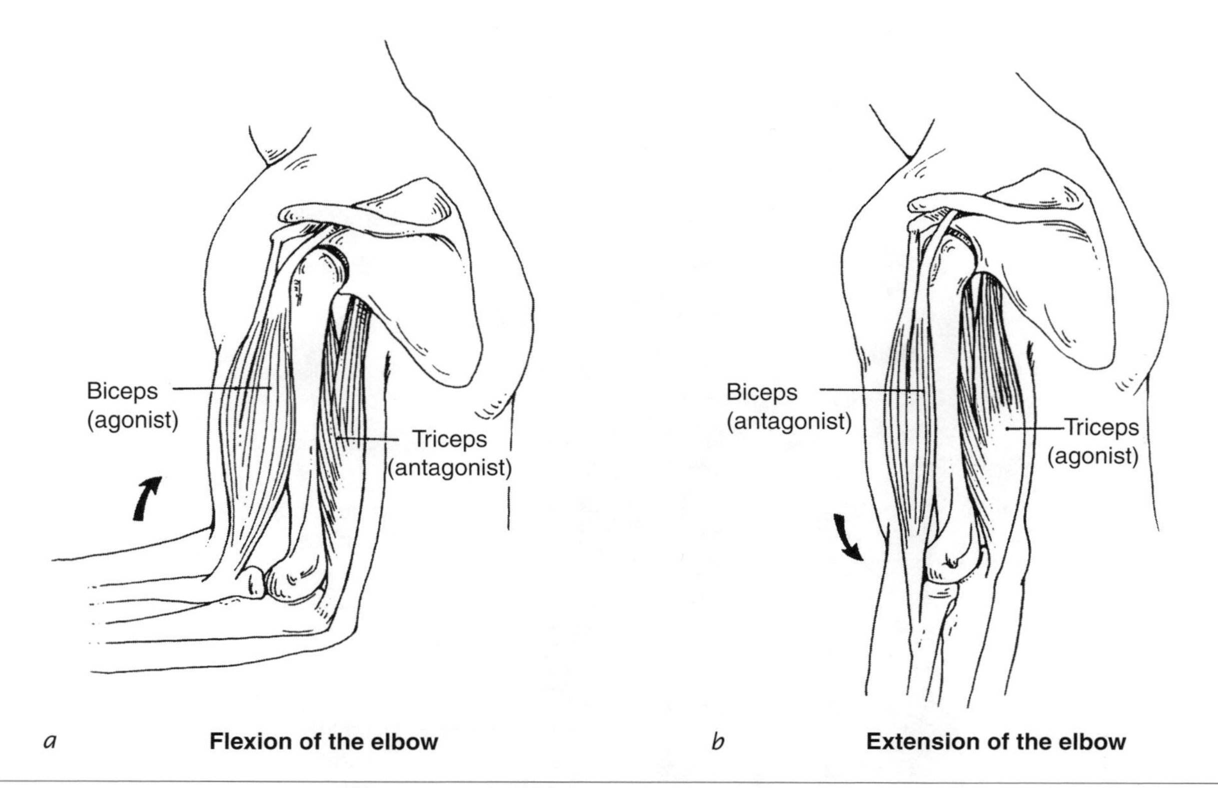

Figure 4.8 (*a*) Reciprocal inhibition; (*b*) reciprocal flexion.

Muscles Used in Common Activities

A variety of muscles are used in everyday activities. The following lists activities and which muscles each type exercises.

- **Walking, jogging, and running.** Walking, jogging, and running have a lot in common; they differ, however, in terms of the muscular force needed to move forward at different speeds. During walking, one foot is in contact with the ground at all times, but in jogging or running there is a period of "flight" when both feet are off the ground. If a period of flight is involved, a greater amount of energy must be expended to both "take off" and "land." The primary muscle groups involved in each phase of these activities include these:

- **Push-off phase.** The push-off uses the concentric contraction of *hip* and *knee extensors*.

- **Bringing push-off leg forward.** The concentric contraction of *hip flexors* initiates movement that is modified by the *lateral hip rotators*. The *knee flexors* first cause knee flexion; then, through an eccentric contraction, control the rate of knee extension before the foot touches down. The foot is *dorsiflexed* before landing.

- **Landing.** The *hip extensors* that initiated the push-off now contract eccentrically to slow the swing of the forward leg. When the foot touches down, the *knee extensors* also contract eccentrically to control the motion of the foot on the ground.

- **Cycling.** Cycling is a restricted activity because the pedals move in a fixed manner; therefore, it should be no surprise that the muscle groups involved in cycling are also somewhat limited. The *hip* and *knee extensors* develop the force to move the pedals downward, and, if toe clips are used by a cyclist skilled in their use, hip and knee flexors are involved in the return to the starting position. Without the use of toe clips, flexor activity is considerably less.

- **Jumping.** The force needed to propel the body off the ground is generated by the *knee* and *hip extensors* as well as the *plantar flexors*. To absorb the forces of impact, these same muscles contract eccentrically.

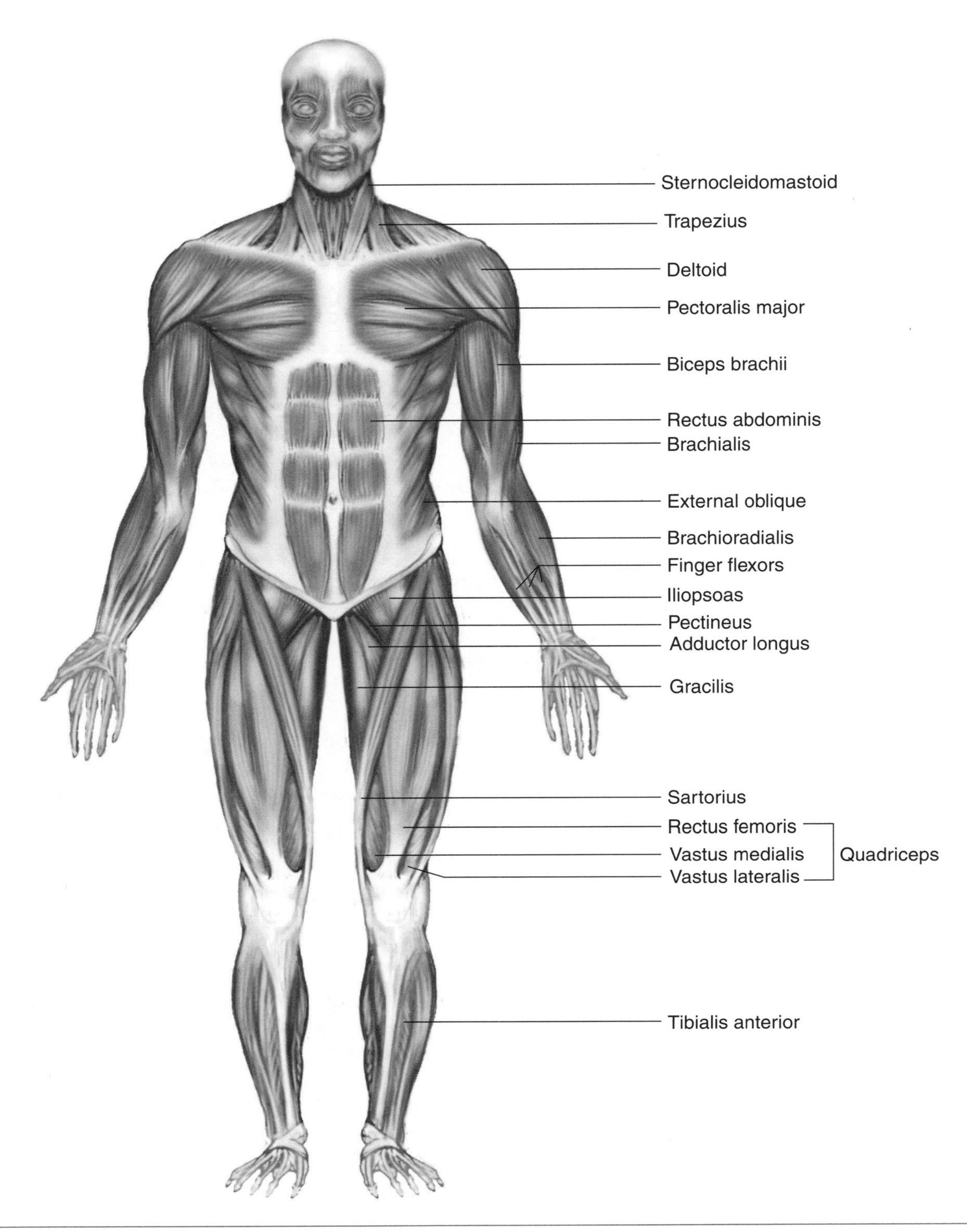

Figure 4.9 Muscles of the human body—anterior view.

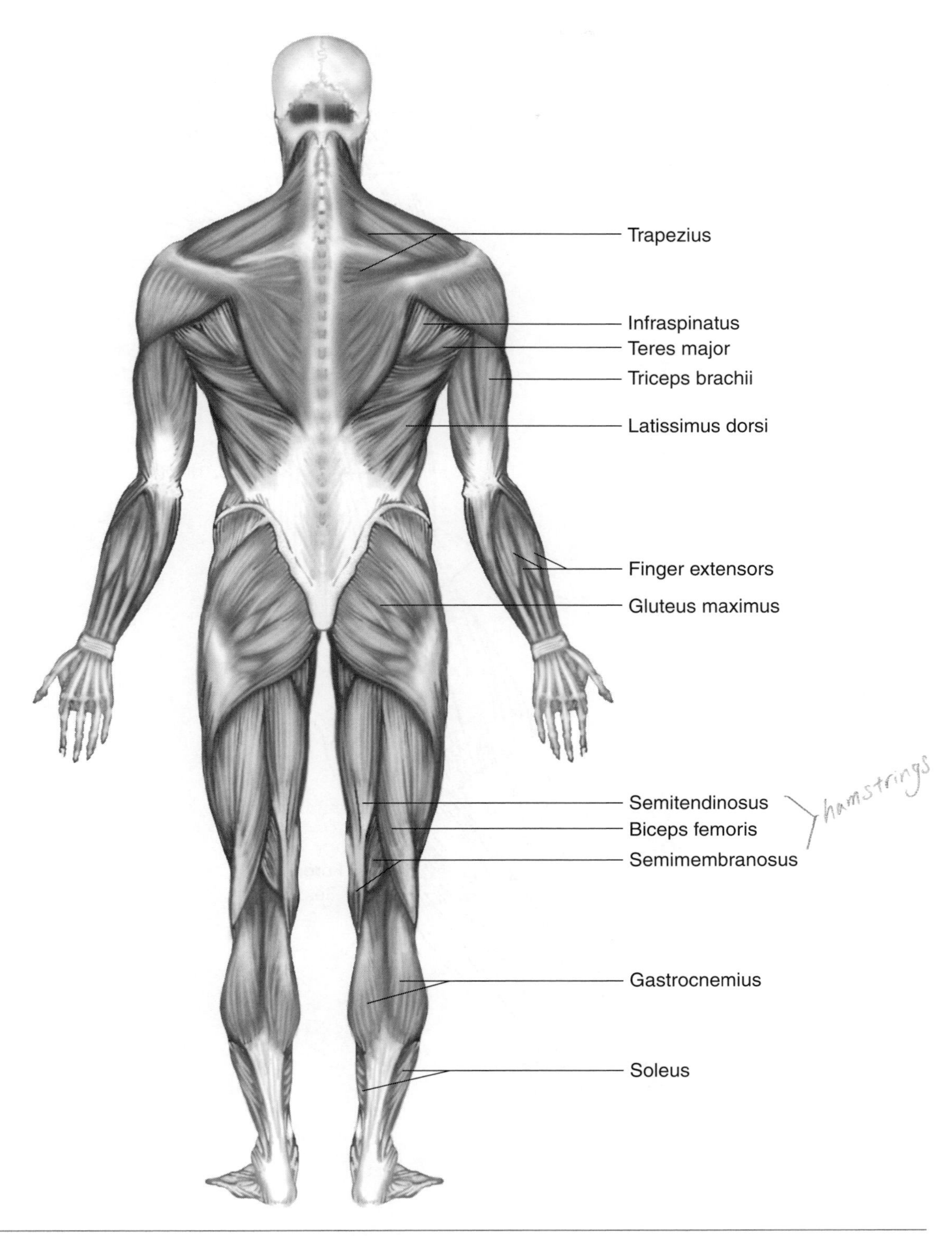

Figure 4.10 Muscles of the human body—posterior view.

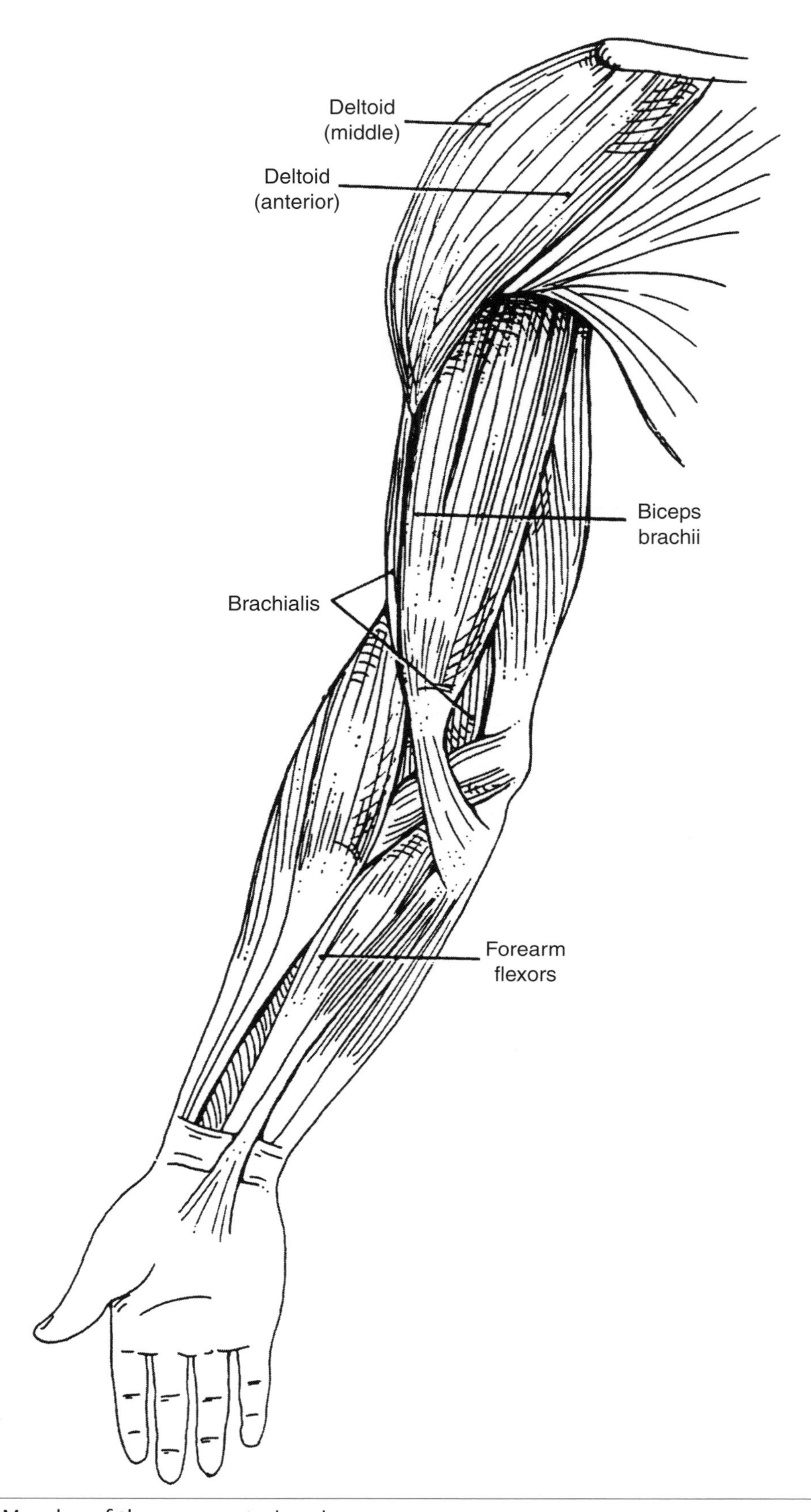

Figure 4.11 Muscles of the arm—anterior view.

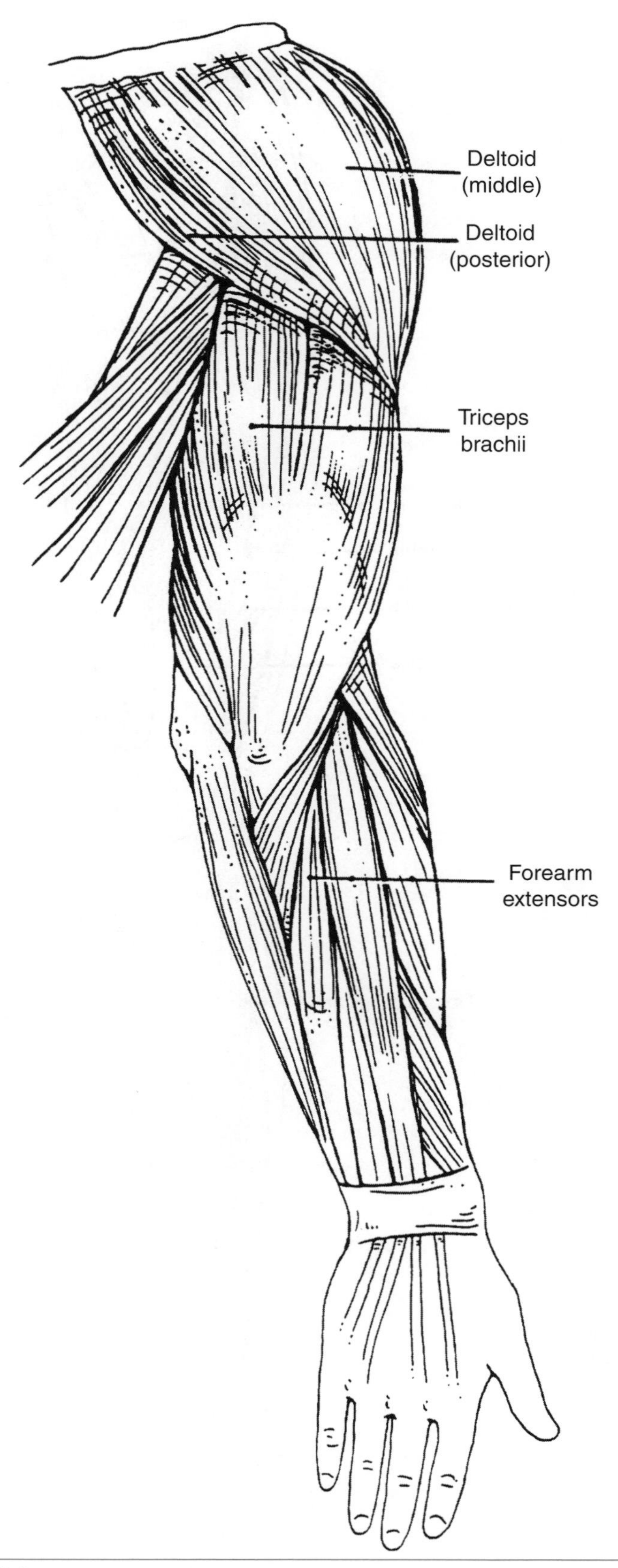

Figure 4.12 Muscles of the arm—posterior view.

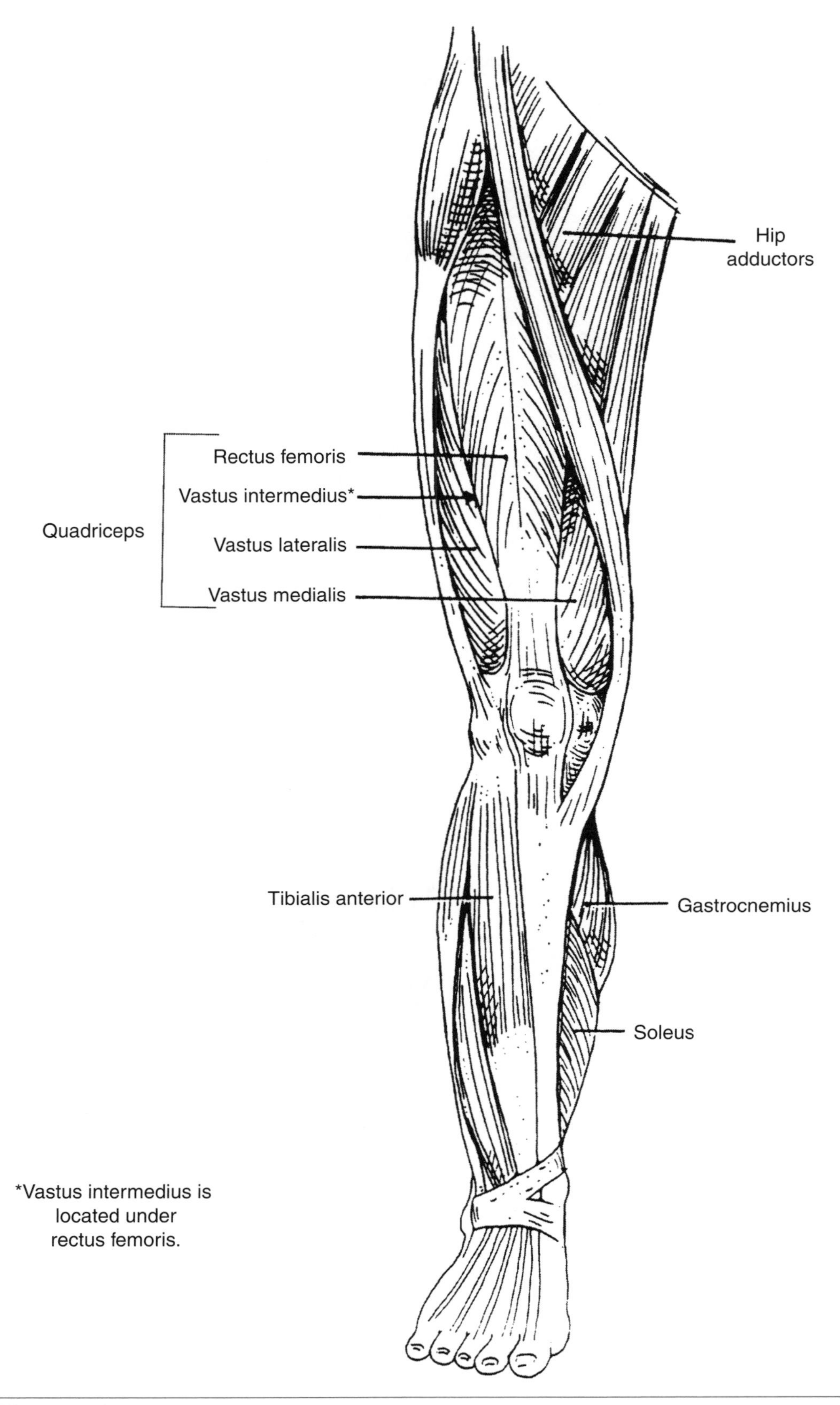

Figure 4.13 Muscles of the leg—anterior view.

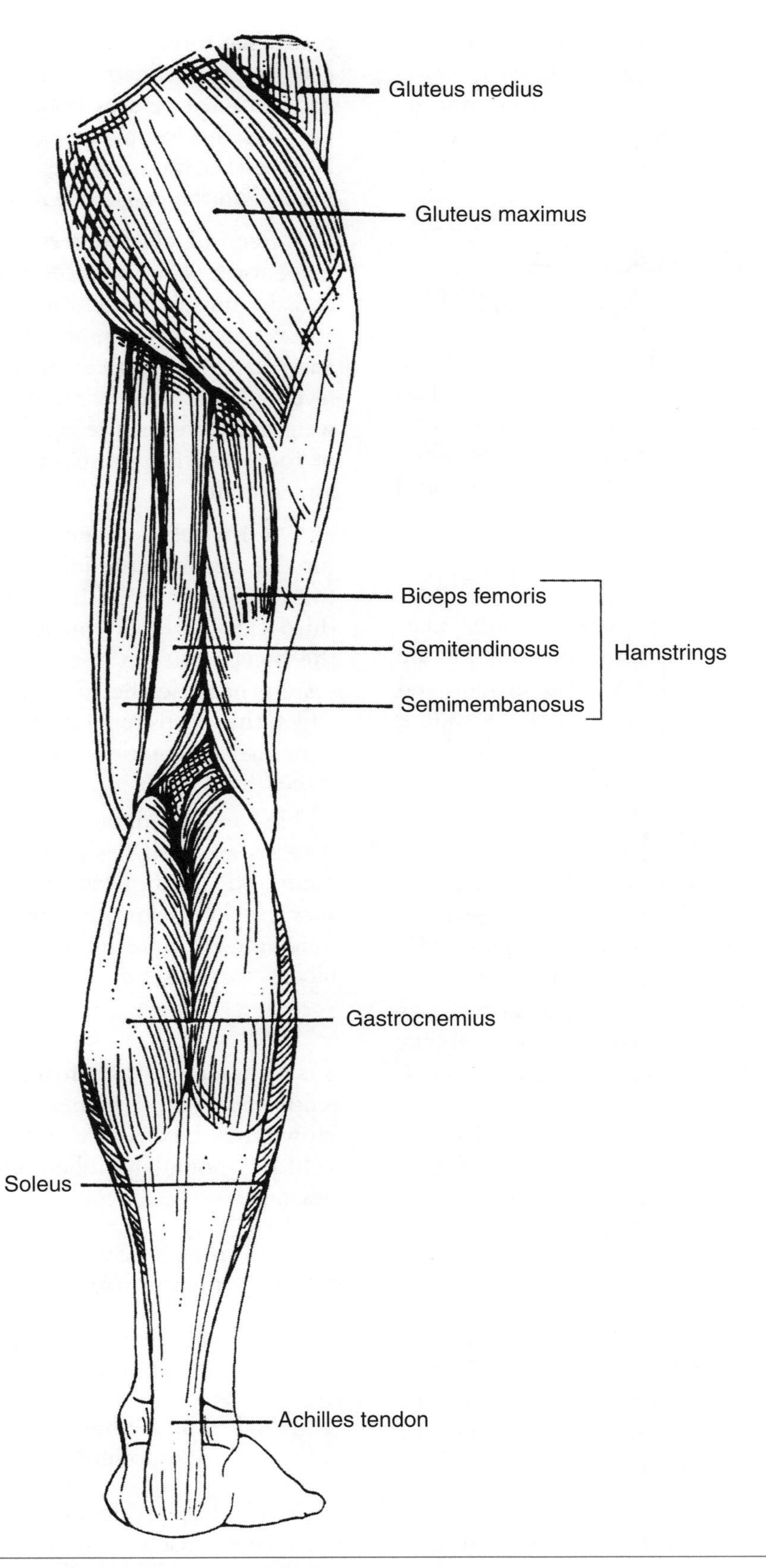

Figure 4.14 Muscles of the leg—posterior view.

• **Lifting and carrying.** When a person lifts an object, the large, strong *knee* and *hip extensors* should be the primary muscles involved, not the muscles in the arms or along the spine. Keeping the object close to one's body reduces the stress on the back.

BIOMECHANICAL CONCEPTS OF MOVEMENT

A variety of basic principles and laws governing the movement of objects and people can, when understood, help you determine proper and improper movements. These include stability, rotational inertia, lever systems, torque, and angular momentum.

Stability

The center of gravity for an average person is near the navel. A person's position is more stable the closer the center of gravity is to the ground and the wider the base of support. A person standing with both feet close together is less stable than when standing with feet spread apart.

Rotational Inertia

The concept of rotational inertia as applied to the body indicates the tendency of a body segment to remain at rest and not rotate around a joint. The larger the body segment and the farther the mass of the segment is from the joint (e.g., arm versus leg), the more rotational inertia the body segment has and the greater the energy required to move that segment through a range of motion. The energy requirement can be reduced by bringing the mass of the segment closer to the joint of rotation; bringing the *flexed* rear leg forward during running is an application of this principle.

Lever Systems

Human movement is possible because of lever systems composed of long bones, joints, and muscles. Muscles produce sufficient force to move bones around a joint's axis of rotation. The systems are divided into three classes: first, second, and third.

• **First-class levers.** Whenever the joint's axis of rotation is between the muscle force and the resistance force, the system functions as a first-class lever. As illustrated in figure 4.15a, the triceps muscle operates as a first-class lever system because the joint's axis of rotation (elbow) is between the muscle force (triceps tendon attachment) and the resistance force (dumbbell).

• **Second-class levers.** Whenever the resistance force is between the joint's axis of rotation and the muscle force, the system functions as a second-class lever. As shown in figure 4.15b, the gastrocnemius muscle operates a second-class lever system because the resistance force (body weight) is between the joint's axis of rotation (ball of foot) and the muscle force (Achilles tendon attachment).

• **Third-class levers.** Whenever the muscle force is between the joint's axis of rotation and the resistance force, the system functions as a third-class lever. As presented in figure 4.15c, the biceps muscle operates a third-class lever system because the muscle force (the point at which the biceps tendon attaches) is between the joint's axis of rotation (elbow) and the resistance force (dumbbell).

The predominantly third-class human lever systems are well designed for range of movement and speed of movement, but they are not very efficient in producing force. Consider the following examples of force relationships in the biceps lever system:

Example

Susan has a 10-inch forearm and her biceps tendon inserts 0.5 inches from her elbow joint. How much biceps force must Susan produce to hold a 15-pound dumbbell at 90 degrees of elbow flexion?

$$\text{Resistance arm} \times \text{resistance force} = \text{muscle arm} \times \text{muscle force}$$

$$10 \text{ inches} \times 15 \text{ pounds} = 0.5 \text{ inches} \times \text{muscle force}$$

$$150 \text{ inch-pounds} \div 0.5 \text{ inches} = 300 \text{ pounds muscle force}$$

Susan must produce 300 pounds of force in her biceps muscle to hold a 15-pound dumbbell at 90 degrees of elbow flexion.

Example

Gayle also has a 10-inch forearm, but her biceps tendon inserts 0.75 inches from her elbow joint. How much biceps force must Gayle produce to hold a 15-pound dumbbell at 90 degrees of elbow flexion?

Resistance arm × resistance force = muscle arm × muscle force

10 inches × 15 pounds = 0.75 inches × muscle force

150 inch-pounds ÷ 0.75 inches = 200 pounds muscle force

Gayle must produce 200 pounds of force in her biceps muscle to hold a 15-pound dumbbell at 90 degrees of elbow flexion. She has a distinct leverage advantage over Susan because of her more favorable point of tendon insertion.

These examples demonstrate that typical human lever systems require relatively high muscle force to overcome relatively low resistance force. They also show that small differences in the point of tendon insertion produce large differences in the muscle force requirements.

Torque

Torque is the effect produced when a muscle contraction (force) causes rotation. Let's look at forearm flexion as an example, with the forearm at a 90-degree angle to the upper arm and a 10-pound weight held in the hand. The resistance is the product of the 10-pound weight and the distance from the center of the weight to the elbow joint.

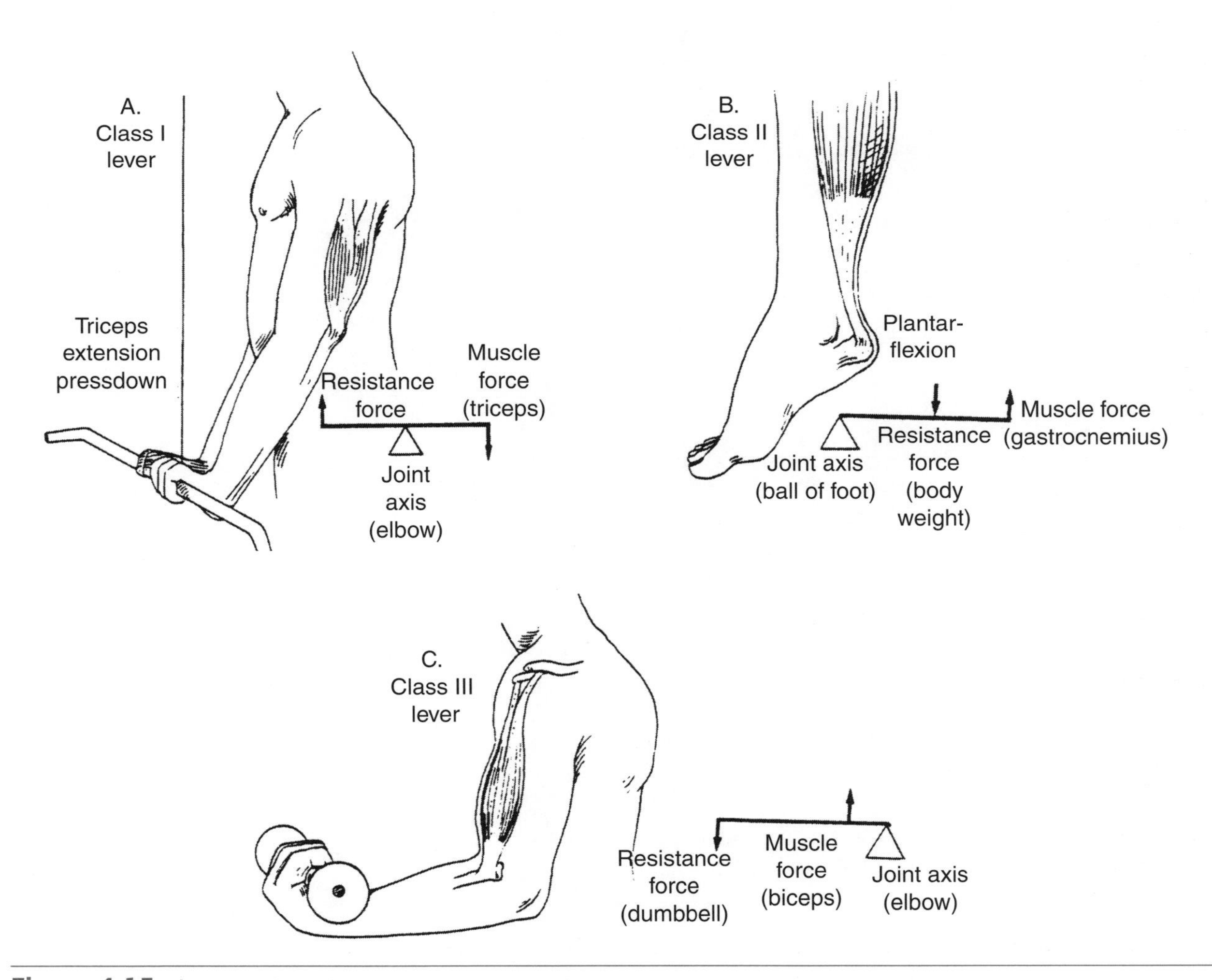

Figure 4.15 Lever systems.

The muscular force needed to move that weight depends on the distance from the elbow to the tendon insertion on the forearm. The closer the biceps' insertion is located to the hand, the smaller the muscular force needed to move the resistance. In the same way, if the 10-pound weight is moved closer to the joint (to reduce the length of the lever arm), less muscular force is needed to move the resistance. This concept can be extended to the act of carrying objects. The reason for carrying an object close to the body is to maintain stability and to reduce the force required by the back muscles to carry the load. If the object is held with arms outstretched, the back muscles must exert more force, which can cause back problems.

Angular Momentum

Angular momentum describes the amount of motion that takes place as a limb moves around a joint or a body rotates; it is equal to the product of angular velocity and rotational inertia. The *conservation of angular momentum* states that once motion is initiated, angular momentum remains constant until an outside force changes it. This means that a decrease in rotational inertia during a movement results in a higher angular velocity. This is best seen when an ice skater spins in place; as the arms move closer to the body to decrease rotational inertia, the velocity of rotation increases.

CHAPTER 5

Strength Training Principles and Guidelines

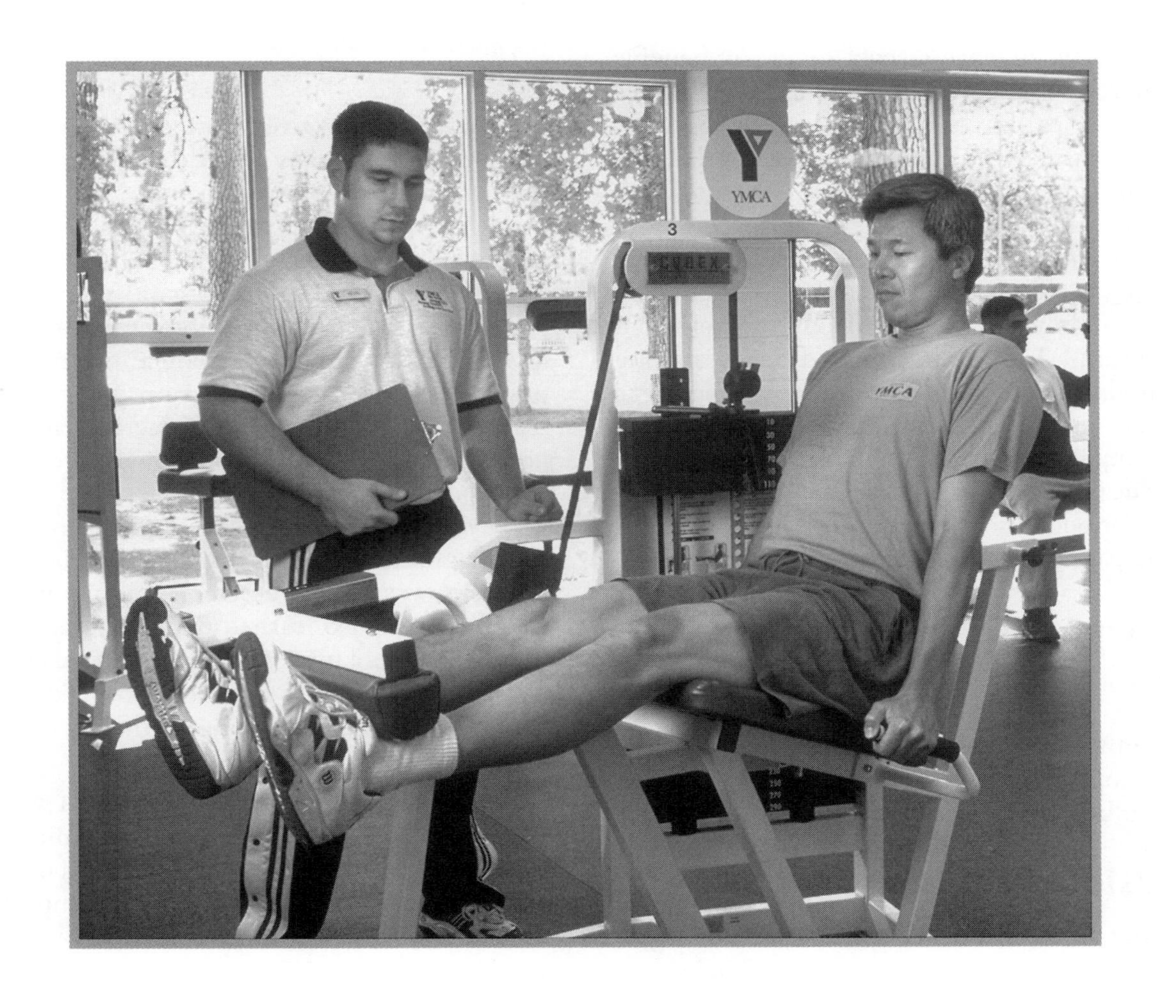

Strength training is a process of systematically applying increasing amounts of stress to muscles. Muscles respond to progressive resistance exercise by gradually becoming larger and stronger. To develop effective strength training programs, you must understand general concepts about how the body adapts to the progressive overload of strength exercises. Strength training is a highly individualized procedure. As a YMCA personal training instructor, you must help your members by designing appropriate programs that will challenge them to develop strength.

In this chapter we discuss the many benefits of and reasons for strength training. We describe the principles of strength training, explain special health considerations and precautions related to training, and dispel myths about training. We then present procedures for performing strength training safely and effectively, describe recommended exercises and how to choose them, and show you how to develop effective and efficient programs. We follow this with advanced training methods that can be used to overcome strength plateaus and a brief discussion of strength training for competitive purposes. Finally, we discuss how to educate members and provide recommendations for beginning, intermediate, and advanced participants, as well as ongoing education.

STRENGTH TRAINING BENEFITS

Strength training has many benefits for exercisers, some physiological, some physical, and some that lead to better overall health.

Physiological Benefits

Regular strength training produces more myofibrils per muscle fiber, more capillaries per muscle fiber, more intramuscular energy stores, and better muscle fiber recruitment. However, the primary response to progressive resistance exercise is an increase in the muscle proteins: actin and myosin. This produces larger muscle fibers with greater structural and contractile strength.

The stress applied to the muscles is transferred to the connective tissue (tendons and ligaments) and bones. This produces more collagen proteins in the tendons and ligaments and more osteoproteins in the bones, increasing the structural strength of tendons, ligaments, and bones. The result is a well-developed musculoskeletal system that is strong and injury resistant.

Physical Benefits

A well-developed musculoskeletal system provides benefits to functional capacity and quality of life. These include athletic power, injury prevention, physical capacity, metabolic function, physical appearance, and benefits to your overall health.

- **Athletic power.** Performance power is the key to success in many athletic activities. Sprinting, jumping, and throwing are examples of power activities. So are driving a golf ball, serving a tennis ball, and hitting a softball. Performance power depends on two factors: movement speed and muscle strength. Slow movement speed or low muscle strength can reduce performance power. The best means for improving performance power is to increase both factors. However, greater muscle strength allows movement with more power, force, and speed.

  Most sports coaches encourage their athletes to strength train in order to enhance their performance power and reduce their injury potential. Coaches have also learned that proper strength training does not hinder movement speed or joint flexibility, and in fact enhances both. All other factors being equal, a stronger athlete is indeed a better athlete.

- **Injury prevention.** It has been widely reported that four out of every five Americans experience low back pain. Most is caused by poor muscle condition. Therefore, it is very important to maintain strong postural muscles to counteract the effects of gravity on the musculoskeletal system. Well-conditioned muscles provide a support system that protects the body from a variety of degenerative processes.

  Musculoskeletal injuries can also be a serious problem for many exercisers. For example, runners and group-exercise participants frequently experience musculoskeletal injuries caused by repetitive landing forces. Swimmers and tennis players often experience overuse injuries caused by using the prime mover muscle groups too much and the antagonist muscle groups too little. Football players and wrestlers are subjected to traumatic soft-tissue injuries as a result of external contact forces.

In all cases, sensible strength training is the best preventive measure. When performed properly, strength training conditions all of the major muscle groups, thereby enhancing the ability both to absorb external forces and to maintain internal strength balance between opposing muscles. Without balanced muscle strength, it is difficult for athletes to avoid overuse injuries and for nonexercisers to delay degenerative musculoskeletal problems. Because the preferred treatment modality for many musculoskeletal injuries and degenerative problems is progressive resistance exercise under the watchful eye of a medical professional, it makes sense that well-designed and well-supervised strength training programs might be equally useful in preventing many of these problems.

- **Physical capacity.** Normally, physical capacity is thought of in terms of cardiorespiratory endurance, and that is certainly an important component of overall fitness. While the heart functions as the fuel pump of the body, the muscles serve as the engine. Muscles use energy to produce movement and are essential to all physical activity. Whereas endurance exercise is necessary for improving cardiorespiratory fitness, it generally has little effect on muscular fitness. Progressive resistance exercise is the key to increasing muscular fitness, which has a major impact on physical capacity to perform work, exercise, and daily activities. Weeding the garden, playing tennis, carrying groceries, and climbing stairs all require muscular strength. Poorly conditioned postural muscles might fatigue quickly, limiting physical capacity and lowering quality of life.

Numerous studies have demonstrated significant improvements in muscle strength after only four to eight weeks of regular strength training. The higher strength levels that result from strength training make almost everything we do a little easier. This is because every physical activity requires a certain percentage of our maximum muscle strength. For example, if maximum biceps strength is 25 pounds, carrying a 25-pound bag of groceries is an all-out effort. If biceps strength increases to 50 pounds, carrying the same bag of groceries requires only half of the available muscle force, making the task much easier.

There is a difference between muscle strength and muscle endurance, even though they are very closely related. Increased muscle strength results in increased muscle endurance, making it possible to perform more work, exercise, and recreational physical activities.

- **Metabolic function.** Muscles are responsible for most of the energy used during vigorous physical activity, and they increase metabolic function as much as 20 times above its resting rate. However, muscles have a major influence on resting metabolic function as well. Muscle is very active tissue that requires continuous energy supplies for ongoing cellular processes such as protein synthesis, maintenance, and building. Even when we are sleeping, skeletal muscles are metabolically active, using more than 25 percent of the total caloric output. In fact, it is estimated that a pound of muscle uses more than 35 calories a day at rest to meet its metabolic requirements. Therefore, muscle mass and metabolic function are closely related. When muscle mass is added, metabolic rate increases, both during activity and at rest. Conversely, when muscle mass is lost, metabolic rate decreases, both during activity and at rest.

Unfortunately, unless regular strength exercise is performed, muscle mass decreases with age. Studies show that after age 25, the average American loses about one-half pound of muscle every year of life because of inactivity. The saying "use it or lose it" definitely applies to skeletal muscles. Without an appropriate training stimulus, muscle fibers gradually become smaller and weaker (atrophy). The gradual loss of muscle tissue is largely responsible for the gradual reduction in metabolic rate that appears to be part of aging. Research reveals that resting metabolism decreases approximately half a percent every year after age 25.

All vigorous physical activity elevates heart rate, blood pressure, and energy metabolism. However, endurance exercise such as jogging, cycling, or swimming increases metabolic rate only during the activity session and for a brief period afterward. Strength exercise increases metabolic rate during the activity session for a relatively long period following the workout and all day after more muscle tissue is developed. Strength training, therefore, has a triple effect on energy utilization. The primary effect is a large increase in metabolic rate during the exercise session. The secondary effect is a moderate increase in metabolic rate for more than an hour after the strength training session. The third effect is a small increase in metabolic rate 24 hours per day, 365 days a year (as long as the person maintains a strength training program).

- **Physical appearance.** One of the most common reason for strength training and the most obvious benefit is improved physical appearance. Muscles are responsible for the overall appearance of the physique. Although few people have the genetic potential to develop extremely large muscles, everyone can enhance their muscle firmness and muscular fitness. Consider an average woman who weighs 126 pounds and is 27 percent fat. Even though she is not overweight by most standards, she definitely has too much fat and too little muscle to look and function her best. A sensible program consisting of progressive resistance exercise, endurance activities, and a prudent diet can improve body composition without changing body weight, as shown in table 5.1.

Of course, it is possible to lose five pounds of fat through dieting or endurance exercise. However, it is unlikely that a person will add five pounds of muscle without performing regular strength exercise. Although the fat loss is certainly helpful, the muscle gain is even more beneficial in terms of physical appearance and physical fitness. Significant changes in body composition and physical appearance are usually observed after just one to two months of regular strength training.

Table 5.1 Example of Body Composition Changes As a Result of Exercise

Preexercise program	Postexercise program
14 lbs bone	14 lbs bone
28 lbs organs and skin	28 lbs organs and skin
34 lbs fat	29 lbs fat
50 lbs muscle	55 lbs muscle
126 lbs and 27% fat	126 lbs and 23% fat

Several studies have found that untrained adults typically gain about three pounds of muscle and lose about four pounds of fat after eight weeks of regular strength exercise. Because the results are apparent to both the exerciser and others, sensible strength training is a reinforcing activity that should become a consistent component of a fitness-oriented lifestyle.

- **Health benefits.** In addition to the more obvious fitness and performance benefits of regular strength training, it enhances overall health in other ways.
  - **Improved body composition.** Body composition can be improved by increasing energy-utilizing muscle tissue and decreasing energy-storing fat tissue. This typically decreases the percentage of body fat (and often decreases body weight), thereby reducing this coronary risk factor.
  - **Decreased blood pressure.** Like endurance exercise, strength exercise tends to normalize elevated blood pressure, thereby reducing this coronary risk factor.
  - **Reduced sedentary risks.** You cannot participate in strength training and remain sedentary, and because sedentary living is a significant coronary risk factor, strength training reduces this risk.
  - **Increased HDL cholesterol.** Research indicates that strength exercise might increase levels of high-density lipoprotein (HDL), or good, cholesterol. Perhaps just as important, people involved in regular strength training tend to be more concerned about proper nutrition and more likely to follow a low-fat diet.
  - **Enhanced overall well-being.** Like most physical activities, strength training seems to enhance overall well-being and has been found to reduce low back pain, decrease depression, and ease discomfort from arthritis. Many strength training practitioners report increased ability to accomplish daily responsibilities, improved job performance, and more meaningful recreational activities.
- **Psychological benefits.** Strength training might help reduce stress, increase success, improve self-confidence, and enhance self-

esteem. Positive changes in physical strength and personal appearance often lead to positive changes in self-image. Without question, strength training is a purposeful physical activity that contributes to self-confidence and personal satisfaction. This might explain why at-risk youth typically respond very well to supervised strength training programs. In addition to improving self-esteem, good strength training programs provide an excellent environment for developing cooperation and leadership skills.

STRENGTH TRAINING AND WELLNESS

We have discussed the physical and practical reasons that people train for strength. Strength training can also contribute to the exploration of the whole person. The whole person combines the physical body, the thinking and rational mind, and the emotional and spiritual being. This is considered viewing the health of a person from a holistic point of view. Strength training can significantly improve one's holistic health. People might begin a strength training program to reach direct and immediate physical or practical goals, but they often continue because of mental and emotional factors, such as

- feelings of self-worth and self-esteem;
- achievement and success;
- acquiring discipline and applying it to other activities;
- substituting a positive habit for a negative one, for example, training instead of overeating; and
- directing motivations such as aggression and egotism into positive and beneficial activities.

Strength training can be a means for self-examination. Dealing with the strenuous nature of the activity involves physical exploration. Performing a number of sets and repetitions in a given amount of time contributes to a person's sense of accomplishment. The worth of the activity is seen in a developing body, which brings about sense of fulfillment and promotes a genuine sense of achievement. The person who trains regularly might go a step further than the physical aspects of training and make strength training a part of his or her philosophical approach to living. It can become a method of looking internally for questions not answered in other areas of life and by other physical activities. Experienced weightlifters, bodybuilders, athletes, and fitness participants express feelings of self-discovery, psychological balance, and spiritual realization.

Advanced strength trainers often attribute their continual training as a quest for personal excellence, self-expression, and self-discovery. The scope of strength training can be limited to the physical act of lifting weights, pulling cables, and pushing machines, or it can be expanded to all aspects of daily living and mental and emotional well-being. Strength training can be the key to physical development, emotional confidence, and spiritual self-discovery, a model YMCA activity that promotes the healthy development of spirit, mind, and body.

PRACTICAL REASONS FOR STRENGTH TRAINING

Besides producing health and fitness benefits, strength training also helps some people with job training and performance and enables them to better defend themselves from attack. It makes daily activities easier, whether those activities are chores or recreational. Finally, for those who work out at strength training facilities, it provides the chance for enjoyable interactions with others who train.

- **Job training.** Many job-training programs incorporate strength training. Police and fire departments use physical fitness testing as part of their evaluation process in hiring. Women who are interested in jobs in fire and police departments might be particularly interested in strength training to develop upper-body strength. The Army, Marines, Navy, and Air Force stress physical readiness and require physical fitness. Forest Service and National Park Service rangers are examples of occupations that require good physical conditioning. Both men and women seek specific strength training programs and information to help them qualify for careers that require physical strength.

• **Job performance.** Improved job performance and increased productivity are important to many workers. Some find physical fitness, and particularly strength, to be a factor in job performance. Those who require physical strength in their jobs directly benefit from strength training programs. But even those in sedentary professions benefit from strength training because physical strength results in less general fatigue, which can maintain and even increase job productivity. Workers who feel better work with more vitality.

• **Self-protection.** A less obvious reason for strength training is the growing awareness and need for self-protection. Self-defense activities require physical strength. Many authorities believe that a strong and confident person is less likely to be approached or attacked. This, along with the practical ability to deal with a variety of emergency situations, motivates many people to develop strength.

• **Daily activities.** Routine daily activities and tasks are made easier with increased muscular strength. A homemaker can complete household tasks with greater ease. Even grocery shopping is easier because carrying heavy packages from the car to the kitchen, especially up stairs, is not as stressful. Lifting heavy objects, doing yard work, and performing dozens of daily tasks can be done more easily and without help. This is particularly relevant for older adults who want to live independently as long as possible. The fear of straining or pulling muscles, hurting the back, or overdoing is lessened with muscular fitness. At the end of the day when work and daily tasks are completed, a fit person is ready and able to participate in hobbies and recreational activities, and once again adequate strength is desirable. Strength training and physical fitness enable people to complete their daily tasks and work, leaving enough strength, endurance, and energy to participate in enjoyable recreational activities.

• **Socialization.** Today's modern strength training facilities are attractive, pleasant places. Strength training and fitness have become a popular way for people to meet and make friends. Most fitness facilities provide a comfortable and inviting atmosphere for people to interact, making physical activity enjoyable and beneficial. The fitness center is a good place to meet people. Strength training participants feel good about being with others who share the same experiences and feel the same physical changes. The interaction between people takes place in a variety of ways, but usually it occurs naturally. The self-confidence and camaraderie found at the fitness facility might encourage people to reach out in other areas, such as with friends and family and in business. Often the social aspect of strength training becomes as important to people as the workout itself.

SPECIAL APPLICATIONS

Strength training can be used to help people rehabilitate from injury or cardiac conditions, and it can also give people the chance to engage in competitive bodybuilding and weightlifting.

• **Rehabilitation from injury.** Strength training is a major component of many rehabilitation programs. Physicians, physical therapists, and athletic trainers use strength training to rehabilitate many injuries. It is also used as therapy for the chronically ill, the injured, and those with disabilities. Strength training programs can have a "cross-training" effect; that is, the uninjured side of the body can be exercised to benefit the opposite, injured side. The muscle training might stimulate all parts of the body; therefore, injured areas can improve because of the general benefits of exercise. The greater blood circulation, oxygen delivery, and innervation that result from strength training enhance the rehabilitation process.

• **Cardiac rehabilitation.** Previously, strength training was not recommended for postcardiac patients. This was based on the assumption that heavy lifting increased the strain on the heart and circulation and increased blood pressure to dangerous levels. However, if the postcoronary patient is to be rehabilitated, the muscular system must be exercised as well as the cardiorespiratory system. Strength training with light weights is, therefore, highly desirable for the postcoronary patient because it is the most efficient way to regain and increase muscle strength. The amount of resistance and the intensity of the exercise should be prescribed by one's personal physician.

- **Bodybuilding.** Bodybuilding is a popular activity that attracts a variety of participants. The bodybuilder concentrates on muscle size, definition, and symmetry. The goal involves aesthetics: a well-formed, well-defined, and well-balanced physique. Bodybuilding requires a well-balanced exercise plan that systematically exercises, strengthens, and develops each muscle group to its maximum. The cosmetic effect has increased bodybuilding's popularity with the general public, although very few participants reach a high competitive level. It has been suggested that bodybuilding is an art form as well as a sport because posing and highlighting muscle groups and physique are important to the activity.
- **Weightlifting competition.** Olympic lifting and powerlifting are the competitive aspects of strength training, and for some people these become a major sport. Olympic lifting is a competitive sport that tests one's ability to lift great amounts of weight in two specific lifts: the snatch and the clean and jerk. Agility, speed of movement, power, flexibility, and technique are all facets of Olympic lifting. The foundation of the sport is, of course, strength, and therefore competitive Olympic lifters train for strength. The same is true for powerlifting. The squat, bench press, and deadlift are the three lifts performed in competition.

STRENGTH TRAINING PRINCIPLES

An unlimited number of strength training routines and programs are available, most of which work to some degree. However, a major problem is that an unacceptable potential for injury is associated with many of them. Not only is it important for a strength training program to be effective, it is essential that it be safe. Several basic training principles should be incorporated into a sensible strength training program. Generally, the probability of experiencing desirable training outcomes depends on how well basic strength training principles are applied to a personal exercise program. The following principles provide the basis for maximizing strength development and minimizing the risk of injury: stress adaptation, building time, movement speed, movement range, muscle balance, training specificity, and exercise breathing.

Stress Adaptation

To stimulate strength development, the muscles must be stressed. However, the amount of stress is critical. If the stress is too little, the muscles will not respond, and their condition will remain essentially the same. If the stress is too great, the muscles will respond undesirably, resulting in tissue damage and strength loss. If the stress is appropriate, the muscles will respond desirably, resulting in tissue building and strength gain. Simply put, the muscles must do more work than they are accustomed to in order to develop more strength.

Of course, it is impossible to outline one specific training protocol that would be ideal for everyone. However, the best guideline is to systematically increase the exercise stimulus so that each training session places just a little more demand on the muscles. This process must be gradual and progressive to achieve desirable results and to avoid the problems associated with abrupt increases in workloads. The key to attaining muscle strength and avoiding tissue injury is a long-range approach to muscle development.

Several training variables influence muscle demands and the resulting stress adaptation: exercise frequency, resistance, repetitions, sets, rest intervals, progression, and periodization.

Exercise Frequency

To some degree, how often a strength training routine is performed is a matter of personal preference and time available. Some exercisers might find a few minutes for brief daily workouts, whereas others might have the time for comprehensive training sessions once or twice a week. The essential factor is the amount of rest necessary for muscles to recover from the training stimulus and build to a slightly higher level of strength. Some people need shorter recovery periods (typically those with a high percentage of slow-twitch muscle fibers), whereas others require longer recovery periods (usually those with a high percentage of fast-twitch muscle fibers). As a general rule, muscles take 48 to 72 hours to fully recover from a strenuous training stimulus and build to a slightly greater strength level.

If too little recovery is taken between training sessions, muscles will not have time to build new tissue and develop more strength. If too much recovery is taken between training sessions, muscles might temporarily build new tissue and develop more strength, but without an appropriately spaced follow-up workout, atrophy will occur and muscles will return to their original condition.

In a study designed to evaluate the effects of different training frequencies on muscle development, 1,132 men and women were placed into two exercise groups (Westcott 1996). Both groups performed one set of 12 exercises two or three days per week over an eight-week training period. The group that trained twice a week attained 88 percent as much muscle gain as the group that trained three days a week. The group that trained three days a week achieved the best results, but twice-a-week training proved to be a highly effective alternative for people with less available time .

Although most studies suggest that two to four days are most effective, the YMCA of the USA recommends training three nonconsecutive days per week for beginners and for general conditioning. In *Designing Resistance Training Programs, Third Edition*, Fleck and Kraemer summarized research that indicated that three training sessions per muscle group per week is the minimum frequency for causing maximum gains (2004).

Most strength exercisers should train three nonconsecutive days per week for best results. Although some people might prefer to train more often, it is not advisable to stress the same muscle groups on consecutive days. If exercise is performed on consecutive days, it might be best to train the lower-body muscles one day and the upper-body muscles the next. As muscles become stronger and experience more stressful exercise sessions, it might take longer for them to recover and build to higher strength levels. Consequently, it is always important to evaluate muscle response to the training program. If a person does not feel at least as strong, and hopefully a little stronger, at each workout, a change in training frequency should be considered. For more information about the effects of rest between exercise sessions, see the section on building time later in this chapter.

Resistance

As is the case with exercise frequency, there is no single specific amount of resistance that has been shown to be most effective for strength development, as this is dependent on many factors. Powerlifters often train with maximum resistance, whereas patients in rehabilitation programs make progress with low resistance. Generally, it is advisable to train between 65 and 85 percent of maximum resistance. A study conducted in 1982 on unconditioned adults concluded that the optimal training for beginners is done with 60 to 80 percent of a person's maximum resistance (Harre 1982). Research shows that at least 65 percent of maximum resistance should be used to attain optimum strength development. Empirical evidence indicates that people have a much higher risk of injury when they use more than 85 percent of maximum resistance. As a general rule, 75 percent of maximum resistance provides an excellent training stimulus. It is heavy enough to produce positive muscle adaptations and light enough to minimize the risk of injury.

Repetitions

The amount of resistance used is directly related to the number of repetitions that can be performed. High resistance necessitates few repetitions, whereas low resistance permits more repetitions. The number of repetitions that can be completed with a given resistance is a genetic characteristic closely related to muscle fiber makeup. Consider the results of a research study on 141 men and women, including several outstanding power athletes and endurance athletes. All of the subjects were evaluated for the number of repetitions they could perform with 75 percent of their maximum resistance in a chest exercise. Most of the subjects completed 8 to 13 repetitions. All of the subjects who performed fewer than 8 repetitions were proficient power athletes who presumably had a high percentage of fast-twitch (low-endurance) muscle fibers. All of the subjects who performed more than 13 repetitions were excellent endurance athletes who presumably had a high percentage of slow-twitch (high-endurance) muscle fibers.

A study by Harre (1982) suggests that beginners should use loads of 60 to 80 percent of maximum with 8 to 10 repetitions in each set. The

American College of Sports Medicine (ACSM) recommends 8 to 12 repetitions for general conditioning. Based on these findings, most men and women can complete 8 to 12 repetitions with 75 percent of their maximum resistance and should typically train within this repetition range. People who have low-endurance muscles should probably train with fewer (5 to 7) repetitions, and people who have high-endurance muscles should probably train with more (13 to 15) repetitions. Generally, training with fewer than 5 repetitions increases the injury risk and training with more than 16 repetitions decreases the strength stimulus.

Sets

An exercise may be performed one time or more during a strength training session. Performing 8 to 12 repetitions of one exercise is referred to as a set. People who prefer shorter training sessions typically perform one set of each exercise. People who prefer longer training sessions generally complete multiple sets of each exercise. Research studies (Atham 1981) indicate that multiple sets work best for strength development and that gains are achieved more quickly than with a single-set system (McDonagh and Davies 1984). However, single-set training effectively stimulates strength development and might be more appropriate for beginners (Fleck and Kraemer 1997).

Another study compared one, two, or three sets of exercise on upper-body strength development as measured by dips and chins with bodyweight (Westcott 1989). The 77 male and female participants trained three days per week for 10 weeks. The subjects who trained with one set of dips and chins improved their performance by 4.8 repetitions. The subjects who trained with two sets of dips and chins improved their performance by 4.1 repetitions, and the subjects who trained with three sets of dips and chins improved their performance by 5.2 repetitions (see table 5.2). There were no significant differences among the three training groups, indicating that one, two, and three sets of exercise were equally effective for improving upper-body strength (as measured by dips and chins with bodyweight). Therefore, the number of sets to perform in a given exercise should be a matter of personal preference. For most purposes, one to three sets per exercise are recommended for improving muscle strength.

For maximum results, finishing a set means attempting to work until no further movement is possible. This point of failure is referred to as momentary muscle fatigue. Submaximal efforts will produce submaximal results; the correct weight must be determined so that maximal results can be obtained with 8 to 12 repetitions. When a set is completed before the point of failure (momentary muscular failure), the maximum number of muscle fibers has not been innervated. For best results, end a set only when another lift cannot be accomplished. This implies modifying the amount of resistance so that the point of failure occurs at the completion of 8 to 12 repetitions.

Rest Intervals

If a single-set program is followed, the amount of rest required between exercises is minimal because each set addresses a different muscle group. However, if multiple sets of each exercise are performed, you should allow longer periods of rest between sets. Powerlifters typically take long rests between sets so they can use heavy weight loads throughout their workout. Bodybuilders generally take short rests between sets to maximize a "muscle pump" during their workout.

Table 5.2 Performance Improvements

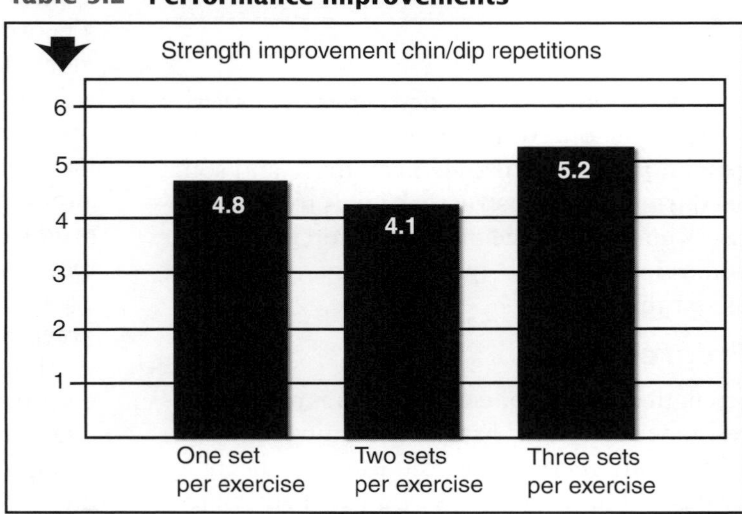

Although many physiological and psychological factors influence exercise intervals, energy replenishment is critically important. The major energy source for strength exercise is creatine phosphate, which is temporarily depleted after a strenuous set of exercise. The half-life of creatine phosphate production is about 30 seconds. That is, after 30 seconds about 50 percent of the creatine phosphate has been replenished. After one minute about 75 percent of the creatine phosphate has been replenished. After 90 seconds about 88 percent of the creatine phosphate has been replenished, and after two minutes about 95 percent of the creatine phosphate has been replenished.

In other words, a two-minute rest between exercise sets permits almost full restoration of the creatine phosphate energy supply (Fox and Matthews 1974). For most purposes this provides an appropriate rest period between exercise sets. A two-minute rest interval is short enough to maintain increased blood flow to the muscle and long enough to train with relatively heavy weight loads. Table 5.3 shows the recommended rest intervals for different types of training.

Table 5.3 Rest Intervals for Various Types of Training

Emphasis	Rest interval
Muscle hypertrophy	1 min or less
Overall muscle development	2 min
Muscle strength	3 min

The amount of rest needed between sets varies for each person. Although two minutes is a good general rule, some people need more and some need less rest. An instructor's job is to help exercisers understand the effects of exercise on their bodies in order to help them judge the amount of rest they need.

Progression

Strength training is often referred to as progressive-resistance exercise. That is, the training resistance is gradually increased as the exerciser becomes stronger. This is one of its significant advantages over bodyweight exercises, such as sit-ups and push-ups, in which the ways to progress with the same resistance are limited to performing more repetitions or changing the angle or speed of contraction. Although these changes are effective up to a point, performing dozens of sit-ups at the same angle or speed of contraction results in minimal strength gains.

It is far more productive to add resistance and exercise for 60 to 90 seconds at a high intensity; that is, to use a resistance heavy enough to cause muscle fatigue within approximately 8 to 12 repetitions. If this training protocol is used, the resistance should increase slightly whenever 12 repetitions can be completed in good form. The average person should increase the weight load in small increments to minimize the risk of injury and to maximize improvement. The increase should be 5 percent or less. For example, if a person can complete 12 biceps curls with 50 pounds, he or she should increase the weight load to 52.5 pounds (or less) for the next workout. Often, a 5-pound increase is the smallest increment available. If this is the case, the participant must choose between a 5-pound increase and fewer repetitions or performing more repetitions at the same weight until the 5-pound increase can be tolerated. A systematic program of gradual progression is perhaps the most important aspect of sensible and successful strength training.

Periodization

The key to muscle development is systematic application of the stress adaptation principle. Theoretically, if each training session is a little more demanding than the last one, the person will continue to gain strength. Unfortunately, the human body does not always respond in this manner. Given the same exercise protocol day after day, muscles become used to the stress and produce little or no adaptation. It is important, therefore, to periodically vary the training program. This type of plan is usually referred to as *strength training periodization.*

Although periodic change of exercise routine is essential for optimum strength results, the exerciser must stay with a given workout routine long enough for it to be productive. For the average lifter, it is advisable to spend three to six weeks on a specific strength training program. A simple and standard form of exercise periodization is a three-month program progressing from higher repetitions and lower resistance to lower repetitions and higher resistance. As presented in table 5.4, the first month's resistance is about 65 percent of maximum with 12 to 16 reps per set. The lower resistance represents a lower percentage of the muscle contractile strength as well as the structural strength of the tendon, ligament, and bone. This provides a lower risk of tissue injury during the initial conditioning stage.

It is particularly important to use high repetitions and low resistance during the first month of a beginning strength training participant's program. During this time, the muscles and nervous system are getting used to the movements and stress of strength training. By performing more repetitions with a relatively low resistance, the body is able to learn the movement patterns and get used to moving with some added resistance through the repetitive movements. Eighty percent of the strength gained in the first month of training is due to motor learning, a concept that is not unique to strength training. The body learns all new movements in a similar fashion, from learning to type to playing a musical instrument. In the early stages of any new activity, the more you perform the movement, the quicker you learn it. This illustrates why it is so important for beginners to learn and practice good technique. They are learning new movements and should learn to do them correctly.

During the second month, resistance is increased to about 75 percent of maximum with 8 to 12 repetitions per set. This is a strength-building period that provides a solid foundation for the final high-resistance stage. In the third month, resistance is raised to about 85 percent of maximum with 4 to 8 reps per set. The near-maximum resistance might provide a more effective strength stimulus and should be well tolerated by the muscle and connective tissue after two months of training.

Table 5.4 shows a sample of a three-month exercise plan.

Following three months of progressive resistance exercise, it is usually advisable to take a week of active rest before repeating the cycle. Active rest refers to substituting non–strength training activities that involve little resistance, such as walking, hiking, jogging, cycling, swimming, racquetball, basketball, tennis, and golf. Although there are numerous periodization variations, the three-month model fits nicely with many seasonal activities. Repeating the three-month training cycle ensures a systematic change in the exercise stimulus, thereby facilitating positive muscle adaptations. Each training cycle should begin at a somewhat higher level of resistance than the previous cycle. Following a planned periodization program is preferred over a day-by-day trial-and-error approach.

Table 5.4 Sample Three-Month Periodization Program

Month	Exercise resistance	Exercise repetitions
First	About 65% max	12-16 reps/set
Second	About 75% max	8-12 reps/set
Third	About 85% max	4-8 reps/set
Active rest	Non–strength training activity for 1 week	

Building Time

The stimulus for strength development takes place during the exercise session. However, muscles do not become stronger at that time. In fact, muscles are weaker after the workout than before the workout. It is only during the recovery period following the exercise session that muscles gradually build to higher strength levels. Building time is an often misunderstood factor that plays a major role in muscle development. According to exercise physiologists, a strenuous strength training session produces some degree of muscle microtrauma (microscopic tissue damage). The time necessary to synthesize actin and myosin proteins and to develop new muscle tissue is called *building time*.

Building time varies among individuals, from 48 to 72 hours. Research at the University of Florida has shown shorter building time for people with predominantly slow-twitch muscle fibers and longer building time for people with predominantly fast-twitch muscle fibers.

As suggested in a previous section on exercise frequency, most people respond well to strength training every other day. However, it is important to carefully monitor progress and evaluate responsiveness. If a participant does not feel a little stronger during successive exercise sessions, building time might not have been sufficient. Table 5.5 indicates the effects of rest time on the strength level attained.

Table 5.5 Effects of Rest Time on Strength

Rest time	Effect
Sufficient	Slightly more strength is attained.
Too little	Muscle does not build more strength and might not reach its previous level.
Too much	Muscle initially builds slightly more strength, but returns to its previous level by the next workout.

One way for participants to monitor progress and assess tissue-building response is through the use of a training or workout log. A workout log contains a record of exercise weight loads and repetitions, and a subjective report of feelings during each workout (see figures 8.2-8.4 for examples).

Movement Speed

Movement speed is an important factor in both strength development and the potential for injury. Although it is not possible to identify an ideal exercise speed, slow lifting movements might be preferable to fast lifting movements for several reasons. These include muscle tension, muscle force, momentum, and injury risk.

- **Muscle tension.** Strength exercise produces muscle tension that stimulates strength development. A slow lifting movement provides a longer period of muscle tension than a fast lifting movement does. For example, performing 10 barbell curls at 5 seconds per repetition requires 50 seconds of muscle tension, whereas performing 10 barbell curls at 3 seconds per repetition requires only 30 seconds of muscle tension.

The YMCA of the USA recommends that exercisers perform all strength training movements in a slow and controlled manner, concentrating on using the prime mover muscles during the exercise. That said, participants, especially beginners, should not move too slowly. Because their muscles are not developed, beginners might place too much pressure on adjacent joints and tendons when performing the exercise too slowly. When the goal of strength training is to enhance sport performance, faster training movement might be appropriate.

- **Muscle force.** Although muscle tension is an important training factor, muscle force provides the primary stimulus for strength development. Muscle force output is directly related to exercise speed and decreases as the movement speed increases.
- **Momentum.** Every movement involves some degree of momentum. Momentum is the quantity of motion determined by an object's mass and velocity. Quick movements generate more momentum than slow movements do. This is significant in strength development because momentum affects the production of muscle force. Experiments with force-recording devices demonstrate that slow barbell lifts require relatively consistent muscle force throughout the movement range. Conversely, fast barbell lifts require high muscle force at the start, but almost no muscle force throughout the rest of the movement range. This is due to momentum.
- **Injury risk.** Quick lifting movements require high levels of force at the beginning of each exercise repetition. This subjects the muscles, tendons, and joints to high stress levels and increases the risk of tissue injury. Slow lifting movements do not require as much force at the beginning of each exercise repetition, which significantly decreases the risk of tissue injury.

Movement Range

Research shows that muscle strength increases only in the movement range in which training occurs. Graves and colleagues (1989) trained four groups using a bilateral knee extension exercise. One group trained the first half of the range of motion, the second trained the second half, the third trained a full range of motion, and a control group did not train. The results showed that the training result was specific to the range of motion trained. The group that trained the full range of motion gained the most strength through the full range. If the goal is to develop muscle strength throughout a full movement range, then training must occur through the full movement range.

Consider how a person's strength typically varies throughout the movement range of the trunk extension exercise. The low back is naturally stronger in a flexed position than in an extended position. If exercise is done on only the first half of this movement range, only the stronger area will be strengthened, creating an even greater strength differential from flexion to extension. The resulting imbalance might cause low back problems.

Exercising through a full range of movement also enhances joint flexibility. For example, in the final position of a back extension exercise, the low back muscles are fully contracted and the opposing abdominal muscles are fully stretched. Full-range exercise is advantageous for strength development, flexibility development, and injury prevention.

In certain populations, such as older adults, a full range of motion is not always possible. This might be due to certain medical conditions, such as arthritis, or to deconditioning. Participants who cannot exercise their joints through a full range of motion should focus on the range of motion that is possible. As they continue to exercise, their range of motion will gradually increase.

Muscle Balance

Balanced strength training is the key to comprehensive muscle development and injury prevention. When a muscle group is disproportionately stronger than its opposing muscle group, muscle imbalance results. This reduces joint integrity and increases the risk of overuse injuries. For example, sprinters typically perform strengthening exercises for their quadriceps muscles. However, if they do not strengthen the opposing hamstring muscles, they probably will experience a muscle imbalance. The stronger quadriceps muscles might overpower the weaker hamstrings muscles as the sprinter drives out of the starting blocks, causing injury to the hamstrings group.

This does not mean that all opposing muscle groups should be equally strong. However, it is important to train all major muscle groups to maintain a desirable muscle balance throughout the body. Although not essential for balanced strength development, it is advisable to train opposing muscle groups in pairs. The following is a suggested sequence for systematically conditioning the major muscle groups in order from larger to smaller.

- Quadriceps
- Hamstrings
- Hip adductors
- Hip abductors
- Chest
- Upper back
- Shoulders
- Biceps
- Triceps
- Low back
- Abdominals
- Neck extensors
- Neck flexors

Individual strength workouts should progress from working the large muscle groups to the smaller, supporting muscle groups. There are several reasons for this.

Because the largest and strongest muscles of the body, the hip and leg muscles, have the greatest potential for developing overall strength and muscle mass and for providing overall stimulation, these muscles should be exercised first. To fatigue the supporting (and generally smaller) muscles first would make them unable to contribute to the many exercise movements of the larger leg and torso muscles.

The order in which the exercises are performed might also affect training effectiveness. In general, exercises that work multiple muscles and joints should be performed before exercises that work a single muscle and joint exercises. For example, it is advisable to do bench presses before triceps extensions. If a person performs the triceps extensions first and fatigues the triceps, he or she would most likely have to use less weight for bench presses, which involve both the triceps and chest muscles. Even though the triceps will experience a good workout, the lighter bench presses might reduce the training stimulus to the chest muscles. Performing bench presses first permits a heavier weight load and increases the training stimulus to the chest muscles. Although the extensions must now be performed with less weight, this should not reduce the training stimulus to the triceps muscles if they are worked to fatigue.

Training Specificity

Bodies respond in a specific manner to a specific training stimulus. For example, long-distance running improves a runner's aerobic capacity by increasing cardiovascular endurance, not by increasing the legs' muscular strength. Conversely, performing heavy barbell squats improves the size and strength of the weightlifter's leg muscles, not the weightlifter's aerobic capacity.

Although a few exercises (such as barbell squats) involve opposing muscle groups (quadriceps and hamstrings), most exercises strengthen only one muscle group. For example, leg extensions strengthen the quadriceps, but not the hamstrings. Conversely, leg curls strengthen the hamstrings, but not the quadriceps. Clearly, strength exercise must be carefully designed to meet specific training objectives. However, it is never advisable to train one muscle group without also training the opposing muscle group. Although a shot putter must strengthen the triceps muscles for peak performance, it is equally important to strengthen the opposing biceps muscles to promote joint integrity and prevent injury. Always combine the principle of training specificity and the principle of muscle balance for maximum muscle development and minimum risk of injury.

Exercise Breathing

It is very important to breathe continuously during every exercise repetition. Holding your breath during resistance training can significantly increase internal pressure in the chest cavity. This situation, known as the Valsalva maneuver, can limit blood return to the heart and elevate blood pressure to dangerous levels. The preferred method of breathing is to exhale during the lifting movement and to inhale during the lowering movement. In this manner, the air pressure decreases as the muscle pressure increases (lifting movement), and the air pressure increases as the muscle pressure decreases (lowering movement).

Although this breathing pattern maintains a better pressure balance, the most essential consideration is to breathe regularly. As long as the breath is not held for more than a moment, the Valsalva maneuver should not be experienced. If beginners have difficulty coordinating breathing with the exercise, tell them to breathe normally. Once they learn the exercise and become more comfortable, they will be able to switch to the breathing pattern described previously.

YMCA of the USA Strength Training Guidelines

The following are the guidelines for strength training in YMCAs.

- Repetitions: 8 to 12
- Sets: 1 to 3
- Intervals: 2 minutes rest between sets
- Resistance: 65 to 85 percent
- Frequency: 3 times per week (full-body workout)
- Building time: 48 to 72 hours rest between workouts
- Progression: 5 percent or less
- Range: Full range of motion or as close as individually possible
- Breathing: Exhale on exertion

SPECIAL CONSIDERATIONS

People just starting strength training often are concerned about how such training will affect blood pressure, heart rate, and body composition. Also, special precautions must be taken when people with disabilities or pregnant women participate in strength training.

Blood Pressure

Many men and women avoid strength training because they are afraid that resistance exercise will adversely affect their blood pressure. Research indicates that these fears are generally unfounded. Adults have been correctly cautioned not to perform strenuous isometric activities such as trying to open a stuck window or attempting to move a stalled car. Activities of this type, including isometric strength training, might cause excessively high blood pressure responses and are potentially dangerous for many people.

It is also true that bodybuilders have recorded very high blood pressures during heavy leg press exercises. However, research indicates that sensible strength training following recommended guidelines does not have a harmful effect on blood pressure. Cardiovascular endurance exercise, strength training for the upper or lower body, and circuit training do not affect blood pressure levels adversely.

- **Cardiovascular endurance exercise.** To place blood pressure response to strength exercise in proper perspective, consider the normal blood pressure response to endurance exercise. In one study, 23 adults were monitored throughout a stationary cycling workout performed at 75 percent of their maximum heart rate. As presented in table 5.6, the results revealed a 35 percent increase in systolic blood pressure from 114 millimeters of mercury (mmHg) at rest to 154 mmHg during the exercise session, considered normal. Whenever vigorous exercise is performed, the heart beats faster and contracts harder to pump more blood to working muscles. The circulatory system adjusts to greater and more forceful blood flow by dilating blood vessels and opening additional capillaries, allowing blood to more readily reach the working muscles.

- **Upper-body strength exercise.** In a study to assess blood pressure response during upper-body strength exercise, 24 men and women performed 10 biceps curls with the heaviest weight possible. Their mean diastolic blood pressure measured 75 mmHg both before and immediately after the exercise set. The mean systolic blood pressure increased gradually from 123 mmHg at rest to 165 mmHg during the final repetition. As shown in table 5.6, this represented a 34 percent increase in systolic blood pressure and was well below the 220 mmHg caution level.

- **Lower-body strength exercise.** Because lower-body strength exercise involves more muscle mass and more muscle force than upper-body strength exercise, another study examined blood pressure response during seated leg presses. Twenty-five men and women performed 10 leg presses with the heaviest weight load possible. The mean diastolic blood pressure measured 73 mmHg before and 61 mmHg immediately after the exercise set. The mean systolic blood pressure increased progressively from 127 mmHg at rest to 190 mmHg during the final repetition. As presented in table 5.6, this represented a 50 percent increase in systolic blood pressure and was well below the 220 mmHg caution level.

- **Circuit strength training.** Another study examined the immediate effects of circuit strength training on blood pressure. The 100 men and women in this study performed one set (8 to 12 repetitions) of 11 different strength exercises. Standing blood pressure was measured 30 to 60 seconds before and 30 to 60 seconds after participants completed the 11-station exercise

Table 5.6 Systolic Blood Pressure Response to Different Exercises

Activity	Subjects	Resting systolic pressure (mmHg)	Peak systolic pressure (mmHg)	Increase
Stationary cycling	23	114	154	35%
Upper-body strength exercises	24	123	165	34%
Lower-body strength exercises	25	127	190	50%

Table 5.7 Blood Pressure Responses Before and After Circuit Strength Training Session

Subjects	Age (years)	Training time (min)	Preexercise blood pressure (mmHg)	Postexercise blood pressure (mmHg)
72 Men	38	29	118/69	119/67
28 Women	34	29	107/62	113/59
100 Total	37	29	115/67	117/65

circuit. As shown in table 5.7, their mean pretraining blood pressure was 115/67 mmHg, and their mean posttraining blood pressure was 117/65 mmHg. That is, their immediate postexercise blood pressure was almost identical to their preexercise blood pressure. The readings both before and after exercise represented excellent blood pressure levels for these people who performed regular strength training.

People who have high blood pressure, heart disease, or other high-risk characteristics should not perform any type of physical exercise without written consent from their physician. These participants should be identified during their first visit to the exercise facility by means of a medical history questionnaire.

Although it is strongly recommended that all adults over age 40 consult their physician before beginning an exercise program, there does not seem to be a reason for healthy men and women to avoid sensible strength training. The studies reviewed in this section revealed acceptable blood pressure responses in normal adults during and after sensible strength exercise. In addition, the mean resting blood pressures for all of the strength-trained subjects were well within normal limits, indicating that sensible strength training does not adversely affect resting blood pressure.

Sensible strength training is characterized by the following:

- Weight loads that can be lifted for 8 to 12 repetitions in good form
- Continuous muscle movement throughout each exercise set
- Continuous breathing throughout each exercise set

Maximum weight loads, isometric contractions, and breath holding should be avoided.

Heart Rate

Like systolic blood pressure, heart rates elevate during vigorous exercise in order to pump more blood to working muscles. And like systolic blood pressure, heart rate increases gradually and progressively throughout each set of strength exercise. Although larger muscle groups use more oxygen, the heart rate response is similar for lower-body and upper-body exercises. Beginning from rest, the heart rate typically doubles during an exercise set of 10 repetitions with the heaviest weight load possible. When brief rests are taken between successive sets of exercise, the heart rate might remain at a high level throughout the training session.

Research indicates that circuit strength training might produce cardiorespiratory benefits (Fleck and Kraemer 1997), such as reduced resting blood pressure, improved lipid profiles, increased muscle capillarization, and enhanced aerobic capacity. However, much greater cardiorespiratory improvement is obtained through traditional aerobic exercise. It is therefore recommended that participants perform strength exercise to develop muscular fitness and endurance exercise to develop cardiorespiratory fitness.

Body Composition

When people are concerned with improving their body composition, they usually think about losing fat by consuming fewer calories and doing more aerobic exercise. Although this approach is effective for reducing fat stores, it might not be the best means for improving body composition because it doesn't address muscle. Muscle is a major factor in body composition and physical appearance. Muscle is especially important as we age, because the average adult loses about half a pound of muscle every year of life. Consequently, a 45-year-old man who weighs the same as he did at age 25 might very well have 10 pounds less muscle and 10 pounds more fat. For him, and most Americans, adding muscle is just as important as losing fat. Gaining muscle provides two benefits. First, additional muscle improves body composition and physical appearance. Second, additional muscle increases resting metabolic rate because muscle is very active tissue with high energy requirements, even at rest. More muscle means more calories are used for tissue maintenance and building functions.

Consider a research study that examined the effects of strength training on body composition. All 72 participants followed the same dietary guidelines and exercised for the same amount of time. Twenty-two subjects performed 30 minutes of endurance exercise, three days a week. Fifty subjects performed 15 minutes of endurance exercise and 15 minutes of strength exercise, three days a week. After eight weeks of training, the subjects who performed only aerobic exercise lost 3 pounds of fat weight and half a pound of lean (muscle) weight (see table 5.8). The subjects who performed both aerobic exercise and strength exercise lost 10 pounds of fat weight and gained 2 pounds of lean (muscle) weight, for a 12-pound improvement in body composition.

This research indicates that strength training is an excellent means of enhancing body composition. Because it is the only activity that reduces fat, replaces muscle, and raises resting metabolic rate, strength training should be a key component in fat loss and body-shaping programs.

Individuals With Disabilities

Strength training can be beneficial for people with disabilities. Carefully screen people with disabilities to determine what type of strength exercise they are capable of. With their physician's written consent and general guidelines, they may effectively participate in appropriately modified muscle-building programs. For those who do not use wheelchairs, it is usually possible to train most of the major muscle groups in a conventional manner. Free weights might offer greater versatility and freedom of movement, whereas resistance machines might provide better support and operational efficiency.

For those who must remain in their wheelchairs, resistance devices are available. In most cases, the participant moves onto a training platform, secures the wheelchair, and performs a variety of exercises for the arms and upper body using cables attached to a preselected resistance. The major concern for strength training among wheelchair users is stabilizing the torso so they can safely and successfully perform the desired exercise movement. Although this might be accomplished by strapping the torso to the seat back, better stability and performance are usually obtained when the instructor holds the participant in place.

Because each person's disability is different, it is difficult to present a specific strength training protocol. It is recommended that staff members collaborate with local agencies and their medical community to effectively plan and implement programs for people with special needs. Once medical clearance and support are obtained, the major emphasis should be providing progressive resistance exercise for all of the functional muscle groups. Participant feedback is perhaps the best means for determining if this objective has been achieved.

Pregnancy

The few studies that have examined strength training during pregnancy have demonstrated a desirable increase in muscular strength and an

Table 5.8 Body Composition Changes for Subjects Performing Endurance Exercise Only and for Subjects Performing Both Endurance and Strength Exercise

Exercise	Subjects	Weight change (lbs)	Fat change (lbs)	Muscle change (lbs)
Endurance exercise only	22	−3.5	−3.0	−0.5
Endurance and strength exercise	50	−8.0	−10.0	+2.0

absence of adverse effects. Nonetheless, certain precautions should be taken when training pregnant women. All pregnant women should obtain their physician's written approval and specific guidelines for participation in all YMCA exercise programs, including resistance exercise programs. The participants should complete health screening and fitness testing to determine an appropriate exercise starting point, taking into account specific guidelines recommended by their physician.

The American College of Obstetricians and Gynecologists provides the following general exercise guidelines:

- Exercise at least three times per week.
- Don't exercise on the back after the first trimester.
- Modify the intensity; listen to the body's signals.
- Don't jeopardize balance.
- Avoid activities with the potential for even mild abdominal trauma.
- Be careful not to overheat, especially in the first trimester.
- Warm up and cool down before and after exercise session.
- Exercise on a resilient floor.
- Don't flex joints excessively or stretch to the limit.
- Eat enough calories for the extra energy needed for both the pregnancy and exercise.
- Don't rotate the trunk while the hips or spine are flexed.

Pregnant women should train with moderate resistance and range of movement to reduce stress on lax connective tissue caused by the release of relaxin and other hormones. They should also drink cold water throughout the exercise session to replace fluids and to cool body temperature. Exercise should be stopped and medical assistance attained in response to the following events:

- Pain (chest, back, abdomen, hip)
- Vaginal bleeding
- Dizziness or weakness
- Headache or nausea
- Decreased fetal activity
- Uterine contractions
- Generalized edema

The goal of strength training for women during pregnancy should be to continue with an ongoing program to maintain muscular strength, not to begin a new program. For more information, refer to the YMCA of the USA's *YMCA Prenatal Exercise Instructor Manual* and related Medical Advisory Committee recommendation.

STRENGTH TRAINING MYTHS

Several myths about strength training have developed over the years. Here are some of those myths and the facts to refute them.

- **Strength training increases blood pressure.** Although it is strongly recommended that all adults over age 40 see their physician before beginning an exercise program, there is no reason for healthy men and women to avoid sensible strength training. The studies reviewed previously in this chapter revealed acceptable blood pressure responses in normal adults during and after sensible strength exercise. Sensible strength training is characterized by the following:

When these guidelines are observed, strength training appears to be a safe physical activity that provides important benefits to our musculoskeletal system.

- **To gain muscle size, free weights, not weight machines, must be used.** The relationship between muscle gain and the exclusive use of free weights has been a misconception since the rise in popularity of resistance-type machines. Many believe that the only way to gain muscle size is to train with free weights. Although many free-weight enthusiasts believe that this is the best method, the type of equipment is, in fact, not the significant variable in muscle hypertrophy. Rather, it is the level of intensity and whether an overload is placed on the muscle that creates the response. As a case in point, in 2004, 15 of the 31 National Football League (NFL) teams trained mostly with high-intensity techniques on weight machines. Obviously, players on all of the teams have developed extremely high levels of strength and muscularity. It is not the type of equipment used, but the progressive overload training that is responsible for the athletes' muscular development. Results are also determined by the individual genetic potential; no matter the type of equipment used, large gains in muscle hypertrophy might not be possible for some people.

- **Strength training decreases flexibility and range of motion.** A properly performed dynamic weight training program does not impair flexibility and can possibly increase range of motion in some muscle joints.

- **Older adults do not benefit from strength training.** A program of resistance exercise can be safely carried out by both older men and women. This type of program significantly increases muscle strength in part because of muscle hypertrophy.

- **Weight belts should be worn at all times.** During movements in which the stress on the lumbar spine is low, little is gained by wearing a tightly cinched weightlifting belt, which might needlessly restrict natural breathing.

- **Protein supplementation is required in order to increase muscle mass.** The American Dietetic Association states that protein requirements are slightly increased in highly active people. Compared to the Recommended Dietary Allowance (RDA) of 0.8 grams per kilogram (g/kg) body weight, protein recommendations for endurance athletes are 1.2 to 1.4 g/kg body weight per day, whereas those for resistance and strength-trained athletes may be as high as 1.6 to 1.7 g/kg body weight per day. These recommended protein intakes can generally be met through diet alone, without the use of protein or amino acid supplements, if energy intake is adequate to maintain body weight (JADA 2000).

- **One set of an exercise is not productive.** ACSM strength training guidelines are based on research that shows that significant strength gains result from one set of exercises. Whether the participant uses free weights, machines, or manual resistance, one set of 8 to 12 repetitions seems to be a good starting point for strength development.

- **When you quit strength training, your muscle turns to fat.** When a person regularly participates in a resistance training program, the common result is additional weight in the form of muscle hypertrophy. This additional muscle combined with the effect of regular exercise sessions increases the body's ability to burn calories and body fat. The result is a lean, well-defined body. If the person continues to participate in the program, his or her chance of remaining lean is very good. However, many fitness enthusiasts are confused about what happens when they stop strength training. Some believe that the muscle turns to fat. Because muscle and fat are two different substances, it is impossible to change one into the other. The result of any type of detraining is muscle atrophy. In addition, people require and expend significantly fewer calories when they are inactive. Therefore, if a person doesn't reduce caloric intake during a period of inactivity, the excess calories are stored as body fat at the same time that muscle atrophy is occurring, creating the perception of muscle turning to fat.

- **Weight training will stunt growth.** Numerous research studies have concluded that a sensibly designed, supervised program of strength training is safe and beneficial for a child's physical growth.

PERFORMING STRENGTH EXERCISES

Participants who perform strength exercises must know the procedures for doing them safely and effectively. They particularly need to be cautious when performing exercises for the low back, knees, and neck. Participants who are knowledgeable about strength training equipment can exercise more safely and comfortably; they also can choose to exercise either alternating limbs or both at the same time. Finally, they often can avoid injuries by using free weights for certain exercises only when spotters are present and by following guidelines for safely using weight machines.

Following are general procedures for performing strength training exercises:

- Perform all movements in a controlled manner, without jerking or bouncing.

- Pause slightly—a momentary hold—between concentric (positive) and eccentric (negative) contractions.
- Do not hesitate or rest between repetitions, and on machine exercises, do not let the weight stacks touch while performing a set.
- Perform the lowering, or negative phase, of each exercise more slowly than the initial, or positive phase, of the exercise; for example, two to three seconds for the positive movement and four to six seconds for the negative portion. Perform the lowering motion in a controlled manner and do not allow gravity to simply "drop" the weight back to the starting position, as many inexperienced lifters do.
- Use a full range of movement during each exercise.
- Do not hold the breath while performing any strength exercises. Exhale on the positive (when raising the weight) when possible.

Strengthening the Low Back, Knees, and Neck

Three areas of the body that typically need strengthening are the low back, knees, and neck. However, these areas are particularly susceptible to injury, so strength training must be performed with certain precautions.

Low Back

It is estimated that more than 80 percent of all people in the United States have experienced some level of low back pain. The vast majority is not related to spinal or other structural damage, but instead to muscular weakness or imbalance. Low back muscles help the body maintain proper posture and body carriage. Along with the abdominal muscles on the front of the body and the oblique muscles on both sides, the muscles of the low back provide a "girdle" of support for the midsection of the body and form a base of support for the spine. Strong low back muscles help people move easily and safely through everyday life, as well as provide support in their daily activities, athletic endeavors, or in emergency situations.

Unfortunately, because many people report back problems, some fitness staff have shied away from including the low back area in exercise routines. However, with guidance from health care professionals, many people with low back problems can effectively exercise their low back muscles, thereby increasing strength and flexibility.

People who have no known back problem should be encouraged to include exercises in their routine to develop and maintain strength and flexibility of the low back muscles. This can be done, in most cases, under the guidance of a certified YMCA Personal Training Instructor.

Following are guidelines for people with low back problems:

- All members who experience low back problems should obtain a physician or health care provider release before participating in a strength training program.
- YMCA staff should incorporate physician or health-care provider recommendations into the member's strength training program.
- Refer individuals who indicate low back difficulties and have no personal physician to the care of a qualified medical practitioner.
- Do not recommend exercises that might be harmful to people indicating back problems. These include squats, leg presses, overhead pressing movements, twisting movements, side-bending exercises, and any exercise movements that cause the body to lean forward or backward unsupported.
- Develop a local Medical Advisory Committee at your YMCA to address program guidelines for people with special needs.
- Begin a YMCA Healthy Back program for people who are unable to perform strength training.

Knees

Exercise involving the knees, when performed correctly, can help prevent injury associated with daily and leisure activity. Exercises performed incorrectly can, themselves, cause injury.

During squatting activities, avoid bending the knee beyond 90 degrees, and don't lock the knee during leg-pressing actions. People with knee pain should consult their physician before performing any type of leg exercises. Do not project the knee beyond the toes in weight-bearing exercises such as squats and lunges.

Neck

The neck is one of the most neglected, yet most used, muscles. The muscles of the neck support a 15-pound head all day, which can lead to muscle fatigue and strain after several hours. Scientific evidence shows that weak neck muscles can cause headaches, migraines, and poor posture.

Strengthening the neck can help prevent this strain and the accompanying pain. Because the neck is a very sensitive area, exercises must be properly executed to prevent injury. When performing neck exercises, participants must prevent sudden, excessive, or inconsistent application of force. Because the neck muscles provide support in all exercise movements, work specifically for the neck should be done last in an exercise session. Fatiguing them early inhibits their ability to be supportive in exercises later in the session.

Strength Training Accessories

The following is a list of common accessories used during strength training. Descriptions of exercises mentioned under Application can be found at the end of this chapter.

Weight Belt

Purpose

Provides back and internal support by increasing abdominal-wall pressure; might be useful in working with heavier weight loads.

Application

Squat, overhead press, standing biceps curl

Note: For a belt to provide support, it must be worn as tight as possible, which might make taking a deep breath difficult. Keeping the belt tight increases intra-abdominal pressure by forming an air pocket, which provides inner support for the spinal erector muscles. This, combined with the external support of the belt, neutralizes the stress of lifting. Wearing a belt improperly might leave a person at risk of injury.

In some instances, weight belts are overused. Exercises such as the squat, deadlift, overhead lifts, and standing curls with heavier weight loads performed with a low number of repetitions might require the use of a weight belt. Using the belt for other exercises might give a person a psychological benefit, but does not prevent injury. There is also the possibility that using the belt might prevent strength increases in the spinal erectors because the musculature becomes dependent on the belt to support the spinal column.

Gloves

Purpose

Provide extra bar-holding ability, protect hands, increase overall comfort of lifting.

Application

Used for all strength training activities as needed or desired.

Wrist Support

Purpose

Provides extra support, improve lifting comfort.

Application

Can be used during all strength training as needed or desired.

Knee Wrap

Purpose

Provides additional support and protection during certain weight training exercises with heavy weights. For healthy knees, knee wraps are not generally recommended or needed. If knee wraps are required because of an injury, the participant should consult with his or her physician or physical therapist for correct application and wrapping procedures.

Application

Squats, lunges

Chalk (Carbonate of Magnesia)

Purpose

Increases bar-holding ability and decreases the likelihood of calluses.

Application

Used commonly by Olympic free-weight lifters to inhibit moisture on the hands, to keep hands from becoming sweaty and making the bar slippery.

Alternating Versus Concomitant Exercise

Exercises can be done either alternating arms or sides or using both arms or sides at the same time (concomitant exercise). Alternating arms or sides increases the ability to concentrate on an individual muscle or side.

Alternating exercise also has these disadvantages:

- Causes greater forearm fatigue
- Takes longer to perform each exercise
- Requires a higher level of aerobic endurance

Concomitant exercise has these benefits:

- Causes less forearm fatigue
- Requires less balance and coordination
- Takes less time to perform each exercise
- Is less confusing for beginners

Spotting

Working with a partner who provides safety, assistance, and motivation is recommended during certain strength training exercises. An effective spotter should

- know how to properly execute the exercise and the appropriate assistance methods;
- focus entirely on the exerciser and be prepared at all times;
- check the bar for even and proper loading;
- be aware of how many repetitions will be attempted;
- decide before the lift how the lifter and spotter will communicate;
- assist with lifting the weight off the rack and returning it as requested;
- always use two hands to ensure balance and safety;
- give the exerciser feedback on form;
- provide motivation and encouragement for the exerciser, but not carry on a dialogue with the lifter or anyone else;
- strongly encourage the use of collars on barbells;
- maintain a solid stance;
- keep hands off of the bench's uprights; and
- above all, use common sense.

The following are spotting techniques:

- **Barbell bench press and incline press.** The spotter stands directly behind the lifter in a ready position. Feet should be planted securely, shoulder-width apart, and arms should be extended in front, palms up, ready to grab the bar if necessary. The moment the barbell stops its upward movement, the spotter grasps the barbell. Using the arms and the legs, the spotter provides enough assistance to complete the lift and return the barbell to the standards.
- **Barbell squats.** The spotter stands directly behind the lifter and moves up and down in tandem with the lifter. The moment the lifter stops the upward movement, the spotter wraps his or her arms around the lifter's upper torso or puts his or her arms under the lifter's arms. Using the legs, the spotter provides enough assistance to complete the lift and return the barbell to the standards.
- **Dumbbell exercises.** The spotter applies assistance directly in line with the resistance force. For example, during the final repetition of the dumbbell bench press, the spotter might best assist by lifting at the exerciser's wrists.

Guidelines for Using Strength Training Machines

Selectorized strength training equipment (weight stack machines with pins used to select a given weight) is popular with many adults seeking to develop and maintain muscular strength and endurance. Use of these machines is considered safer, particularly for beginners, as the weights are fixed on the machine. However, not every participant can execute exercises on certain types of equipment with proper form. This is because some machines cannot be adjusted to match the limb lengths of every participant, especially youth, women, and older adults. General guidelines follow. However, encourage participants to suggest other adjustments to their trainer if needed. This particularly applies to participants who require rehabilitation, have disabilities, and face other special or medical circumstances.

- Use each machine in the manner the manufacturer recommends. Do not try alternative applications for which the machine is not intended.

- Use belts and straps if provided by the manufacturer.
- Adjust seat heights to ensure proper body alignment on all machines by aligning the machine's axis of rotation or cam center with the participant's joint axis.
- Do not allow the moving weight stack to touch the stationary weight stack during the exercise.
- Do not drop weight plates or allow them to slam onto the weight stack.
- Use the appropriate pin in all selectorized machines.
- Focus on proper exercise form, which is more important than the amount of weight lifted.
- Use additional seat pads when limb length or body size do not fit the machine dimensions.
- Grasp exercise handles lightly and don't use excessive grip force.
- Concentrate on performing each exercise with the prime mover muscle and don't engage assisting muscles.
- Use as full a range of motion as comfortably possible.
- Staff should regularly check equipment to make sure machines are working correctly and teach members to report repair needs.

RECOMMENDED STRENGTH TRAINING EXERCISES

This section lists strength exercises for each major muscle group of the body, using both free weights and machines. It also describes how to choose the right exercises and how to train effectively and efficiently. Generic descriptions of exercise machines are used because a variety of brands exists. The exercises listed were chosen based on the types of equipment commonly found in YMCAs, and to best match the needs of the majority of YMCA members. Descriptions of other equipment and exercises can be found in other strength training resources.

Descriptions and photographs of the strength training exercises can be found in table 5.9 and at the end of this chapter. They are listed by parts of the body.

Choosing the Right Exercises

The challenge for YMCA personal training instructors is selecting appropriate exercises to design a strength training program that covers all of the major muscle groups and allows the member to attain his or her goals. Table 5.10 on page 105 is a sample basic workout that is appropriate for most adults seeking to develop overall muscular fitness and conditioning.

Training With Effectiveness and Efficiency

When designing a strength training program, make sure it is effective by choosing exercises that will produce the desired results. An efficient program is one the participant can complete in the time he or she has available.

Although any system of progressive-resistance exercise will produce at least minimal strength gains, some programs are more effective than others. Strength development depends on applying the strength training principles discussed earlier; however, many people and equipment manufacturers believe that the type of exercise equipment plays a more significant role in training effectiveness than it actually does. For example, some people prefer free weights to machines and vice versa. Of the machine advocates, some prefer weight stacks, whereas others favor compressed air, hydraulic, or electronic resistance. For the majority of participants, the type of resistance has less influence on muscle response than the way resistance is applied. A prime consideration is the degree to which the resistance force matches the muscle force throughout the movement range.

For example, dumbbell flys are intended to strengthen the chest muscles, and they are reasonably effective for this purpose. However, dumbbell flys do not match resistance force and muscle force very closely throughout the entire movement range. Because of leverage factors, the bottom position is characterized by relatively high resistance force and relatively low muscle force.

Table 5.9 Strength Training Exercises

Exercise	Muscles involved
Upper leg	
Barbell squat	Quadriceps, hamstrings, gluteus maximus
Dumbbell squat	Quadriceps, hamstrings, gluteus maximus
Dumbbell lunge	Quadriceps, hamstrings, gluteus maximus
Leg extension machine	Quadriceps
Leg press machine	Quadriceps, hamstrings, gluteus maximus
Leg curl machine	Hamstrings
Low cable–crossover adduction	Hip adductors
Ankle weight adduction	Hip adductors
Hip adduction machine	Hip adductors
Low cable–crossover abduction	Hip abductors
Ankle weight abduction	Hip abductors
Hip abduction machine	Hip abductors
Buttocks	
Low-cable hip extension	Gluteus maximus, hamstrings
Lower leg	
Weighted toe raise	Anterior tibialis
Low-cable dorsiflexion	Anterior tibialis
Supported single-leg dumbbell heel raise	Gastrocnemius, soleus
Seated calf apparatus	Soleus, gastrocnemius
Standing calf apparatus	Gastrocnemius, soleus
Calf press using leg press machine	Gastrocnemius, soleus
Chest	
Barbell bench press	Pectoralis major, anterior deltoid, triceps
Dumbbell bench press	Pectoralis major, anterior deltoid, triceps
Incline barbell press	Upper pectoralis major, triceps, anterior deltoid
Incline dumbbell press	Upper pectoralis major, triceps, anterior deltoid
Dumbbell fly	Pectoralis major, anterior deltoid
Chest press machine	Pectoralis major, anterior deltoid, triceps
Chest cross machine	Pectoralis major, anterior deltoid
Incline press machine	Pectoralis major, anterior deltoid, triceps

Exercise	Muscles involved
Middle back	
Dumbbell bent row	Latissimus dorsi, teres major, middle trapezius, posterior deltoid, rhomboids, biceps
Lat pull-down	Latissimus dorsi, biceps
Chin-up	Latissimus dorsi, biceps
Pullover machine	Latissimus dorsi, teres major
Seated rowing machine	Rhomboids, posterior deltoid, latissimus dorsi, teres major, middle trapezius
Pull-down machine	Latissimus dorsi, teres major, biceps
Upper back	
Barbell shrug	Upper trapezius, levator scapulae
Dumbbell shrug	Upper trapezius, levator scapulae
Shoulder shrug machine	Upper trapezius, levator scapulae
Shoulders	
Dumbbell lateral raise	Middle deltoid
Dumbbell shoulder press	Anterior deltoid, middle deltoid, triceps, upper trapezius
Barbell shoulder press	Medial deltoid, anterior deltoid, triceps, upper trapezius
Dumbbell front raise	Anterior deltoid
Lateral raise machine	Deltoid
Shoulder press machine	Anterior and middle deltoid, triceps, upper trapezius
Upper arm	
Dumbbell curl	Biceps
Barbell curl	Biceps
Incline dumbbell curl	Biceps
Standing cable curl	Biceps
Biceps machine	Biceps
Triceps press-down	Triceps
Dumbbell kickback	Triceps
Seated dumbbell triceps extension	Triceps
Triceps machine	Triceps
Seated dip machine	Triceps, pectoralis major, anterior deltoid

(continued)

Table 5.9 *(continued)*

Exercise	Muscles involved
Lower arm	
Reverse forearm curl	Forearm extensors
Weighted forearm roll	Forearm flexors, forearm extensors
Reverse cable forearm curl	Forearm extensors
Cable forearm curl	Forearm flexors
Forearm curl	Forearm flexors
Midsection	
Trunk curl (unweighted and weighted)	Rectus abdominis
Hip flexor apparatus	Hip flexors
Abdominal machine	Rectus abdominis
Twisting trunk curl (unweighted and weighted)	Obliques, rectus abdominis
Cable or dumbbell side bends	Obliques
Rotary torso machine	Obliques
Back	
Seated low-pulley back extension	Erector spinae, hip extensors
Floor back extension	Erector spinae
Low back machine	Erector spinae
Neck	
Supine weighted neck flexion	Sternocleidomastoid
Prone weighted neck extension	Upper trapezius, levator scapulae
Neck machine	Upper trapezius, levator scapulae
Shoulder and rotator cuff	
Cable internal rotation	Pectoralis major, latissimus dorsi, subscapularis, anterior deltoid
Cable external rotation	Infraspinatus, teres minor, posterior deltoid
Dumbbell abduction	Supraspinatus, deltoid

Conversely, the top position is characterized by relatively low resistance force and relatively high muscle force. In contrast, some variable-resistance exercise machines match resistance forces and muscle forces better by means of a counterleverage system. Through a system of cams or levers, the resistance is reduced in positions of low muscle force and increased in positions of high muscle force, resulting in what some argue to be a more effective exercise.

Another consideration with respect to exercise effectiveness is external friction. Although free weights meet virtually no external friction, machines provide varying levels of frictional force because of the movement of chains, cams, and the weight stack. It is therefore essential to

Table 5.10 General Strength Training Program for Adults

Muscle groups	Free-weight exercise	Machine exercise
Quadriceps, hamstrings, gluteus maximus	Dumbbell squat, dumbbell lunge	Leg press machine
Calves (gastrocnemius and soleus)	Dumbbell heel raise	Calf press using leg press machine
Pectoralis major, anterior deltoid, triceps	Barbell or dumbbell bench press	Chest press machine
Latissimus dorsi, teres major, middle trapezius, posterior rhomboids, biceps	Dumbbell bent row	Pull-down machine
Anterior deltoid, middle deltoid, triceps, upper trapezius	Dumbbell shoulder press	Lateral raise machine
Biceps	Dumbbell curl	Biceps machine
Triceps	Dumbbell kickback	Triceps machine
Rectus abdominis	Trunk curl	Abdominal machine
Erector spinae	Floor back extension	Low back machine

Select either free-weight or machine exercises, or combine.

reduce friction as much as possible by cleaning weight stack guide rods, for example. Guide rods that are rough produce more friction, making it more difficult to lift the weight stack (concentric movement) and easier to lower the weight stack (eccentric movement). This is opposite of muscle force output, which is lower during concentric contractions and higher during eccentric contractions. All sprockets, chains, pulleys, and cables should also function as smoothly as possible to reduce external friction.

For many people, strength training is a viable fitness activity only when it can be accomplished in a time-efficient manner. Training two hours a day might be acceptable for athletes, but is impractical for most adults. The average person is more likely to participate in a strength training program when it requires less than 30 minutes per session, three times per week. Fortunately, in the area of strength development, training effectiveness and training efficiency go hand in hand. Whereas cardiorespiratory endurance is best developed through exercise of low intensity and long duration, muscular strength is best developed through exercise of high intensity and short duration. In addition, research has demonstrated that brief strength training sessions can significantly improve body composition. Studies have shown a three-pound muscle gain and a four-pound fat loss after two months of strength training for 30 minutes per session, three sessions per week.

While successful bodybuilders perform many sets of different exercises, few of us have either the ability or the time to train in this manner. Although numerous training protocols provide an efficient workout, two basic exercise formats work for most people: one set of multiple-muscle exercises or several sets of single-muscle exercises (see table 5.11). When training a beginner, design a 30-minute workout consisting of single-muscle exercises. These exercises are easier to learn than those that work several muscle groups at once, and recovery is quicker. When the participant is ready for a more comprehensive training program, it is easy to build on the solid foundation of basic exercises by adding sets of multiple-muscle exercises.

ADVANCED STRENGTH TRAINING PRINCIPLES AND TECHNIQUES

After participants have performed the same strength training exercises for a while, they probably will reach a plateau, at which point progression ceases. Some of the techniques described in

Table 5.11 Sample Exercise Circuits

Single-muscle exercises—Perform one set each of 10 to 12 exercises.

Exercise	Muscle worked
Leg extension	Quadriceps
Leg curl	Hamstrings
Chest cross	Pectoralis major
Pullover	Latissimus dorsi
Lateral raise	Deltoid
Biceps curl	Biceps
Triceps extension	Triceps
Trunk curl	Rectus abdominis
Back extension	Erector spinea
Neck flexion	Sternocleidomastoid
Neck extension	Levator scapulae, upper trapezius

Multiple-muscle exercises—Perform three sets of 4 to 5 multiple-muscle exercises.

Exercise	Muscle groups worked
Squat	Quadriceps, hamstrings, gluteus maximus
Bench press	Pectoralis major, triceps, anterior deltoids
Pull-down	Latissimus dorsi, biceps
Shoulder press	Deltoid, triceps
Weighted trunk curl	Rectus abdominis, sternocleidomastoid

this section can help participants get past these plateaus and continue making progress.

Some participants might also become interested in the competitive sports of bodybuilding or weightlifting. Some of the basics of these sports and how they differ from general strength training are explained here.

Strength Plateaus

During the first few weeks of strength training, progress occurs relatively quickly with noticeable strength improvement occurring almost every exercise session. However, the rate of strength gain typically slows during the second and third months of training as strength levels off and little additional progress is observed. This is referred to as a *strength plateau*, and it indicates that the training program needs to be modified to facilitate further progress.

Strength plateaus appear to be a normal result of continued training and should not be cause for discouragement. Every strength training program eventually becomes stale if it remains unchanged. Sensible and systematic changes in the training program should help overcome a strength plateau and achieve further muscle development. Following are suggested modifications that can be made to a strength training routine when a plateau is reached:

- **Change training exercises.** The first training modification probably should be to select different exercises. As muscles become accustomed to performing the same exercises, the stimulus–response pattern becomes less and less effective. The same muscle fibers are activated in the same recruitment pattern, which becomes routine and unproductive.

  By changing the training exercises periodically, different muscle fibers are activated in different recruitment patterns, which fosters positive stimulus–response adaptations. For example, after six weeks of standing barbell curls, the biceps muscle's response to this exercise is lessened. When a new biceps exercise is substituted, such as incline dumbbell curls, different muscle fibers are stimulated in a different recruitment order, and positive adaptations are likely to occur. When the muscles become accustomed to incline dumbbell curls, a return to standing barbell curls or another biceps exercise should prevent another plateau and continue progress.

- **Change training frequency.** As muscles become stronger and able to lift heavier resistance, they might require longer recovery and building periods between training sessions. For example, if training each muscle group every other day ceases to be productive, it might be necessary to switch to training every third day. One example of such a program is to perform back and biceps exercises on Mondays and Thursdays, chest and triceps exercises on Tuesdays and Fridays, and leg and shoulder exercises on Wednesdays and Saturdays. In this manner, each major muscle group is trained twice a week with at least three days of recovery and building time between workouts.

- **Change training sets.** The number of sets performed per exercise is a significant factor in muscle development and strength gains. People who perform multiple sets of an exercise might gain little additional strength, but experience a lot of muscle fatigue from the high-volume training. They might obtain better results by cutting down the number of sets and training with greater intensity. On the other hand, single-set training might not produce maximum benefits for many people. For those who have difficulty training at a high intensity, less weight or fewer repetitions or both might be beneficial. Generally, the more exercises a person performs, the fewer sets per exercise he or she needs to do.
- **Change training repetitions.** Repetitions and resistance are inversely related. Heavier resistance limits repetitions, and less resistance allows more repetitions. Periodically changing the repetition and resistance relationship might produce further strength development. For example, performing 8 repetitions with 160 pounds provides a different muscle stimulus than completing 12 repetitions with 140 pounds. It is therefore advisable to consider occasional repetition variations to overcome both physical and mental staleness.

Another effective way to address strength plateaus is to use various techniques to increase training intensity. An exercise can be made more difficult in several ways, but some techniques carry a high risk of injury. The following high-intensity training methods—breakdown training, assisted training, super-slow training, superset training, and negative training—are safe and effective when used properly and can help participants move beyond strength plateaus.

A safety note: When increased resistance is used, the role of the spotter becomes even more important. When using methods such as assisted training or negative training, the spotter is crucial to the success, safety, and motivation of the lifter.

Breakdown Training

Let's assume that Pedro has 100 fibers in his biceps muscles and that each fiber can produce 1 pound of force. Theoretically, he could curl a maximum weight of 100 pounds. If he trains with 75 pounds, he might complete 10 repetitions before the weight exceeds his muscle force and he must stop. At this point he has fatigued at least 26 of his 100 muscle fibers, and there are not enough fresh fibers to lift the weight load. If he rests for about two minutes, most of the fatigued muscle fibers will recover and he can perform a second set of 9 or 10 curls. He will again fatigue the same 26 muscle fibers, at which point he must terminate the exercise set. In this manner, his biceps muscles are pushed to the limit once during each exercise set.

Suppose that at the completion of Pedro's last repetition with 75 pounds, a training partner reduces the weight load by 10 pounds. Because Pedro still has 74 functioning muscle fibers and only 65 pounds of resistance, he can complete two or three additional repetitions and fatigue 10 more muscle fibers before stopping the exercise set. Perhaps more important, his biceps muscles are pushed to the limit twice during the extended exercise set.

This type of high-intensity exercise is referred to as breakdown training because the starting weight load is "broken down" to permit more repetitions. This is a demanding training technique that causes temporary discomfort and requires additional recovery and building time. An example of breakdown training is to perform 10 repetitions to failure in a given exercise, let's say 100 pounds in the leg extension exercise. Immediately after completing the final repetition, the lifter reduces the weight load by about 15 percent (lifting 85 pounds) and performs as many additional repetitions as possible. The additional two to four repetitions make a big difference in the fatigue level and the strength-building stimulus.

Breakdown training is effective for stimulating muscle development, as long as it is not overdone. It is not usually advisable to break down the weight load more than once per exercise or to perform breakdown training more than once per week for a particular muscle group.

Assisted Training

Like breakdown training, assisted training, or forced reps, involves a small reduction in exercise resistance at the point of muscle fatigue. But unlike breakdown training, forced reps reduces the resistance only during the lifting (concentric) phase of the exercise. Let's assume Karen has performed 10 repetitions in the leg curl, and her hamstring muscles are unable to complete another lift. Her training partner assists her just enough to lift the weight load, but allows her to lower the weight load on her own because her eccentric force output is greater than her concentric force output. Assisted training allows her to perform additional repetitions that would not be possible otherwise.

Generally, two to four assisted repetitions are sufficient to stimulate the desired muscle response. Like breakdown training, this is a demanding form of exercise that should not be overdone. One assisted training session per week is probably enough for a given muscle group.

Super-Slow Training

Slow exercise movements minimize the role of momentum and produce increased muscle tension. Simply slowing the exercise speed is therefore a highly effective means for increasing the training stimulus. Super-slow training is usually conducted with a 10-second lifting movement and a 5-second lowering movement. At 15 seconds per repetition, four to six super-slow reps require 60 to 90 seconds of continuous muscle tension. This might be the most demanding and productive form of high-intensity training. It is also a very safe exercise technique as long as the exerciser breathes continuously.

Superset Training

Performing two or more sets of the same biceps exercise activates the same muscle fibers in the same recruitment pattern. Performing two or more sets of different biceps exercises activates different muscle fibers in different recruitment patterns, and is referred to as superset training. This becomes particularly effective when the exercises are performed in close succession.

For example, a set of barbell curls could be followed immediately by a set of incline dumbbell curls. Both exercises target the biceps muscles, but require different muscle fiber recruitment patterns. Involving different muscle fibers in a different activation order seems to enhance the training stimulus. Once again, it is not advisable to carry superset training to extremes. This could result in overtraining. One superset session per week per muscle group is a reasonable high-intensity training technique.

Negative Training

As indicated in the description of assisted training, emphasizing the negative (eccentric) movement is an excellent way to stimulate muscle development. Generally, a person can lower (negative movement) about 40 percent more weight than she or he can lift (positive movement), producing a highly effective muscle stimulus. Unfortunately, for the same reason, negative training also carries a high risk of tissue injury.

The safest method of negative exercise is assisted training in which the exerciser works to fatigue, then receives help on the lifting movement but not on the lowering movement. The most risky method of negative exercise requires a training partner to lift a heavier resistance than the exerciser can manage. The exerciser then lowers the resistance slowly to emphasize eccentric muscle contraction. If the exerciser loses control midway through the lowering movement, muscle tissues could be damaged.

Negative training can be useful for exercises using one's body weight, such as chin-ups and bar dips. For example, after five chin-ups, Tonya can no longer lift her body to the bar. However, she can use a prop to step up to the top position and then slowly lower her body. The lowering (negative) movement uses the same muscles as the lifting (positive) movement and provides an excellent training stimulus. Be aware that forceful negative exercise typically produces delayed onset muscle soreness a day or two after the exercise session. While uncomfortanble, this usually is not harmful, but it underscores the need to use negative training prudently. A little negative training goes a long way and should never be overdone or performed carelessly. One negative training session per muscle group per week should be sufficient.

STRENGTH TRAINING FOR COMPETITIVE PURPOSES

Many people pursue strength training for the purpose of becoming competitive bodybuilders or weightlifters. Although this might be an admirable goal, for most it is unrealistic because very few people possess the genetic potential to develop really large and strong muscles. One's basic body type, predominant muscle fiber (fast twitch, slow twitch), skeletal structure (small frame, large frame), biomechanical advantage (tendon insertion points), relative muscle length (short, medium, long), and hormone balance (testosterone level) all affect the capacity to become big and strong. For every bodybuilder featured in a magazine, there are thousands of dedicated strength trainers who achieve very modest results by comparison. Too often, some believe that training harder and longer will produce the physique they desire. Unfortunately, this typically leads to overuse injuries, frustration, and discontinuation of their exercise program.

Although there is nothing wrong with pursuing a bodybuilding or weightlifting program, one should be aware of the genetic factors and time commitment necessary to achieve competitive success in these sports. If someone understands these requirements and still wants to pursue a competitive goal, it is advisable to begin with a well-balanced training program that is substantially less demanding than those of competitive athletes. If the initial results are positive, then more exercises, more sets, and more resistance may be progressively added. If the initial results do not justify the time and effort, if there is undue fatigue and muscle soreness, or if there is high incidence of injury, then perhaps the exercise routine should be modified and scaled down.

Both bodybuilders and weightlifters exhibit large and strong muscles. However, bodybuilders train primarily for muscle size and typically look strong because of increased muscle definition. Conversely, weightlifters train primarily for muscle strength and usually are stronger than they look. Although they both train with weights for two or more hours per day, their exercise routines are different. Training specialization is most evident in the amount of rest bodybuilders and weightlifters take between exercise sets.

Bodybuilders use a variety of techniques to achieve their goals. A common technique is for bodybuilders to take very brief breaks (15 to 45 seconds) between sets to achieve "pumped-up" muscles. The muscle pump is actually a temporary increase in muscle size as a result of blood accumulation. By quickly repeating the exercise sets, fluid is trapped in the muscle tissue, thereby producing the pumped-up look. Because short rests allow only partial muscle recovery, bodybuilders must train with relatively low percentages of their maximum resistance. For example, a bodybuilder who is able to bench press 400 pounds might perform six sets of 10 reps with 250 pounds during a given workout. The short recovery periods force him to train with about 65 percent of his maximum resistance.

Weightlifters, on the other hand, take relatively long rest periods (three to six minutes) between sets to permit the use of heavy weight loads. The longer rest interval enhances muscle recovery between sets and allows weightlifters to train with relatively high percentages of their maximum resistance. For example, a powerlifter who is able to bench press 400 pounds might perform a pyramid workout such as the following:

150 pounds × 8 reps
200 pounds × 7 reps
250 pounds × 6 reps
300 pounds × 5 reps
350 pounds × 3 reps
350 pounds × 3 reps
350 pounds × 3 reps

The long recovery periods permit the powerlifter to train with about 90 percent of his or her maximum resistance.

Although bodybuilders and weightlifters train for more than two hours per workout, bodybuilders complete a much greater volume of work during each exercise session. Table 5.12 provides typical training protocols for bodybuilders and weightlifters.

Few activities are as physically demanding as bodybuilding and weightlifting. However, successful bodybuilders and weightlifters appear to have two genetically related training advantages: They tolerate stressful workouts with relatively few injuries, and they respond to training stimuli with greater muscle size and strength than the average person. People interested in bodybuilding or weightlifting should work with trained instructors to develop a sound and systematic approach to attaining their competitive goals.

Table 5.12 **Typical Training Protocols for Bodybuilders and Weightlifters**

	Bodybuilders (muscle size)	Weightlifters (muscle strength)
Exercises	3-5 per muscle group	1 or 2 per muscle group
Sets	4-6 per exercise	6-8 per exercise
Repetitions	6-15 per set	2-8 per set
Resistance	60-75% max	80-95% max
Rest between sets	15-45 sec	3-6 min

EDUCATION

Member education is an ongoing process that begins with an orientation program presented by trained, knowledgeable instructors. It requires a planned member communication strategy.

Orientation

This section provides guidelines for providing strength training participants with a thorough orientation if they are not working with a personal training instructor. Each YMCA should recommend that all members participate in a strength training orientation before beginning an exercise program, regardless of their previous experience with strength training. Here are ideas for designing orientations appropriate for beginning, intermediate, and advanced participants.

Beginners

The first step is to screen for various health risks. People who have arthritis, heart disease, low back pain, knee pain or injury, or high blood pressure; who are pregnant; or who have recently undergone surgery should not participate without a physician's permission. If they do participate, they might need to follow their physician's recommendations for safe participation.

Recommend performing one set every other day; the number of sets depends on the type of equipment used. Suggest 8 to 12 reps for the set, although more might be necessary (with lower resistance) as they first learn how to perform the exercise. If the training intensity and pace are right, the last two reps of each set should be difficult as the participant nears muscle failure.

Select specific exercises and equipment according to what is available, the participant's previous experience with weights, and his or her body weight. Design a workout that has one exercise for each major muscle group. Start participants with a submaximal weight that they can lift for 8 to 12 reps. Beginners should not do more than 12 exercises during a session.

Give beginning participants a tour of the strength training facility, showing them the various equipment and stations. Teach beginners how to perform exercises using the correct technique and form. It is often helpful if beginning participants have a support partner, someone who counsels them and ensures that they perform the exercises correctly. In many cases this function can be performed by facility staff.

Check each person's progress once every four to six weeks. Examine each of the following check points:

- Heart rate
- Height and weight measurements
- Body composition
- Blood pressure
- Appearance
- Strength increase, measured by retesting

After checking, acknowledge progress that has been made and suggest appropriate modification to the program. This type of support can help participants feel good about themselves and about the YMCA.

Intermediates

Briefly discuss items in the beginners' program that need review. At the intermediate level, participants can still benefit from a training partner—someone who assists them, watches to see that they perform correctly, and perhaps also trains with them. This could be another knowledgeable strength training participant or an instructor. Review the following techniques for intermediate-level participants to try:

- *Strict reps* are repetitions performed in a way that isolates the muscle so that no assistance is supplied by any other body part or muscle group.
- *Forced reps* (assisted training) are repetitions in which a training partner manually helps the participant move through a desired range of motion when the participant can't do it alone.
- *Negative training,* which emphasizes the eccentric contraction, is the lowering of resistance against gravity through a desired range of motion.
- *Breakdown training* is doing a set at a given weight to muscle failure, then having the weight immediately reduced by 15 to 20 percent by a training partner, and performing another two or three reps.
- *Isolation* is much like strict reps; it emphasizes a specific body part or muscle group and doesn't allow assistance from another part of the body. It is usually done with dumbbells or cable exercises.
- *Pyramiding* is increasing weight and decreasing repetitions in successive sets.

Following are two systems for designing intermediate-level workouts:

- *Supersets* are sets in which an exercise is done for a particular muscle group and then followed by a different exercise for the same muscle group. For example, with barbells, concentration curls would follow arm curls.
- *Split routines* are workout schedules that emphasize particular muscle groups on certain days. For example, the chest and shoulders would be exercised on Mondays and Wednesdays and the legs and back on Tuesdays and Thursdays.

Advanced

Briefly discuss items in the orientation programs for beginners and intermediate participants that need review. Following are techniques you might want to teach advanced participants:

- *Priority training* emphasizes conditioning programs for a specific or immediate need, such as for a particular sport. For example, off-season and in-season sports training will differ.
- *Advanced isolation* is doing two exercises instead of one for a particular body part.
- *Continuous tension* means that the resistance remains the same throughout the complete range of motion during an exercise.
- *Preexhaustion* is exercising a muscle with a single isolated muscle movement before a compound movement that uses the same muscle group.
- A *varied tempo* means adjusting the speed at which the participant progresses from exercise to exercise.
- *Cycling* (periodization) is gradually increasing resistance in a series of exercises over an extended time. Note that it is sometimes necessary to decrease repetitions as the resistance increases.

The following are three training methods for advanced-level participants:

- *Diminishing sets* is a method of performing three sets of a specific exercise for a particular muscle or muscle group. The sets are done as follows: A set of 10 reps is completed. Then 20 to 25 percent of the weight is removed and a second set of 4 to 6 reps is performed. Again, 20 to 25 percent of the weight is removed, and a third set of 4 to 6 reps is done.
- *Compound sets* are groups of two or three exercises for the same body part in which each is performed for 8 to 12 reps. Up to two minutes of recovery time is allowed between exercises. For example, for the chest, the exercises can be the bench press, dumbbell flys, and dips.
- *Trisets* are compound sets in which there is no rest between exercises. This is a more intense effort.

Ongoing Education

Few health and fitness areas are in greater need of our educational efforts than strength training.

There is a general lack of understanding regarding strength training benefits and a widespread misunderstanding of strength training principles. This is partly due to the large number of self-proclaimed experts with no credentials and bodybuilding magazines that promote an almost unlimited number of training routines.

Strength training education should therefore be one of our professional priorities. One thing we can do to better educate our members is provide well-written strength training materials using information from this textbook and appropriate article reprints. A frequently updated strength training bulletin board is also helpful. Another effective means for sharing information is through strength training seminars and workshops. These should be conducted regularly for both instructors and members. Better understanding leads to better training, which leads to better results. When members learn and practice the strength training principles, they become models for other participants, and the cause of sensible strength training is advanced.

UPPER LEG

Barbell Squat

Muscle Group

Quadriceps, hamstrings, gluteus maximus

Begin with barbell supported across upper back. Hands should have a firm overhand grip. Feet should be shoulder-width apart and toes pointed slightly outward as if sitting into a chair. Lower hips until thighs are parallel to the floor (or as far as comfortable without going beyond parallel). Keep the head up and torso erect. Raise hips to standing position and repeat.

Note: Do not let knees extend beyond the toes. The barbell squat should be performed with a spotter who wraps his or her arms around the lifter's torso and helps the lifter stand up, if necessary.

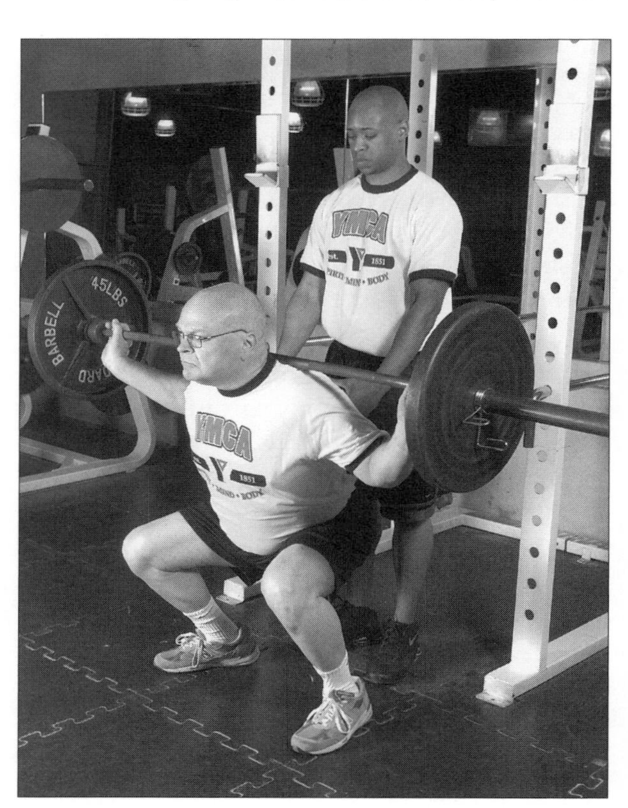

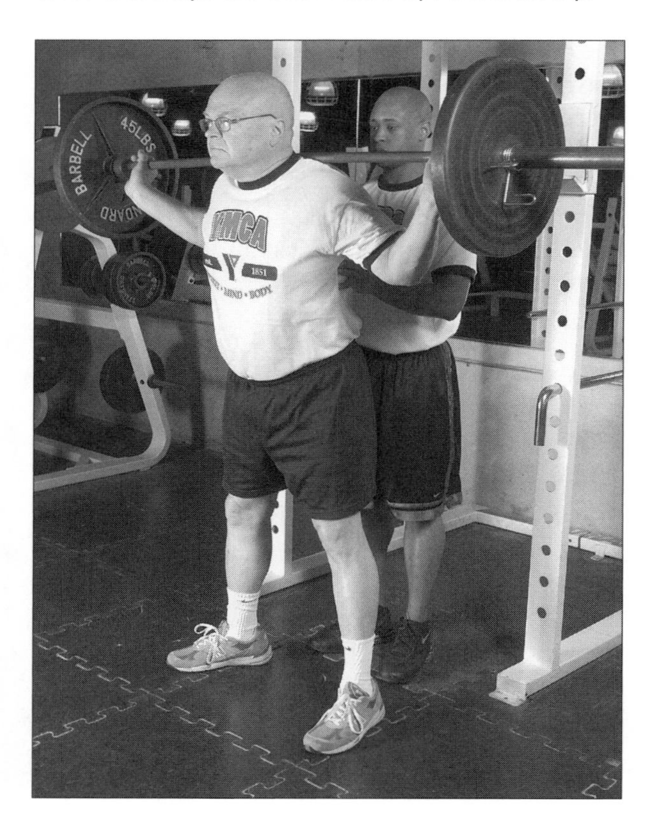

Dumbbell Lunge

Muscle Group

Quadriceps, hamstrings, gluteus maximus

Begin by holding dumbbells at the sides, feet hip-width apart. Take a large step forward with one leg, landing heel first. Bend the forward leg until the knee is directly over the foot and the rear knee is close to the floor. Pause. Push up to the starting position, keeping the head up and torso erect. Repeat. Continue exercise with other leg.

Note: Move in a controlled manner to reduce landing forces and joint stress.

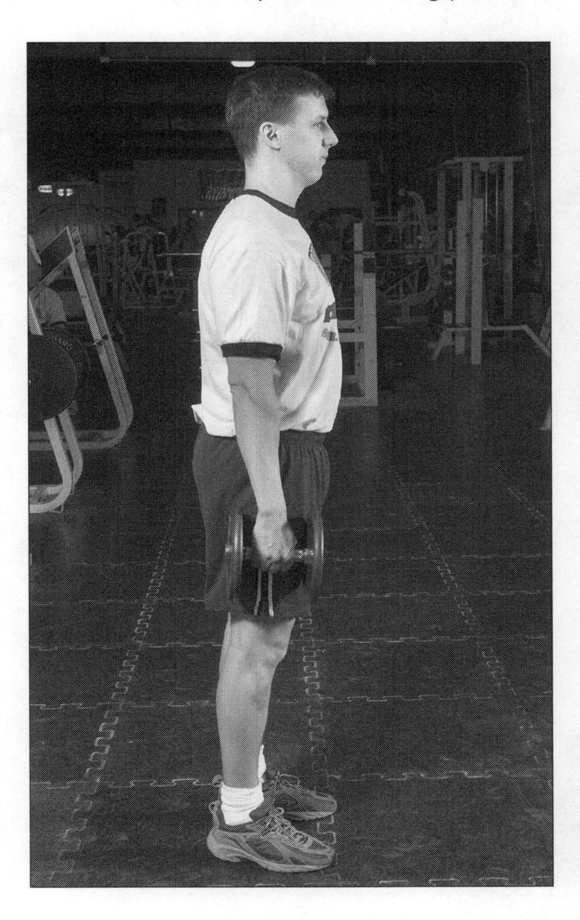

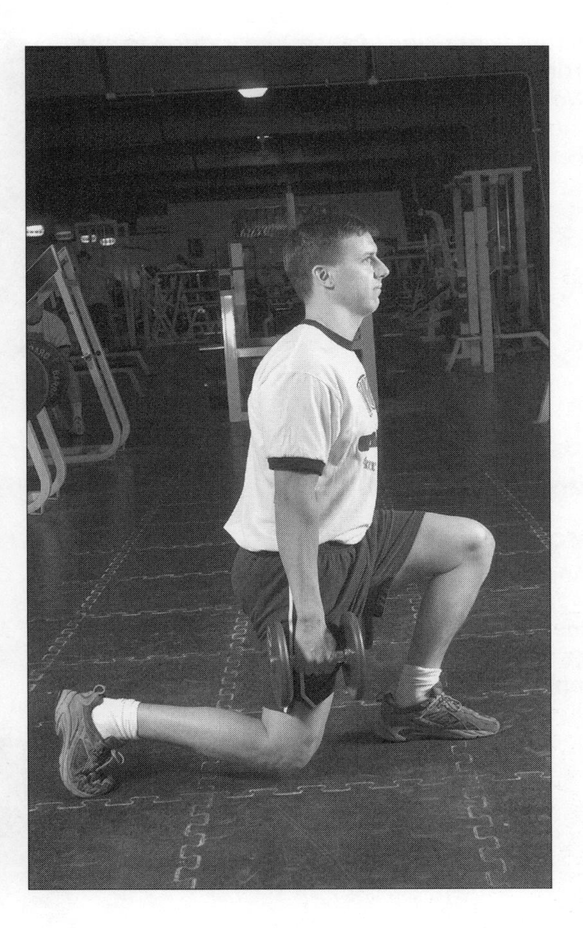

Leg Extension Machine

Muscle Group

Quadriceps

Sit on machine with low back touching back support pad. The bend of the knee should fall at the end of the seat, and the knee joint should line up with the machine's axis of rotation. The rollers or pads should touch just above the ankle. Extend the lower leg to a fully extended horizontal position. Pause and return to the starting position. Repeat.

Note: Keep constant tension on the muscle. Do not allow the weight stacks to touch during the exercise.

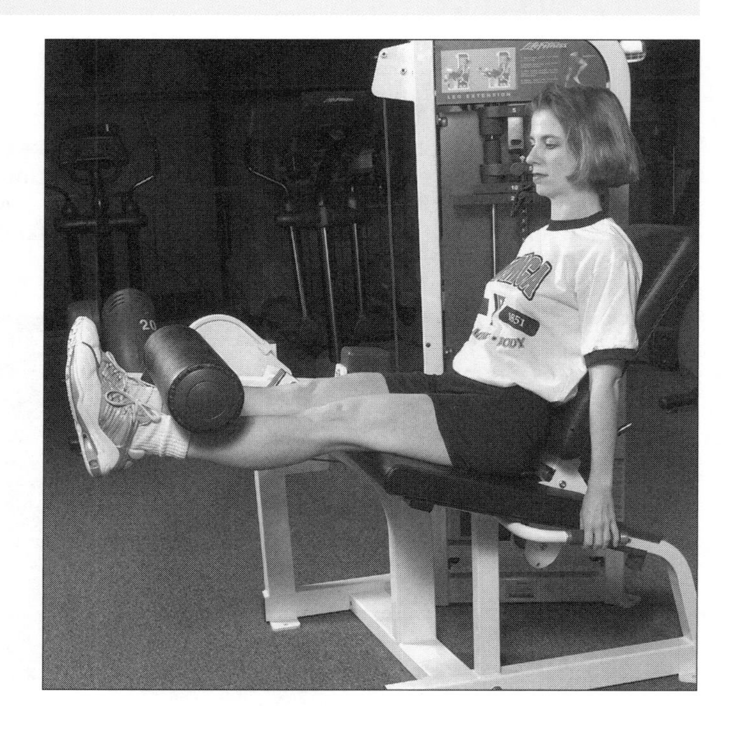

Leg Press Machine

Muscle Group

Quadriceps, hamstrings, gluteus maximus

Adjust seat to allow a 90-degree angle of the knee. Place full foot on foot pedal. Press both feet forward, stopping just short of knee lock or straight leg. Bend knee again and return to starting position. Repeat. Do not allow gluteals to rise off seat.

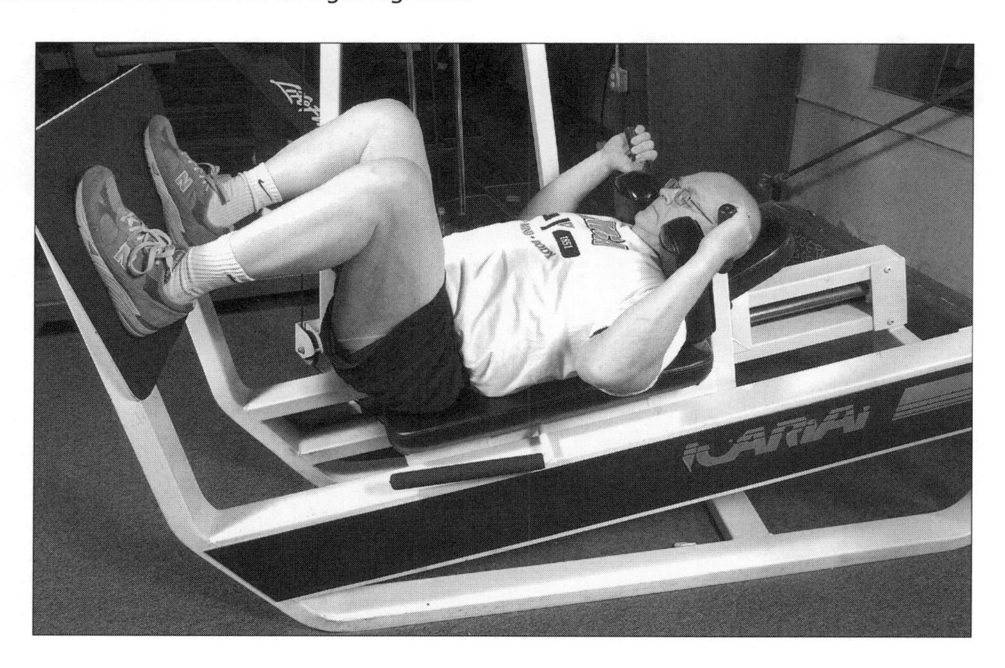

Leg Curl Machine

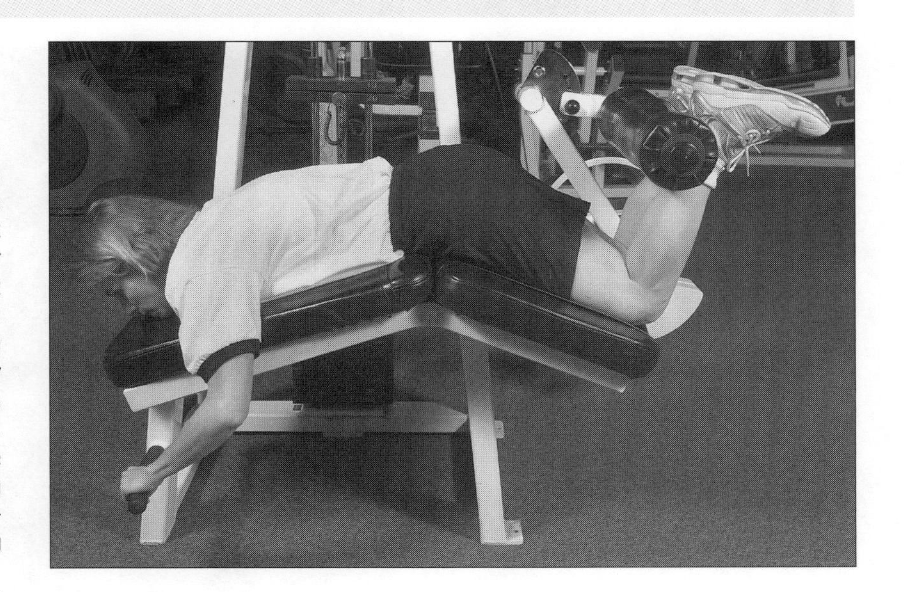

Muscle Group

Hamstrings

Lying facedown, place heels under pads or rollers. Align knees with the point of rotation of the machine's resistance arm (the point where the arm holding the pads for the ankle and the machine connect and rotate). Move the heels toward the buttocks, keeping the upper leg stationary (hips may rise slightly off the pads). Grasp the handles below the bench for stability only. Avoid excessively squeezing the handles. Stop leg flexion with heels one to two inches from buttocks. Pause and return to starting position. Repeat.

Note: Feet should remain at right angles to lower leg.

Low Cable–Crossover Adduction

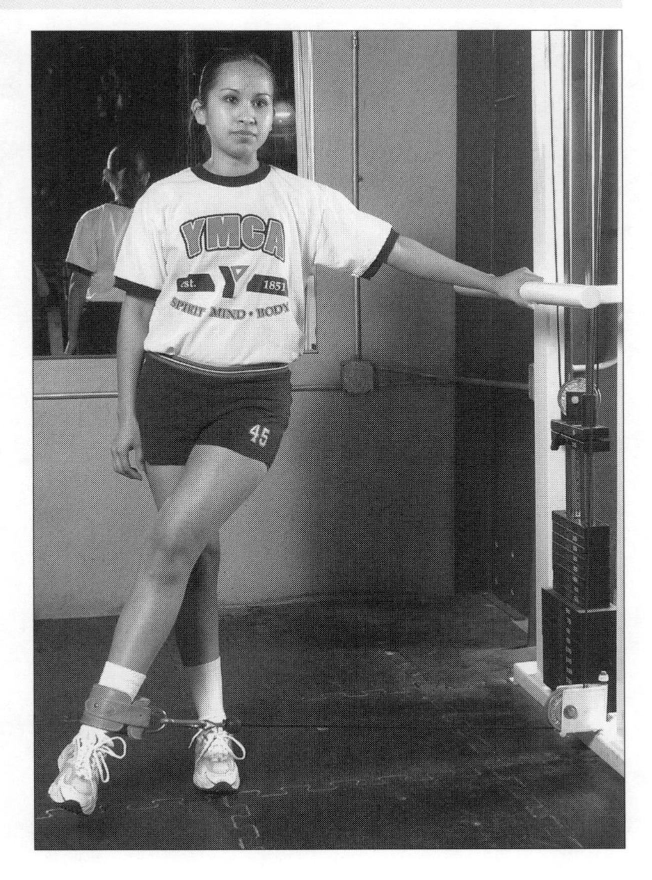

Muscle Group

Hip adductors

Sit or stand sideways with ankles in line with pulley, legs straight, and feet 12 to 18 inches apart. Place strap over ankle nearest pulley and move strapped ankle toward other ankle. Pause and return to starting position. Repeat.

Note: Keep torso in neutral position. Avoid shifting or twisting movements.

Low Cable–Crossover Abduction

Muscle Group

Hip abductors

Sit or stand sideways with ankles in line with pulley, legs straight, and feet together. Place strap over ankle farthest from pulley and move strapped ankle away from pulley to the fully contracted position. Pause and return to starting position. Repeat.

Note: Keep torso in neutral position. Avoid shifting or twisting movements.

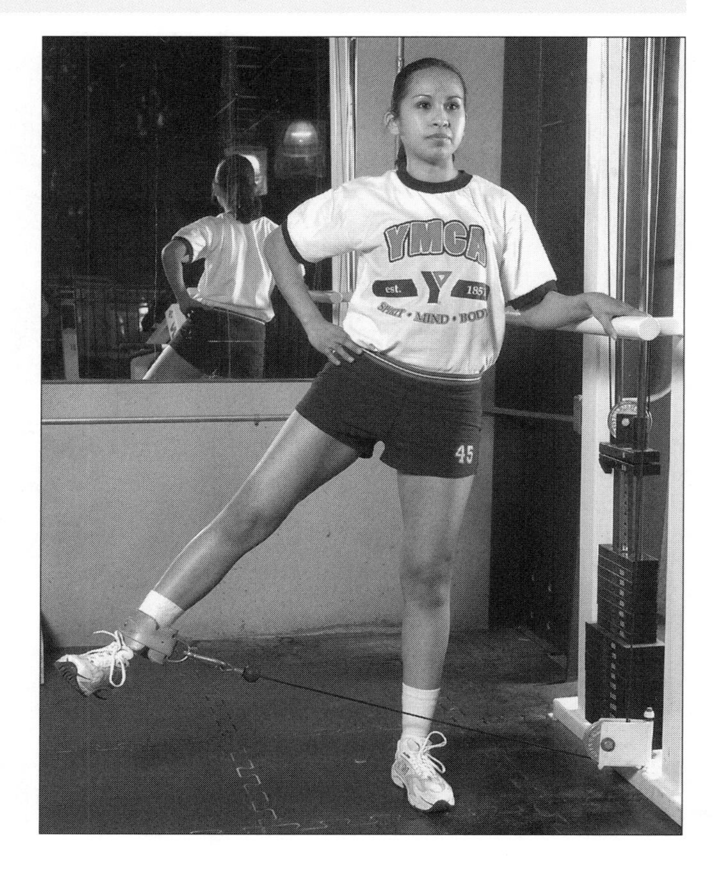

BUTTOCKS

Low-Cable Hip Extension

Muscle Group

Gluteus maximus, hamstrings

Place strap over right ankle and stand facing weight stack. Using arms for support, move right leg backward (straight, not locked) to fully contracted position. Keep back in neutral position. Pause and return to starting position. Repeat. Continue exercise with left leg.

Note: Avoid shifting or twisting motion. Keep back in neutral position.

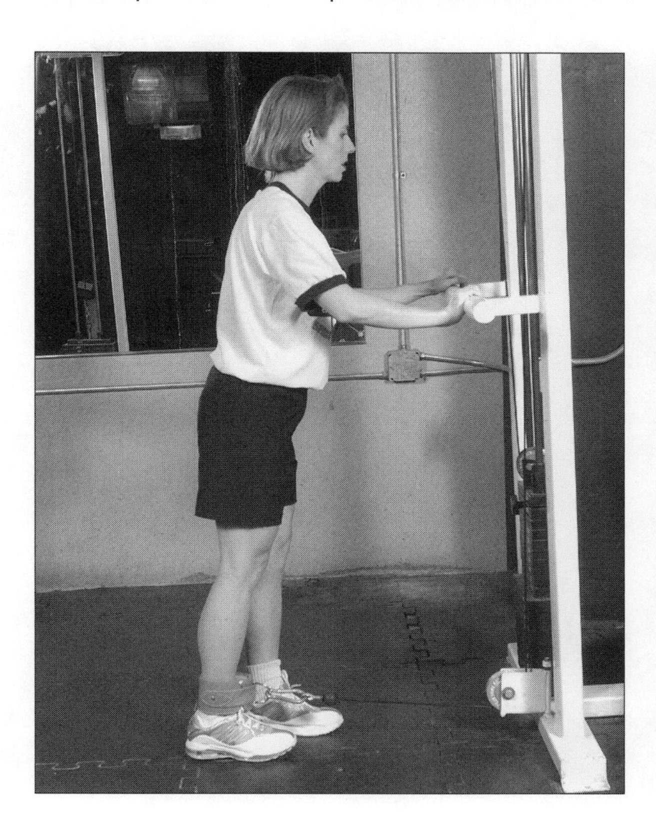

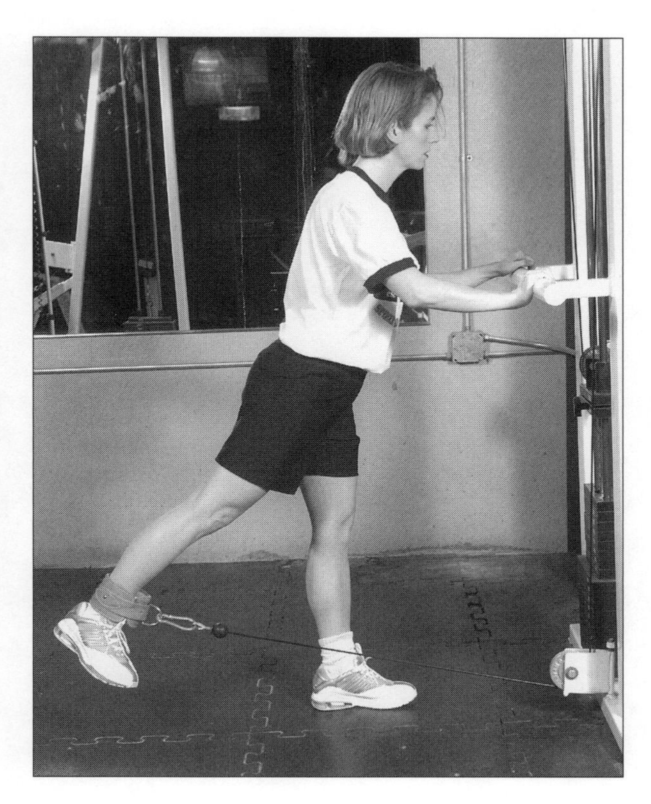

LOWER LEG

Standing Calf Apparatus

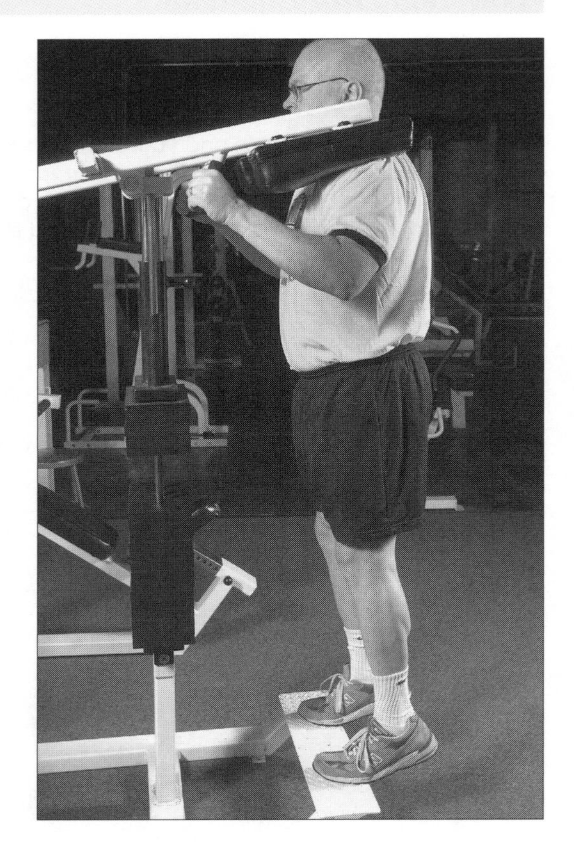

Muscle Group

Gastrocnemius, soleus

Stand with toes on platform and adjust loading pad for full movement range. Keeping toes on platform, lower heels until calf muscles are fully stretched. Raise onto toes until calf muscles are fully contracted. Pause. Slowly return to starting position and repeat.

CHEST

Barbell Bench Press

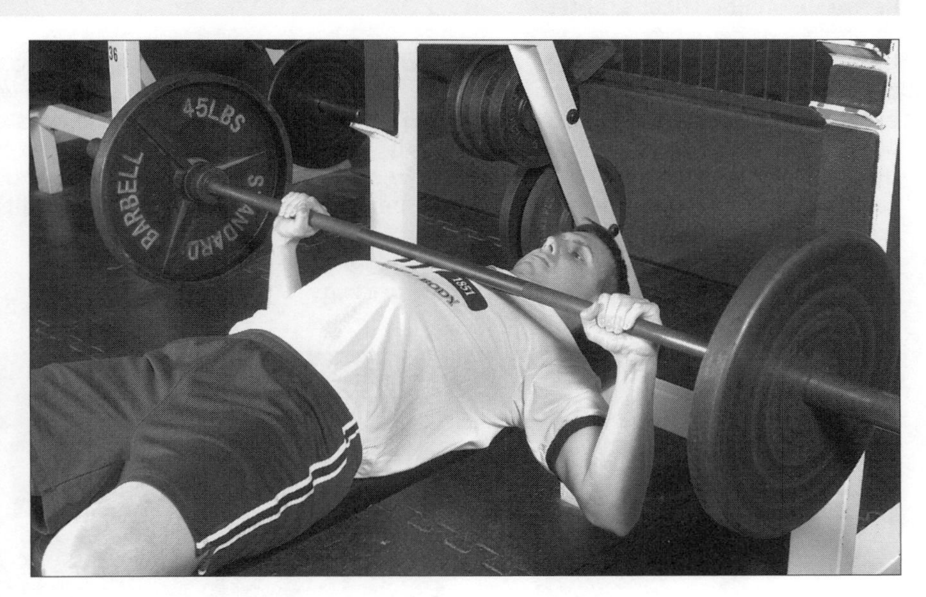

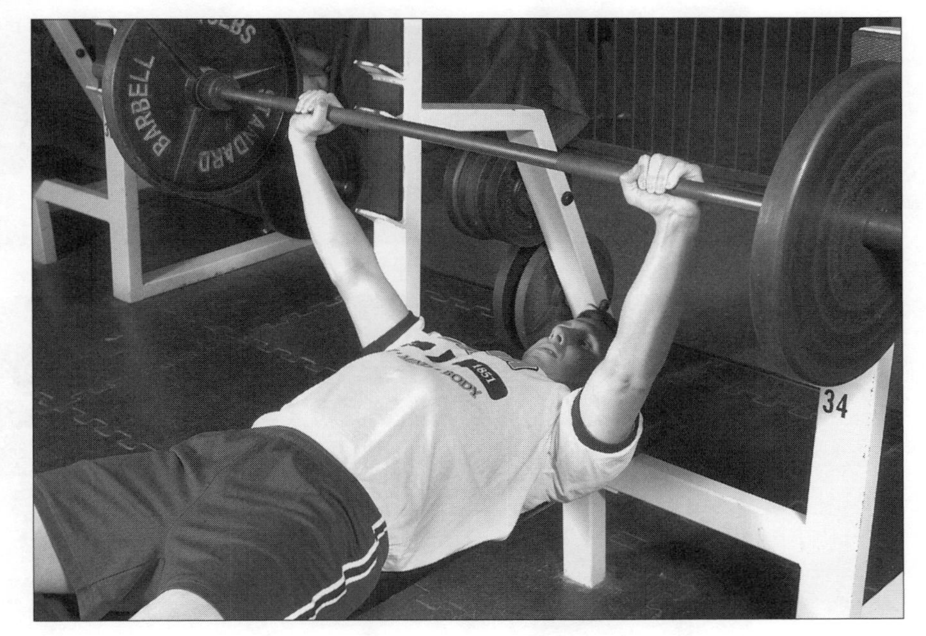

Muscle Group

Pectoralis major, anterior deltoid, triceps

Lie faceup with head, shoulders, and hips on bench and feet flat on floor or support stand. Remove barbell from standards and hold above shoulders. Lower barbell slowly to thickest part of chest and pause. Press barbell to full elbow extension (do not lock) and repeat. After final repetition, replace barbell on standards.

Note: Grasp bar with secure (thumb-around) grip, a little wider than shoulder-width so that forearms are perpendicular to the floor when the bar is at the chest. Distance between hands will be different for each person. This exercise should always be performed with a spotter who helps lift the barbell from and return it to the standards and assists whenever the lifter experiences difficulty.

Incline Barbell Press

Muscle Group

Pectoralis major, triceps, anterior deltoid

Lean back with head, shoulders, and hips on bench and feet flat on floor or support stand. Remove barbell from standards and hold above chin. Lower barbell slowly to top part of chest (slightly lower than collarbone). Press barbell to full elbow extension (do not lock) and repeat. After final repetition, replace barbell on standards.

Note: Grasp bar with secure (thumb-around) grip, a little wider than shoulder-width so that forearms are perpendicular to the floor when the bar is at the chest. This position will be different for each person. When possible, this exercise should be performed with a spotter who helps lift the barbell from and return it to the standards and assists whenever the lifter experiences difficulty.

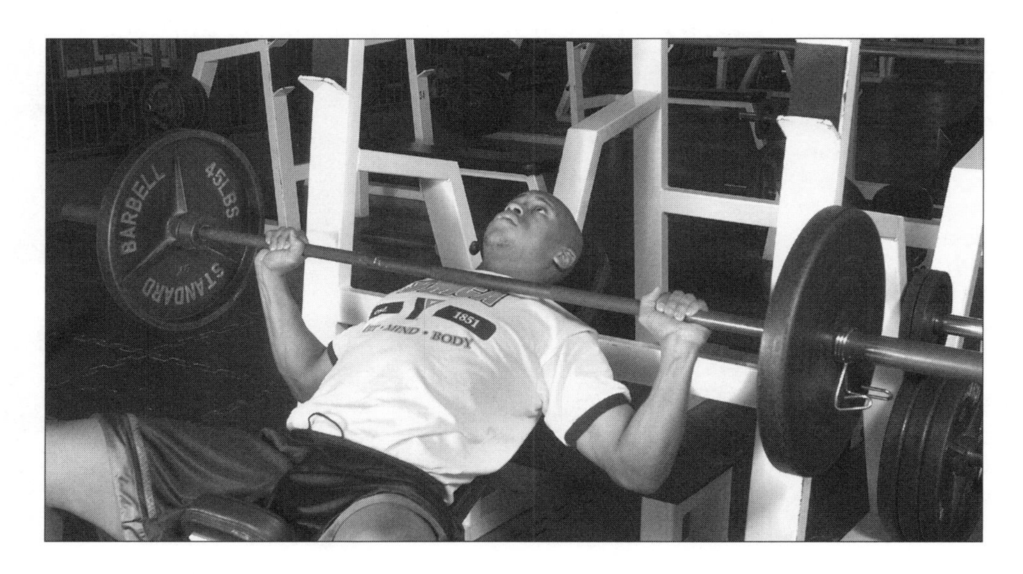

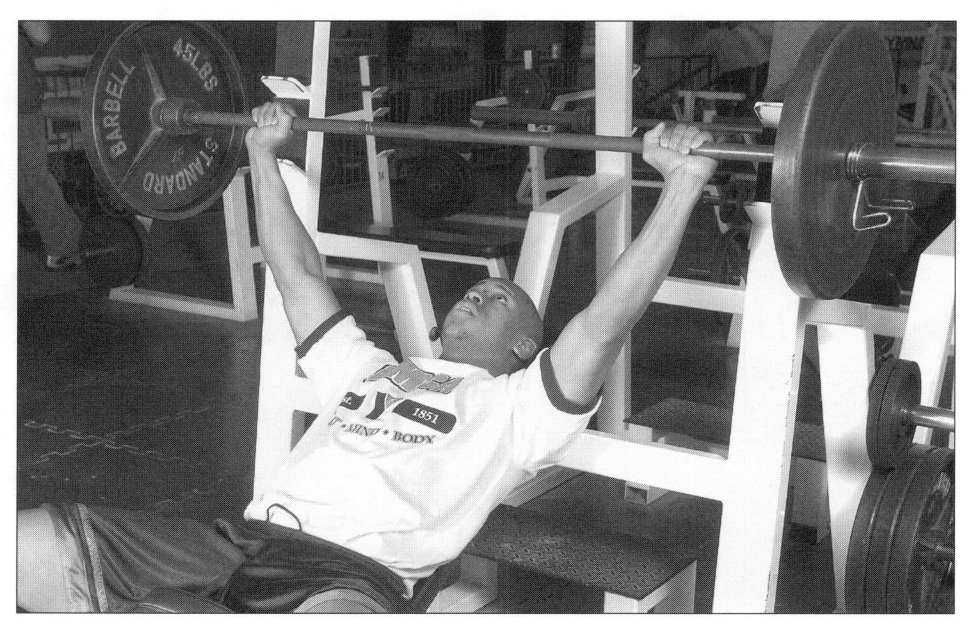

Dumbbell Fly

Muscle Group

Pectoralis major, anterior deltoid

Lie faceup on a flat bench. Start with arms extended and dumbbells directly above the shoulders with elbows slightly bent. With slow and controlled movement, lower arms to the side until they are parallel to the floor. Slowly raise the dumbbells to the starting position. Pause. Repeat.

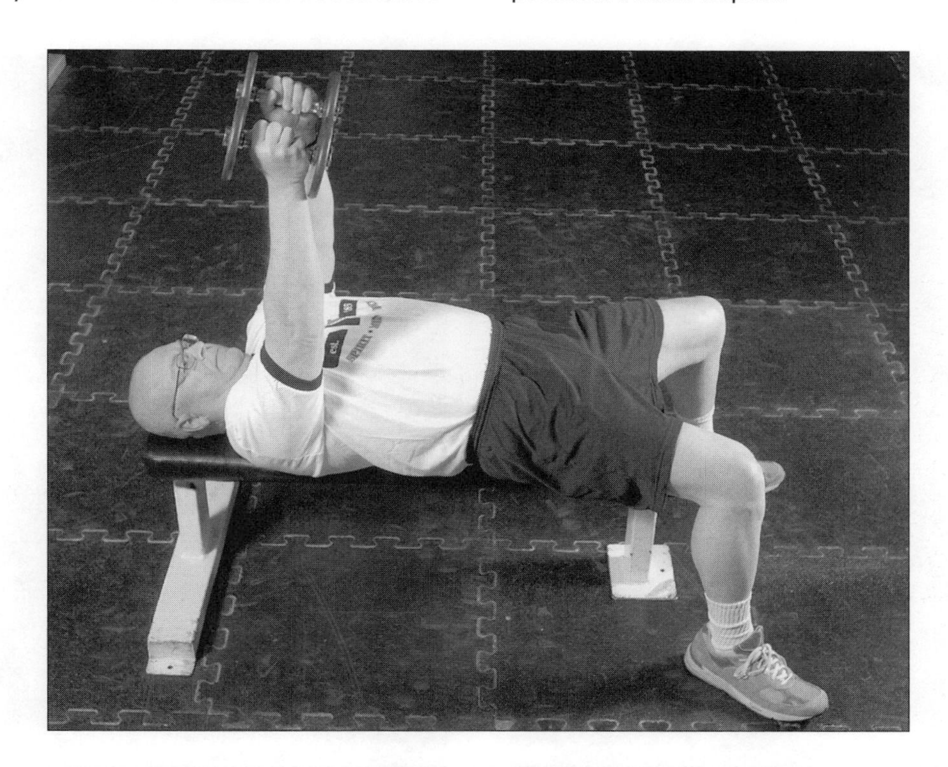

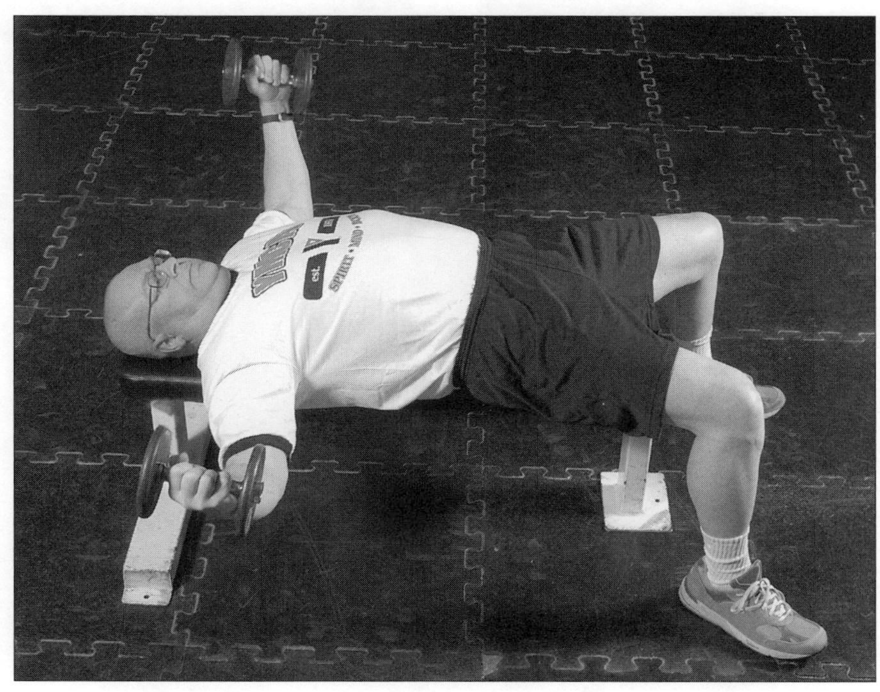

Chest Press Machine

Muscle Group

Pectoralis major, anterior deltoid, triceps

Adjust the machine to fit each person. Use belts if provided by machine manufacturer. Align the middle of the chest with the movement arm or handles. Grasp handles lightly while pushing the movement arm away to full extension (do not lock elbow). Pause. Slowly lower the movement arm. Repeat.

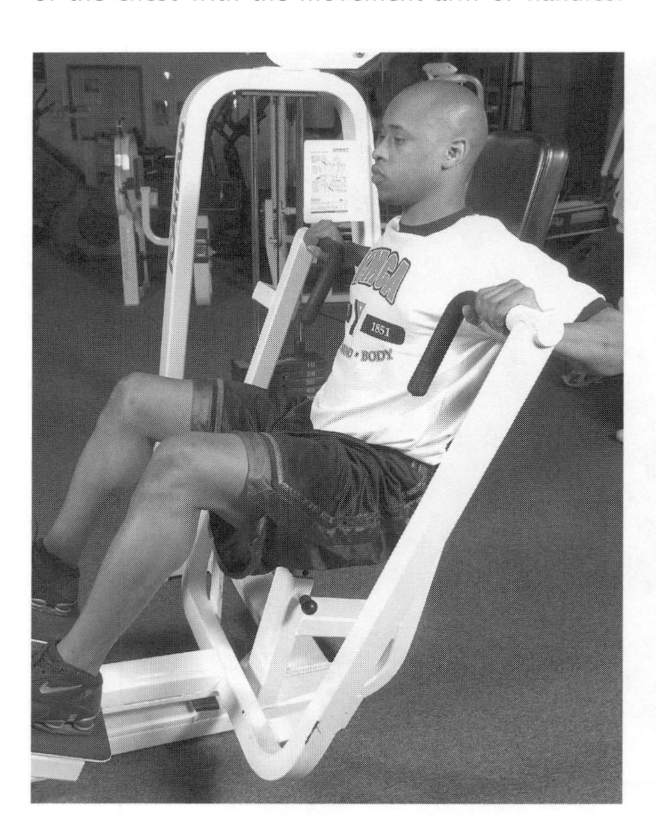

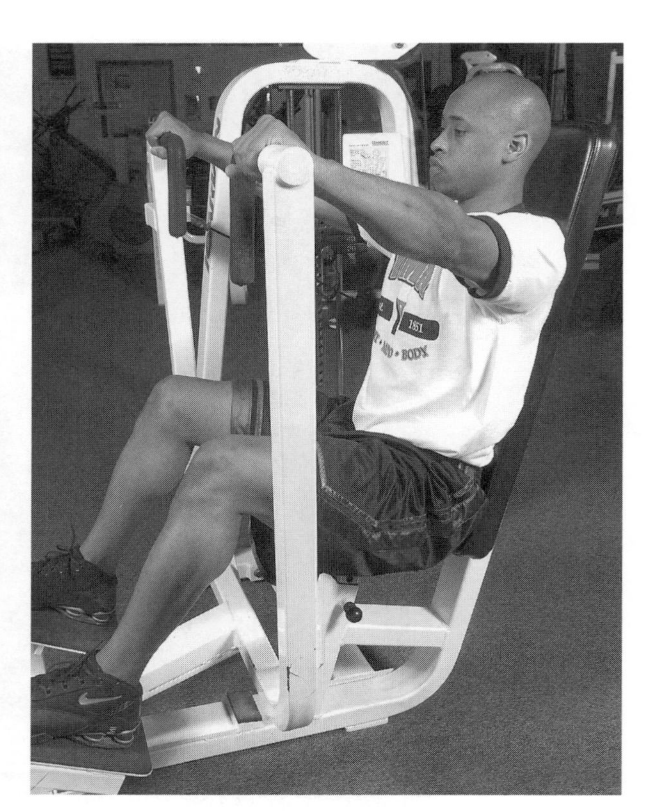

Pec Deck Machine

Muscle Group

Pectoralis major, anterior deltoid

Adjust the seat so that the arms are parallel to the ground when the hands grasp the handles and the forearm is at a 90 degree angle at the elbow. Push the handles forward and together in front of the chest. Pause and return to a stretched position. Repeat.

Note: Keep back pressed firmly against back pad and head in a neutral position during entire movement.

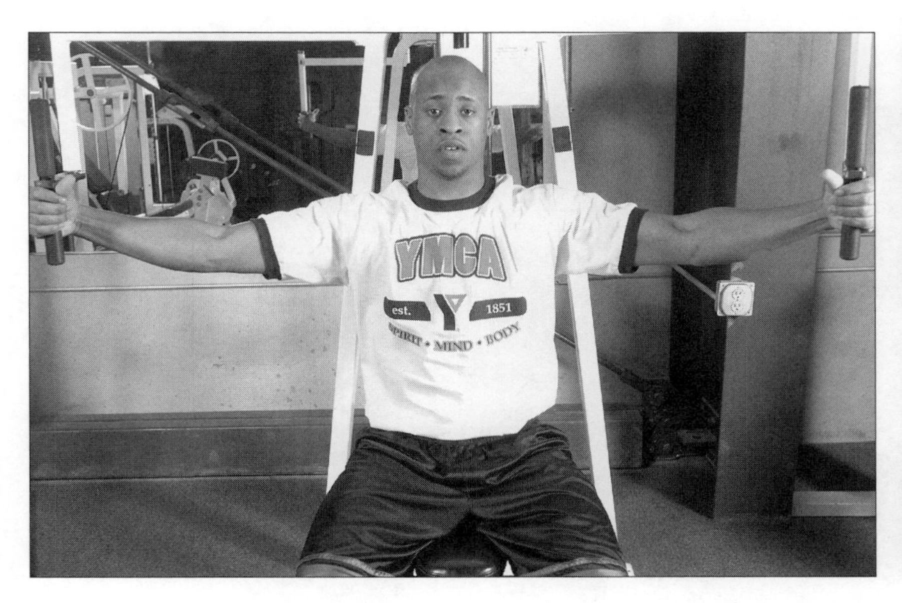

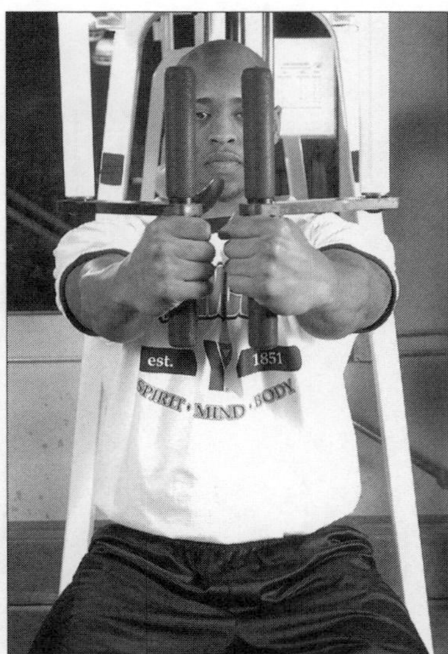

Incline Press Machine

Muscle Group

Pectoralis major, anterior deltoid, triceps

Sit on machine with seat adjusted so that handles are at chest level. Grip handles and press them forward and up until arms are nearly extended. Pause and return slowly until hands are at chest. Repeat.

Caution: To avoid excessive stress on the shoulder joint, do not allow hands to move too far backward.

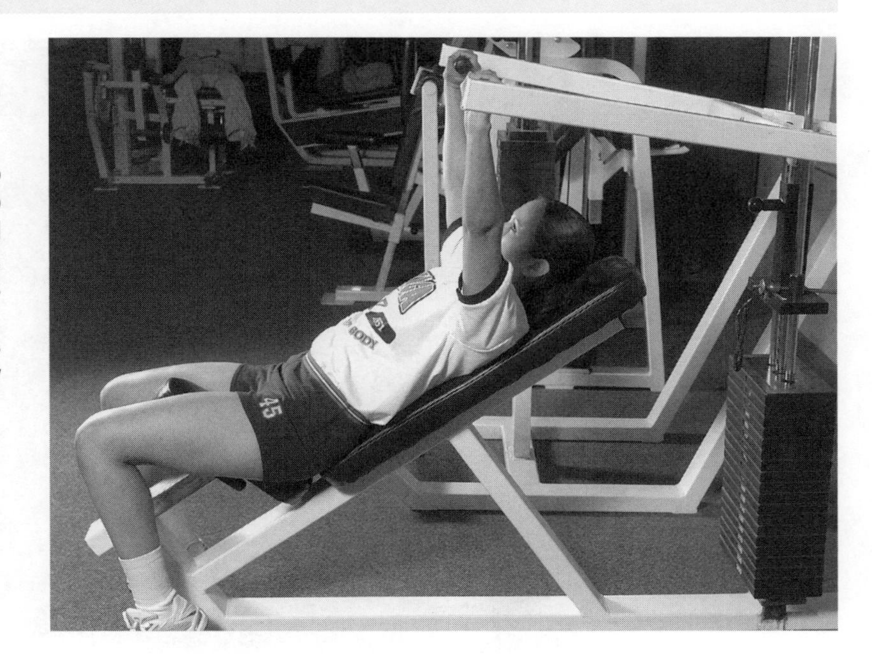

MIDDLE BACK

Dumbbell Bent Row

Muscle Group

Latissimus dorsi, teres major, middle trapezius, posterior deltoid, rhomboids, biceps

Support the body with one hand or one hand and knee on a bench. Hold the dumbbell with the other hand. Bend the elbow, lifting the weight close to the side to approximately shoulder height. Pause. Slowly return to starting position. Repeat. Repeat exercise on opposite side.

Note: Keep pelvis square to the floor throughout movement. The farther the elbow is from the side of the body, the more the posterior deltoid is involved.

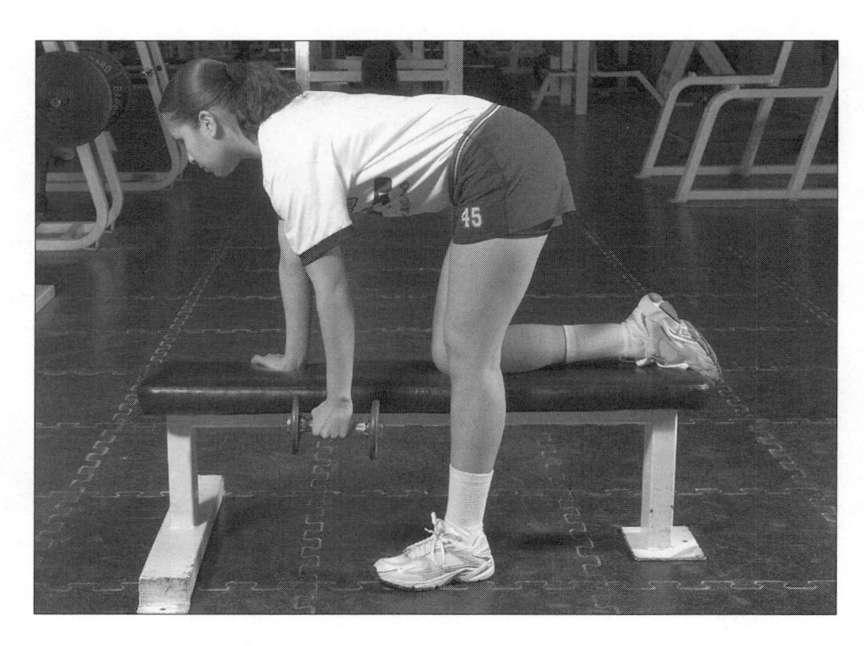

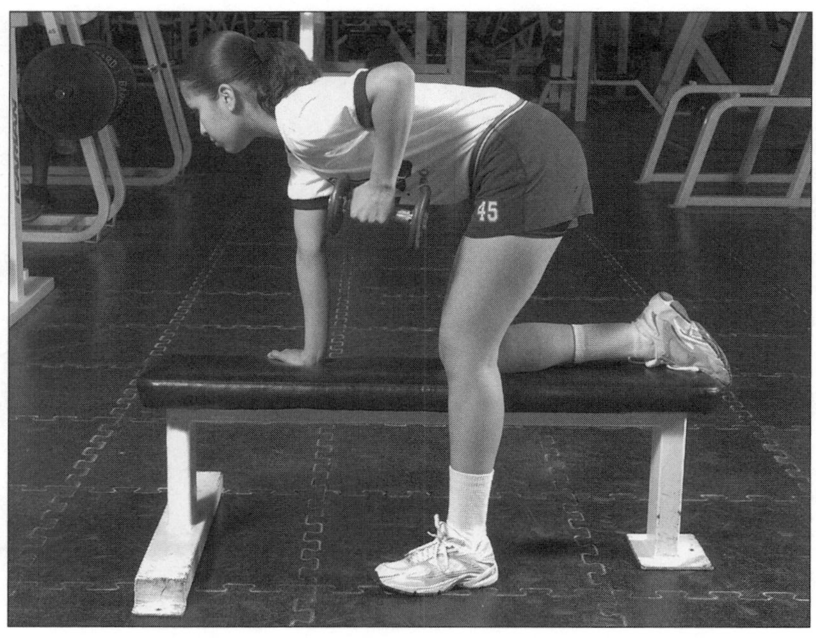

Lat Pull-Down

Muscle Group

Latissimus dorsi, biceps

Hand positions vary: palms in, out, or facing each other. For the palms-in position, use a shoulder-width grip. For the palms-out position, use a slightly wider than shoulder-width grip. If the palms face each other, use a grip approximately shoulder-width apart. Grip the bar above the head. Slowly and with control, pull the bar in front of the head to the chest (palms in, palms out, or palms facing each other). Pause. Return the bar to the extended position, allowing a slight bend in the elbow. Repeat.

Note: On machines equipped with an adjustable knee pad, adjust to body size.

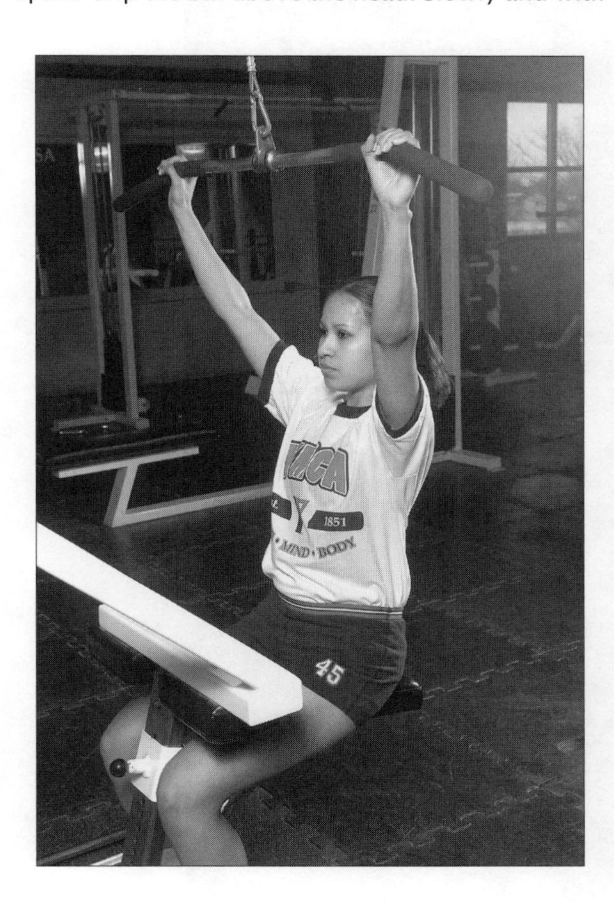

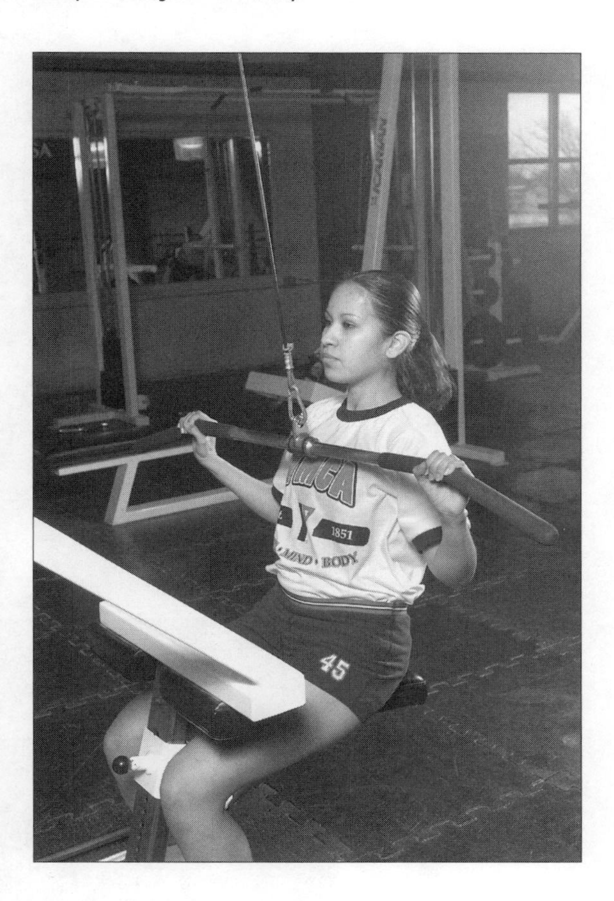

Seated Rowing Machine

Muscle Group

Rhomboids, posterior deltoid, latissimus dorsi, teres major, middle trapezius

Adjust seat so that the shoulders and machine handles are at the same height and the handles are just within reach. Grasp handles and bend the elbows to pull toward you as far as possible while keeping the chest against the supporting pad. Pause, slowly return to starting position. Repeat.

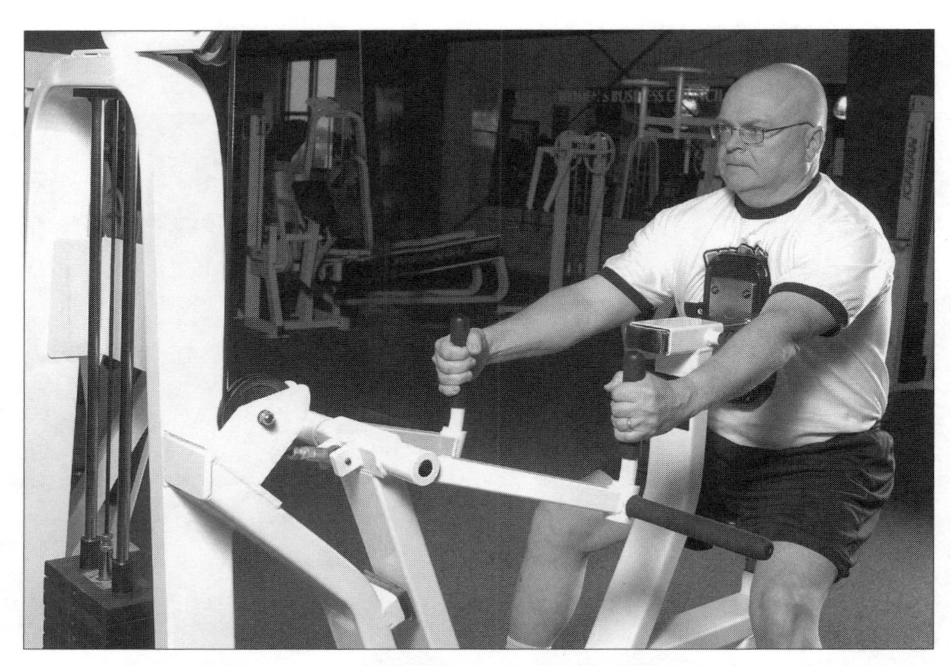

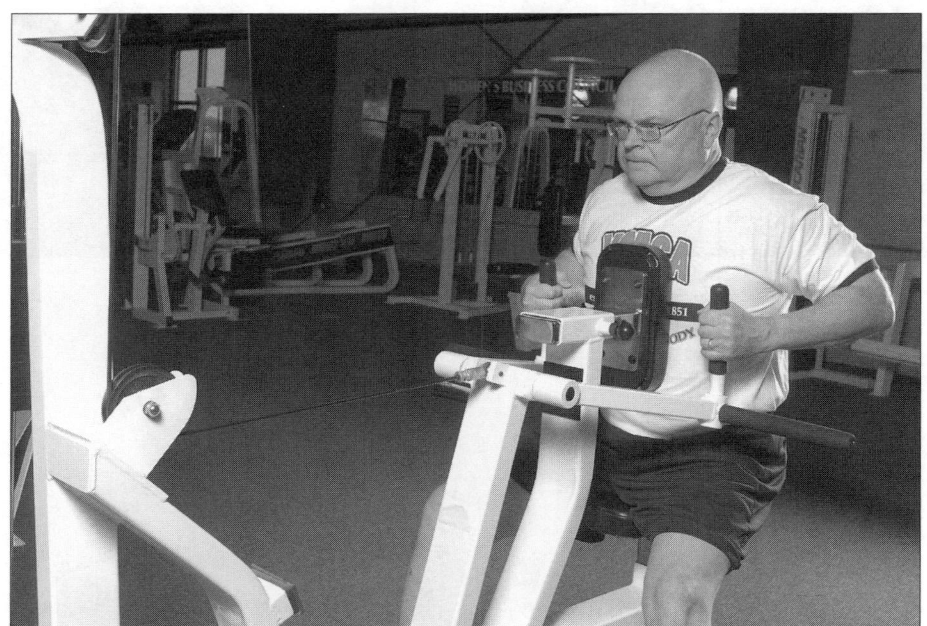

SHOULDERS

Dumbbell Lateral Raise

Muscle Group

Middle deltoid

Sit or stand with a dumbbell at each side, palms facing the body. Raise the dumbbells directly to the side to shoulder height, keeping the arms slightly bent throughout. Hold at the top position for a second. Lower and repeat.

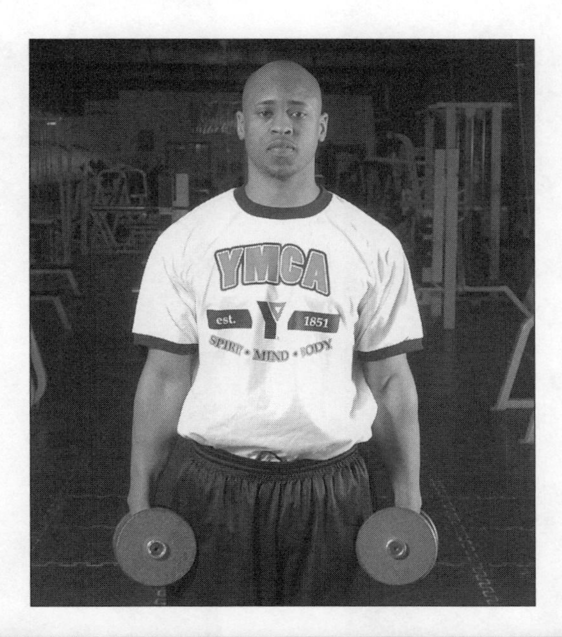

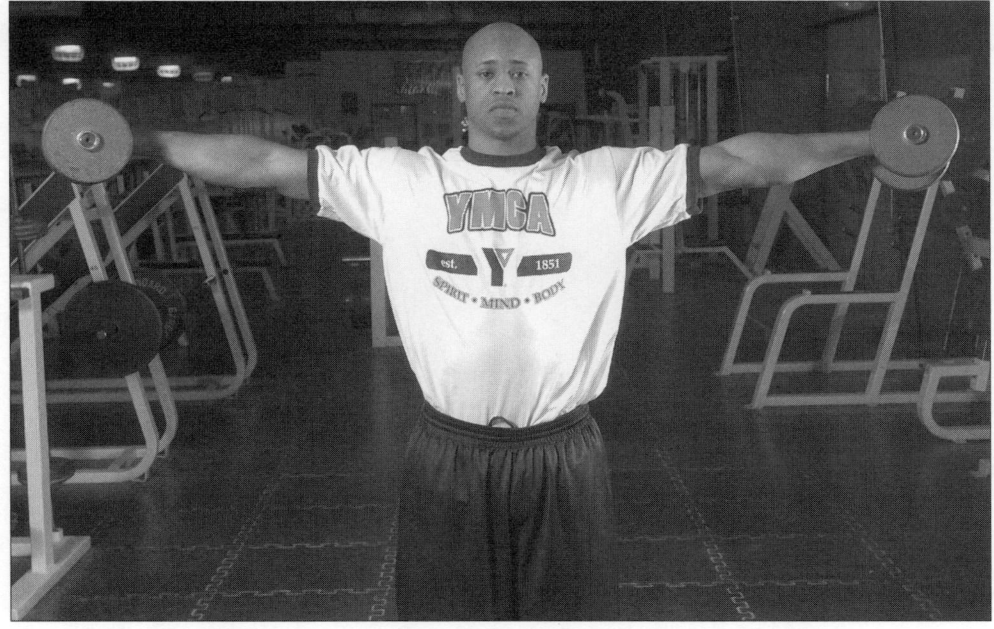

Dumbbell Shoulder Press

Muscle Group

Anterior deltoid, middle deltoid, triceps, upper trapezius

Sit with dumbbells at shoulder level with palms facing forward (overhand grip). The dumbbells should start at the corners of the shoulders and travel overhead to a point where the dumbbells almost touch when pressed overhead. Return to starting position and repeat.

Note: Keep the back straight and shoulders back.

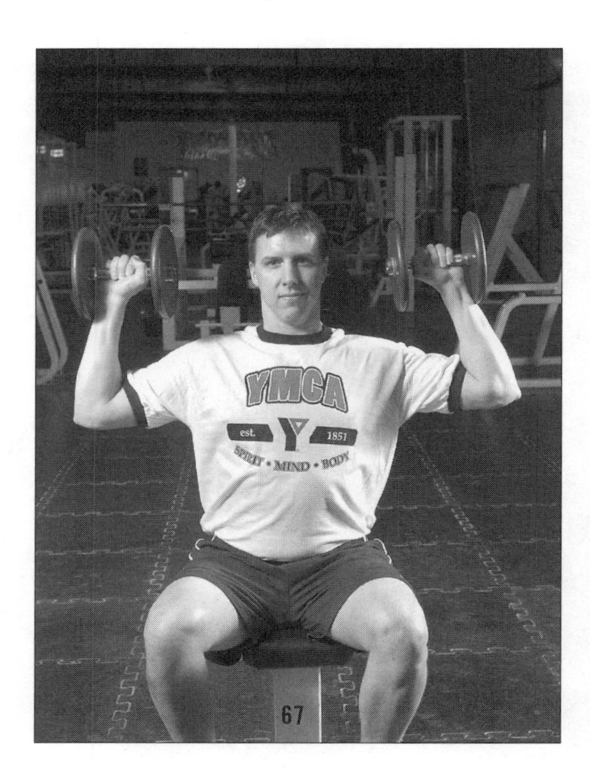

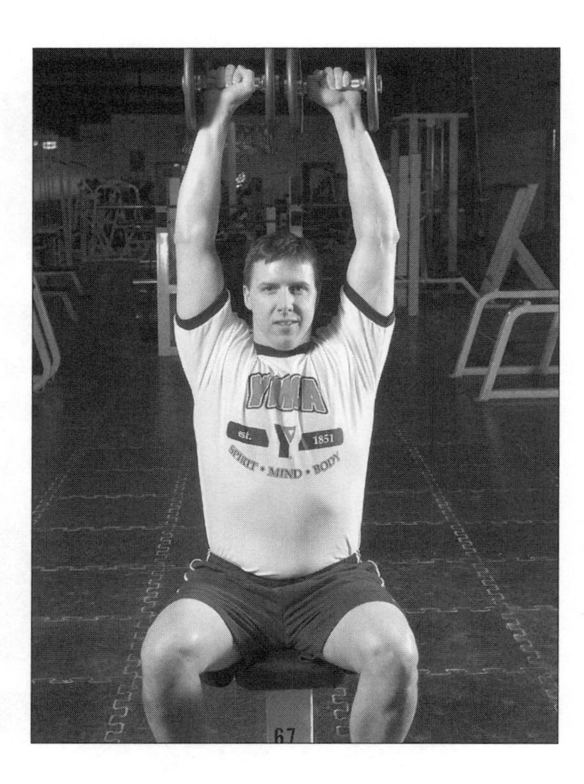

Dumbbell Front Raise

Muscle Group

Anterior deltoid

Stand with a dumbbell at thigh level with palms facing thighs. Raise dumbbells alternately with wrist slightly flexed and elbow slightly bent. Raise dumbbell to eye level, hold for a second, lower, and repeat alternately with other arm.

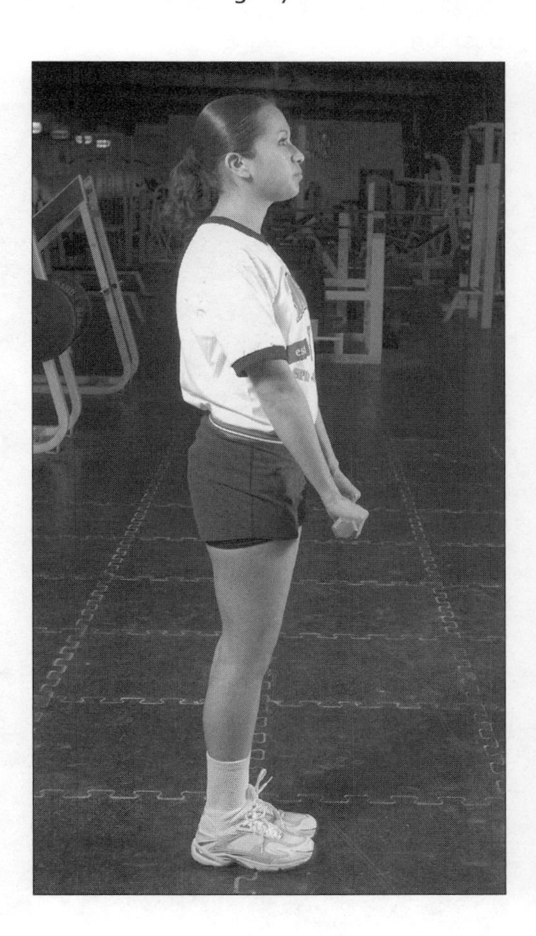

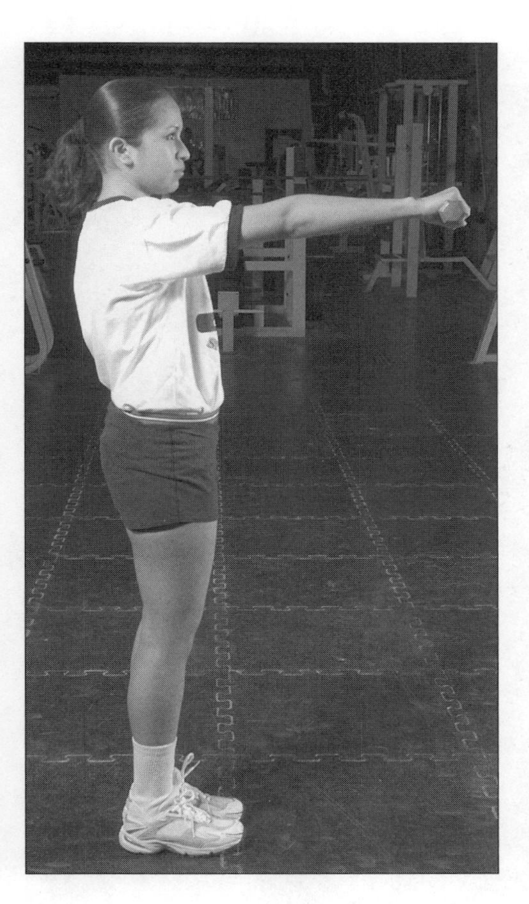

Shoulder Press Machine

Muscle Group

Anterior and middle deltoid, triceps, upper trapezius

Position body in the machine so that the seat height allows a full range of movement. This is accomplished when the movement arms are allowed to stop just before touching the shoulders and when the weight stacks do not touch. Lightly grasping the movement handles and keeping the back flat against the supporting pad, slowly press the movement arms directly overhead to full arm length. Do not lock elbows. Pause. Slowly lower to the starting position. Repeat.

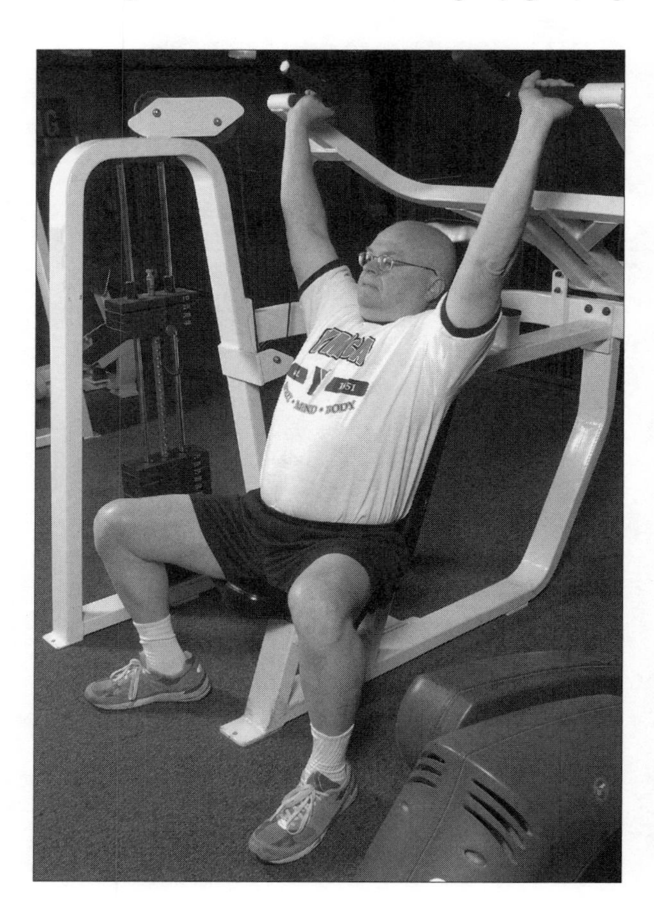

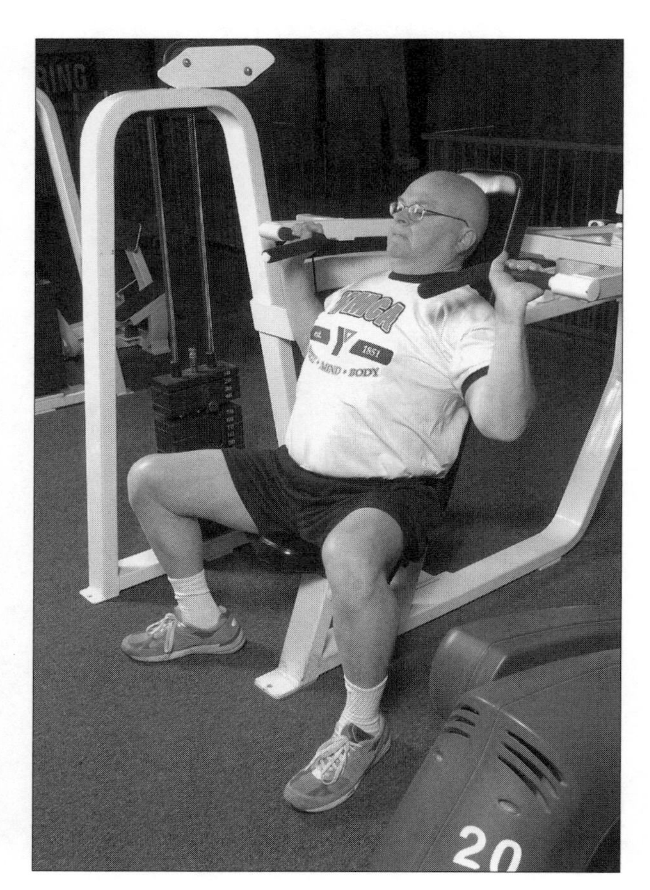

UPPER ARM

Dumbbell Curl

Muscle Group

Biceps

Sit or stand using underhand grip, keeping a neutral back, and holding elbows close to sides. Alternately raise dumbbell toward the shoulder. Pause at the top of the movement. Lower and repeat with other arm.

Note: Keep upper arm in vertical position close to sides through full range of movement.

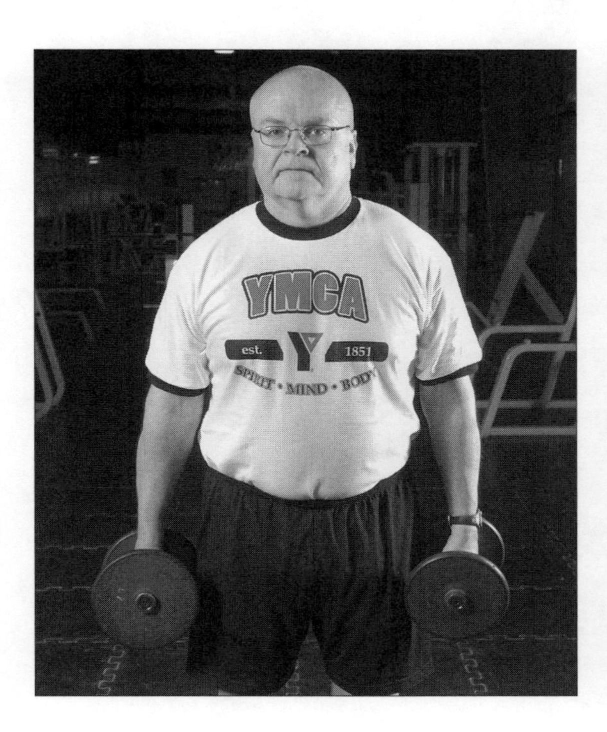

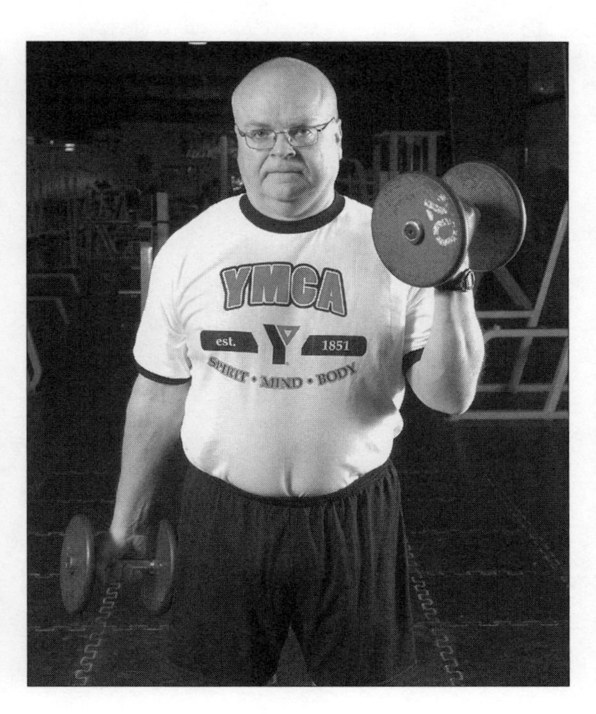

Standing Cable Curl

Muscle Group

Biceps

Using an underhand grip and with arms at full length, lean slightly back, making sure that the arms are in line with cable. Bring hands toward shoulders, keeping upper arm stationary. Pause at top of movement and return to starting position. Repeat.

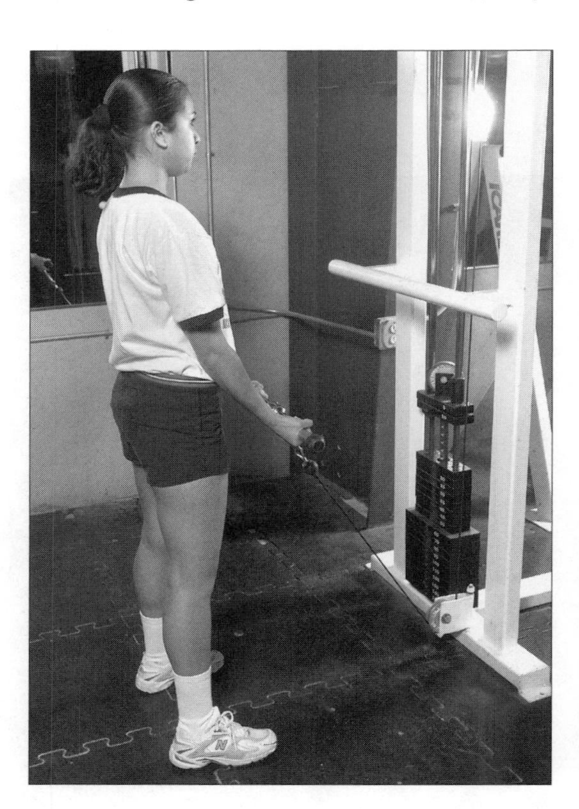

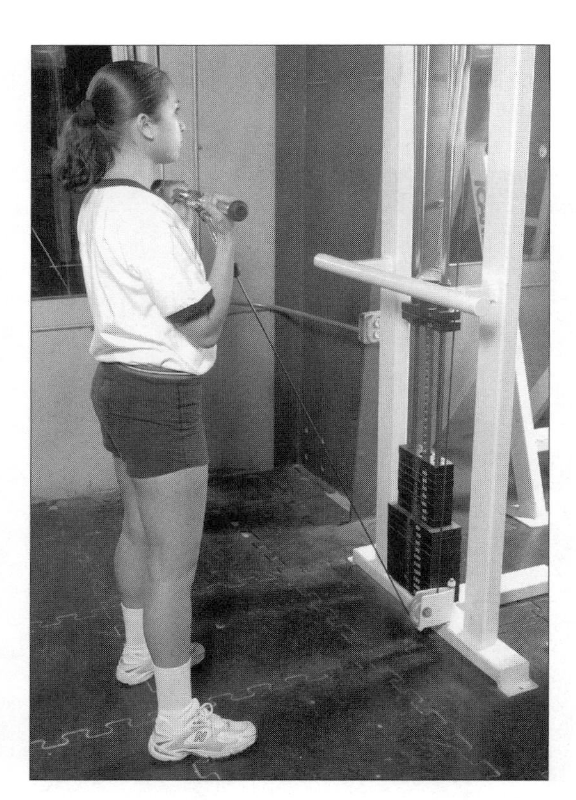

Biceps Machine

Muscle Group

Biceps

Adjust seat so that elbow joints align with machine's axis of rotation and so that elbows, when resting on pad, are even with shoulders. Extend forearms and lightly grasp machine handles. Pull hands toward shoulders as far as possible. Pause and return to starting position. Repeat.

Note: Wrist should remain in neutral position throughout movement. Elbows higher than shoulder may cause hyperextension.

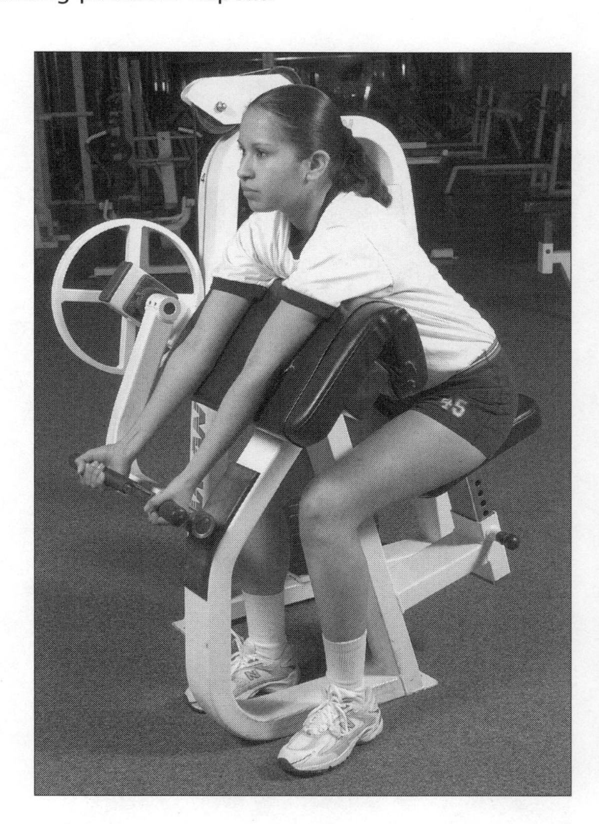

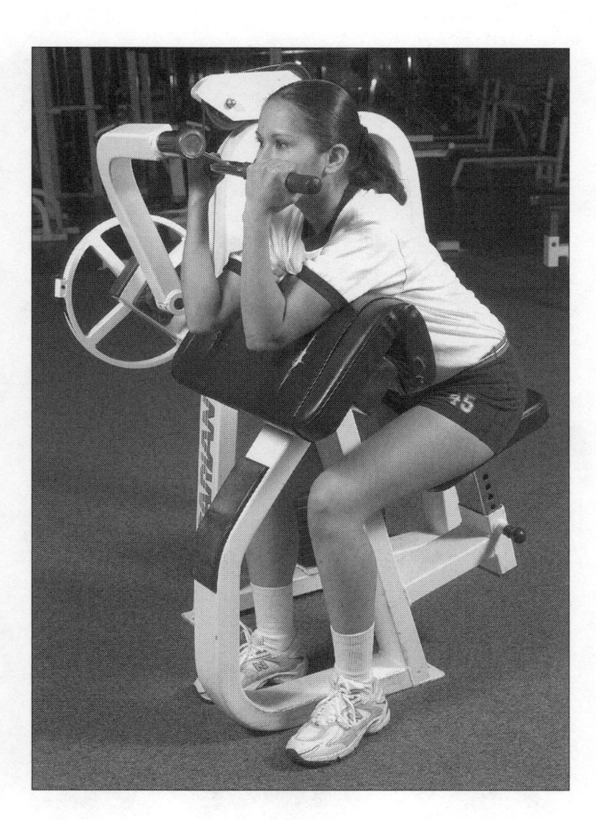

Triceps Press-Down

Muscle Group

Triceps

Grasp cable bar with close-spaced (six to eight inches apart), overhand grip, feet shoulder-width apart, knees slightly bent. Begin with hands at chest level. Keeping elbows firmly pressed against sides and wrists in neutral position, push cable bar down until elbows are fully extended (do not lock). Pause and return slowly to the starting position. Repeat.

Note: Do not let the cable bar go above chest level. Using a V-bar or ropes instead of a straight bar places the wrists in a less stressful position and might allow for a slightly greater range of motion. Wrists should be kept in a neutral position.

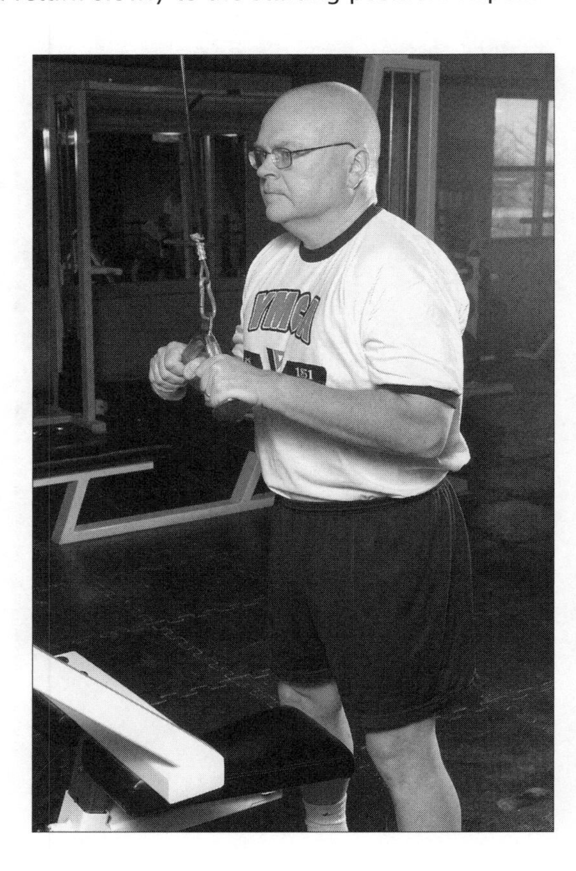

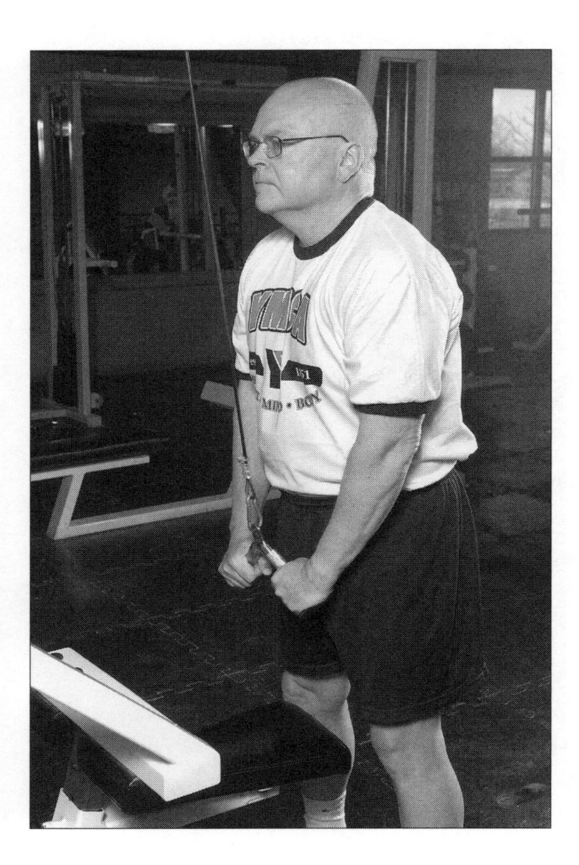

Dumbbell Kickback

Muscle Group

Triceps

Support the body with one hand or one hand and knee on a bench. Hold dumbbell in other hand, palm facing body, upper arm tight to the side and parallel to floor. Extend forearm until arm is straight. Pause and return to starting position. Repeat.

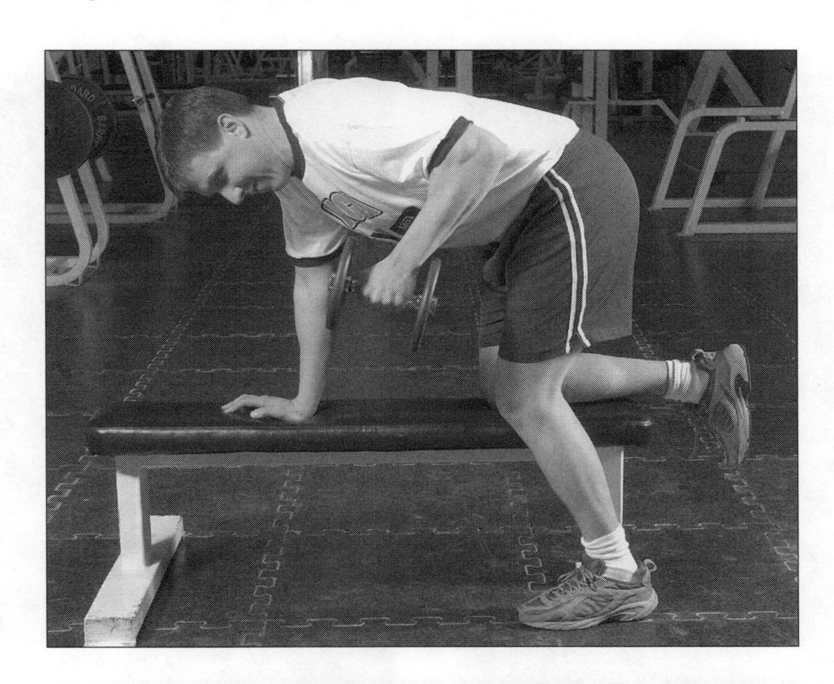

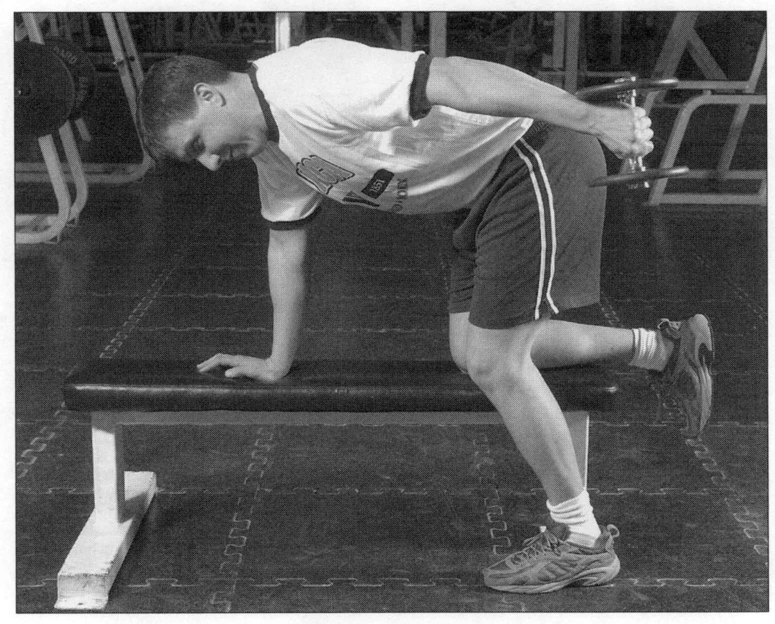

Seated Dumbbell Triceps Extension

Muscle Group

Triceps

From a seated position, hold a dumbbell in both hands and extend arms straight overhead (palm facing in). Keeping upper arm stationary, lower dumbbell to a point immediately behind the head. Pause at bottom of movement, and extend elbows to a straight arm position (do not lock joints). Lower and repeat movement.

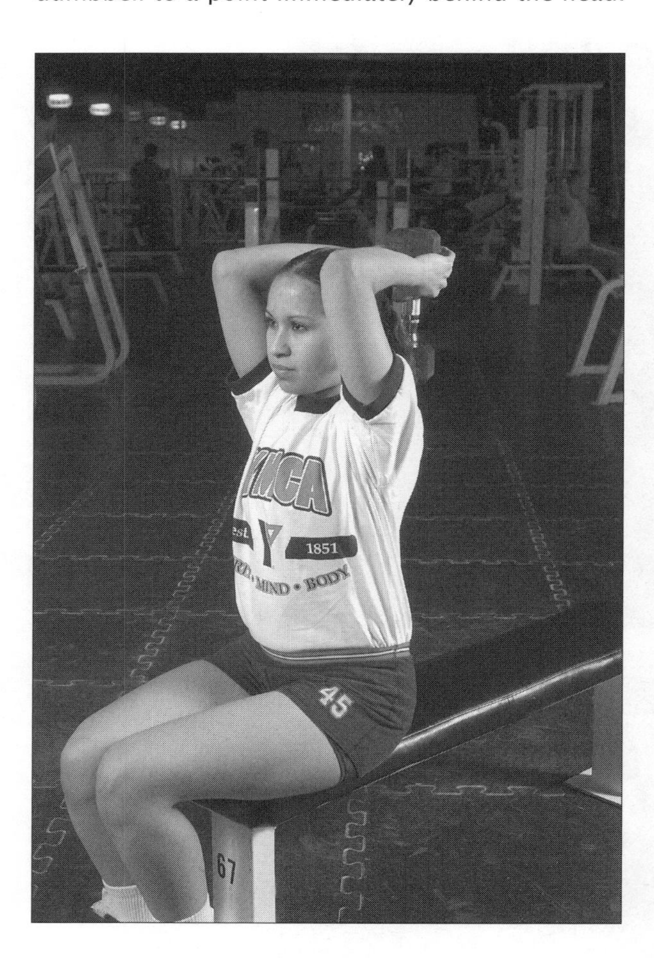

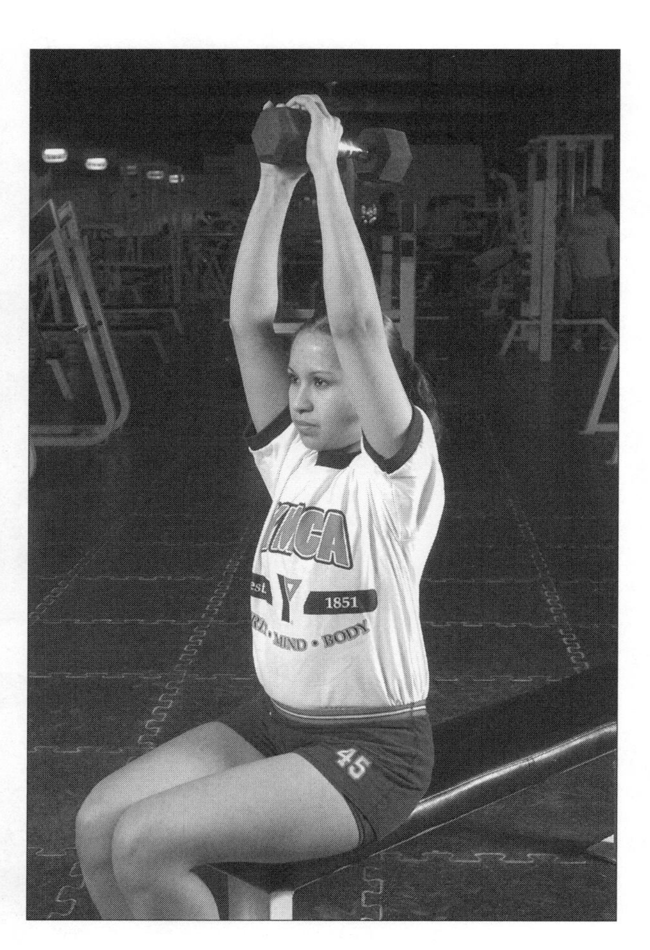

MIDSECTION

Trunk Curl

Muscle Group

Rectus abdominis

Lie in a supine position. Place both feet flat on the floor with knees bent. Cross both arms over the chest. Slowly curl the head, neck, and shoulders up off the floor, keeping the low back in contact with the floor at all times. Pause. Lower slowly to the starting position, attempting to keep the head from touching the floor. Pause. Repeat.

Note: Keep the head and neck in a neutral position throughout the exercise.

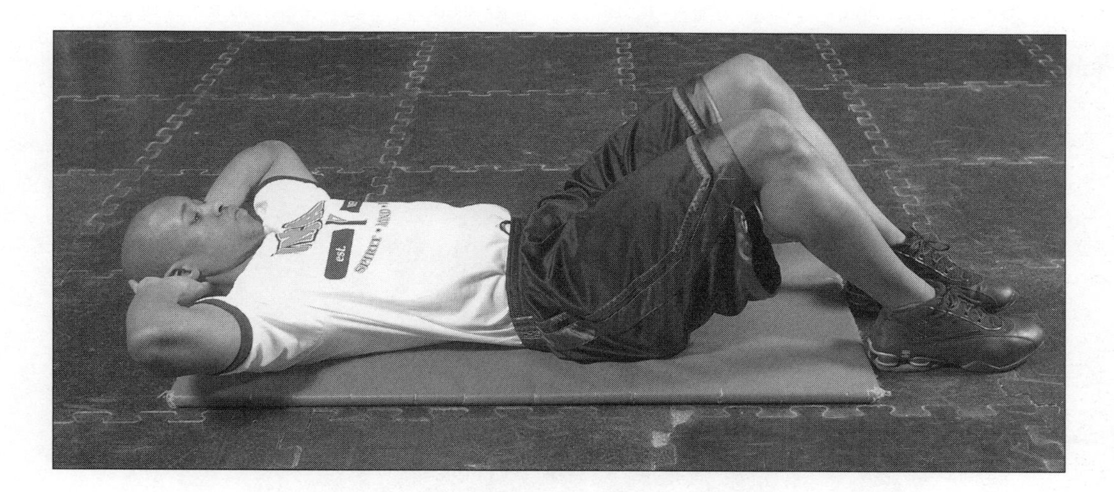

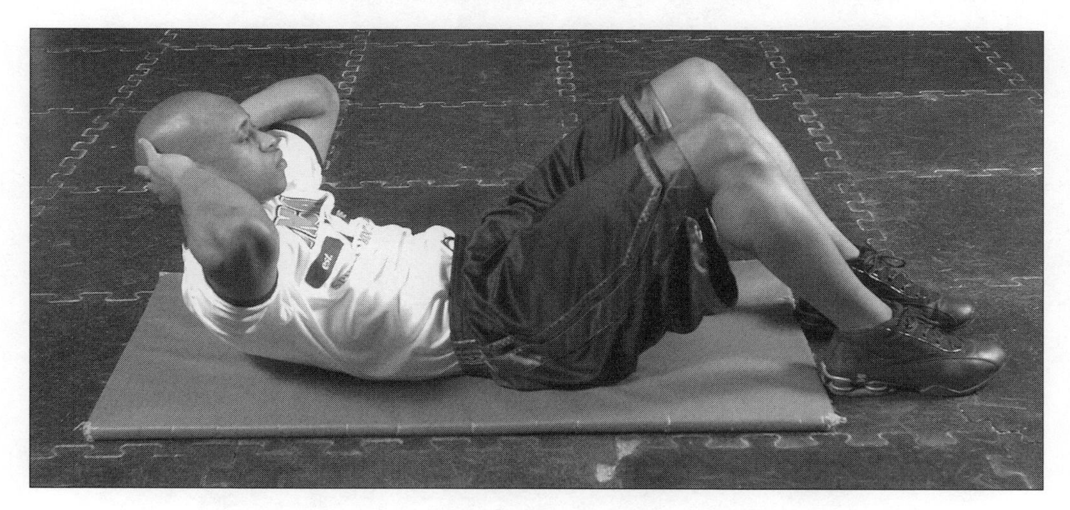

Abdominal Machine

Muscle Group

Rectus abdominis

Although machines vary, generally the axis of rotation of the body (the navel or midsection) should be aligned with the axis of rotation of the machine. This is usually done by adjusting the seat height or length, and the position of the feet. Place the hand and feet in a position so they do not assist the movement. Keep the head and shoulders in alignment, and start with the spine in neutral alignment. If there are handles, grasp them lightly with a closed grip. Exhale and slowly flex the trunk by contracting the abdominals, pulling the bottom of the rib cage toward the hips. Keep arms in the starting position and the head aligned over the shoulders. Contract abdominals through the full range of motion, about 30-35 degrees of flexion. Pause. Slowly return to starting position. Repeat.

Note: Avoid attempting to handle too much weight. Concentrate on using the abdominal muscle to initiate and control the entire movement slowly and steadily. Work with control, keep tension in the abdominals, and maintain proper head and neck alignment throughout the exercise.

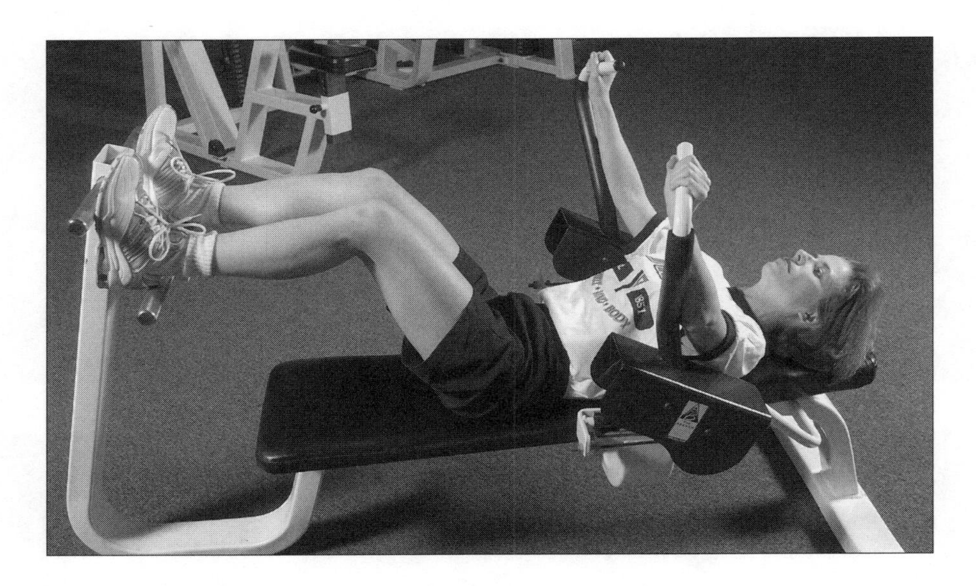

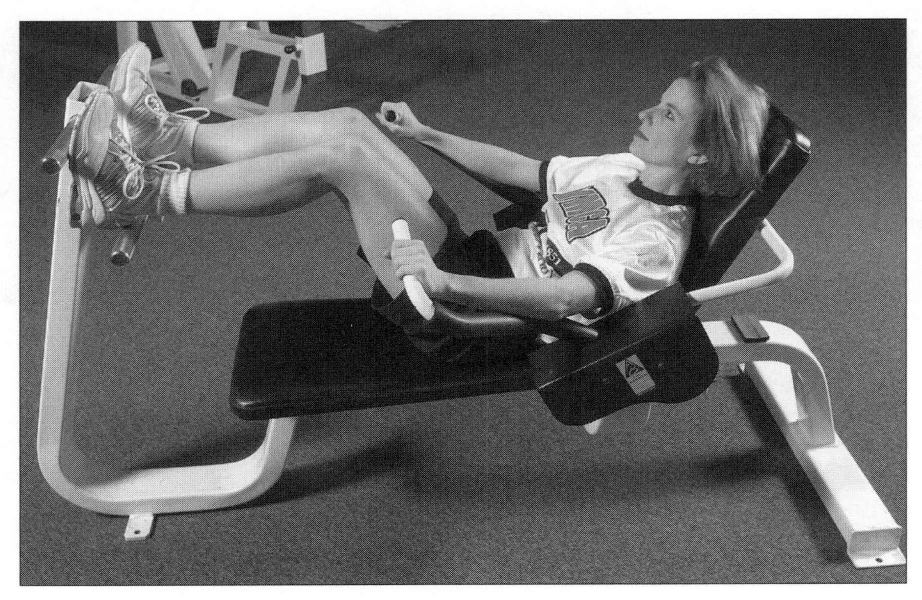

Cable or Dumbbell Side Bends

Muscle Group

Obliques

Stand with one side of the body facing a low pulley station. Grasp the pulley station handle or dumbbell securely. Place the opposite hand against the back of the head. Slowly bend the body sideways toward the weight station or dumbbell as far as possible without compromising the direct sideways movement (i.e., Do not lean the body forward or backward). Slowly return to the starting position, allowing a full range of motion to stretch the oblique area, which has just been contracted. Pause. Repeat. Change weight or pulley station handle to opposite side and repeat. Start leaning toward resistance and move to upright position.

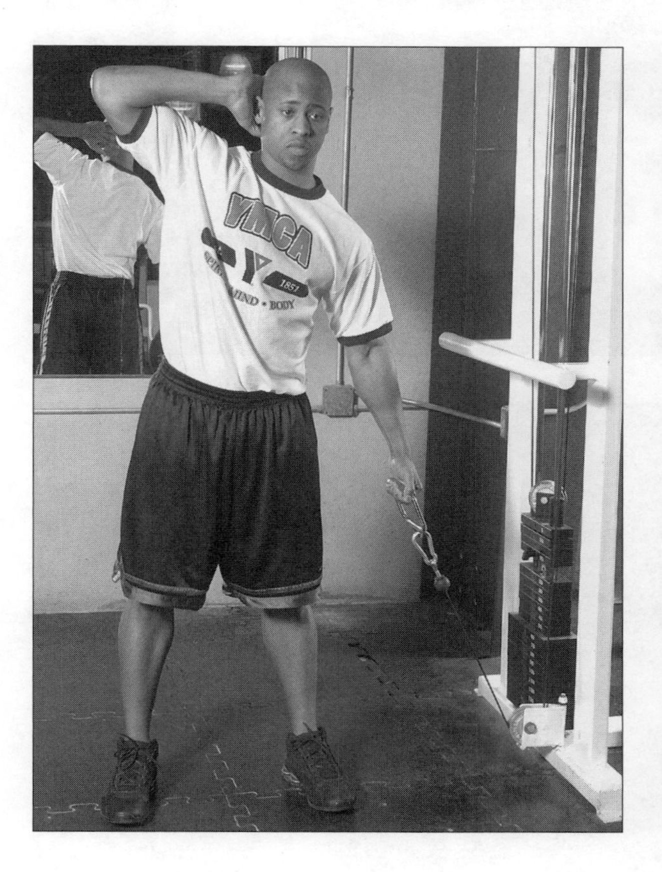

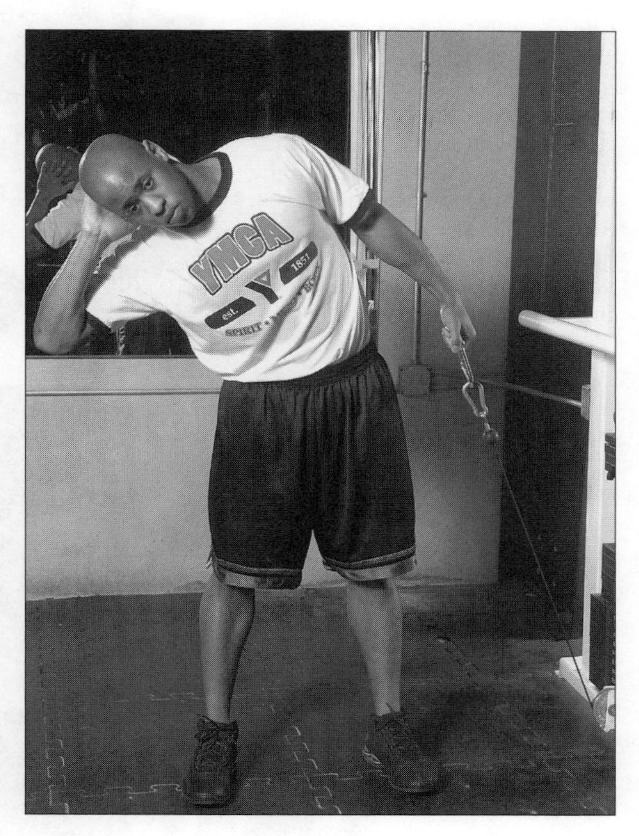

BACK

Seated Low-Pulley Back Extension

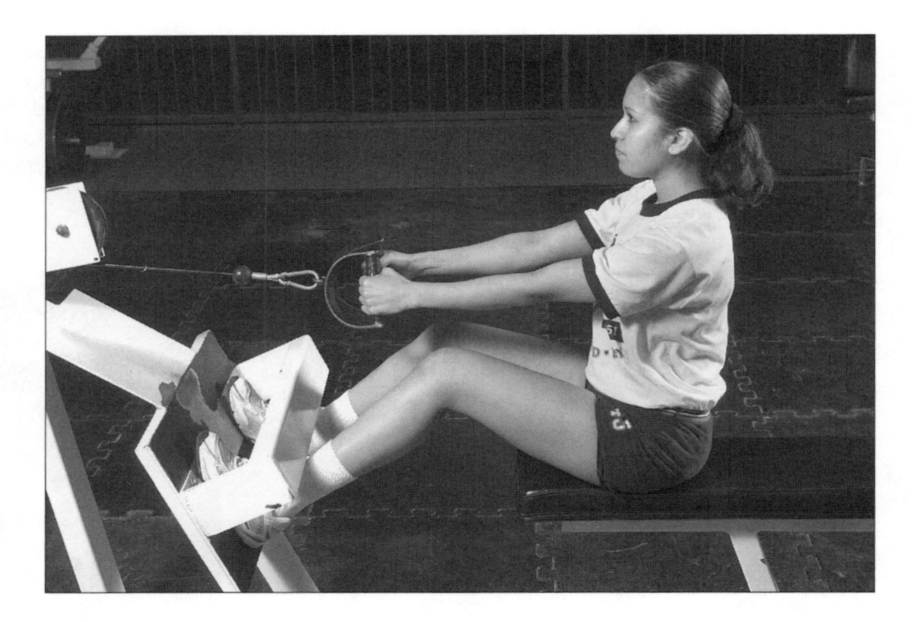

Muscle Group

Erector spinae, hip extensors

Sit on the floor facing a low pulley station. Grasp both handles firmly. Place the bottoms of the feet against the base of the weight station (or a box or platform). Keeping the knees slightly bent and arms straight, lean back to nearly full extension, pausing just before the low back area touches the floor. Slowly return to the starting position, pausing before the weights touch the weight stack. Repeat.

Note: Keep the back and spine in their neutral positions throughout the exercise.

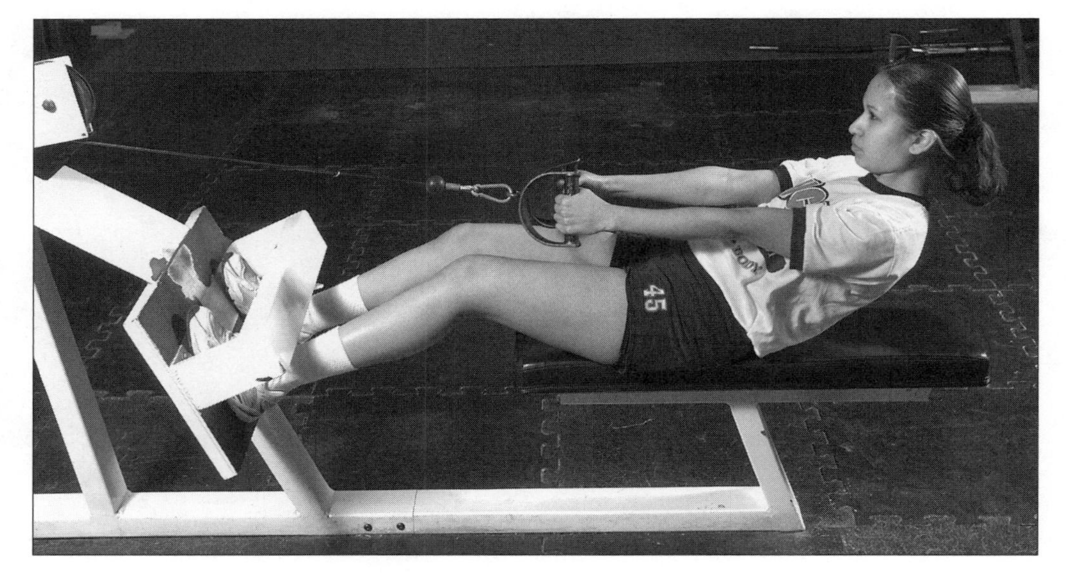

SHOULDER ROTATOR CUFF

Cable Internal Rotation

Muscle Group

Pectoralis major, latissimus dorsi, subscapularis, anterior deltoid

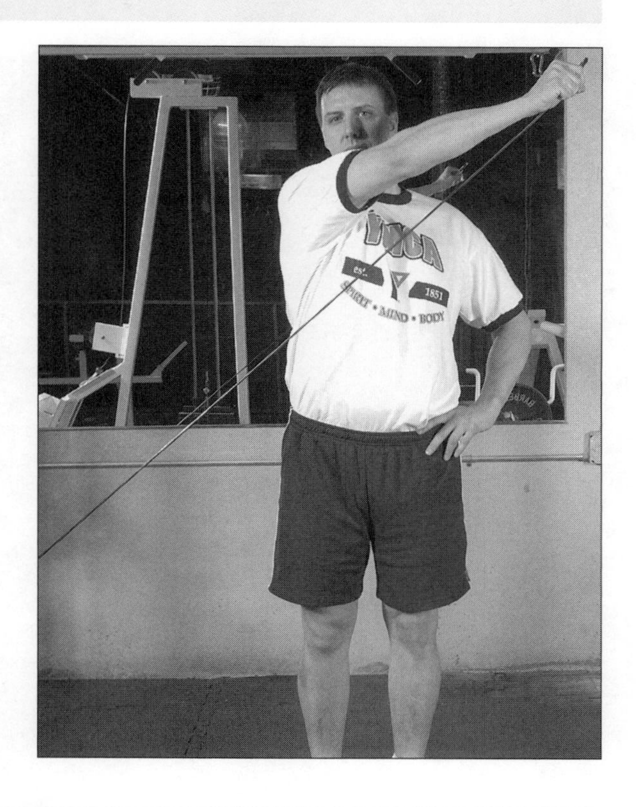

Stand with right side to cable resistance and grasp cable handle with right hand. With upper arm vertical against side, allow lower arm to rotate backward horizontal to floor. Slowly move lower arm forward as far as comfortable (internal rotation). Pause, slowly return to starting position, and repeat.

Note: Perform the same exercise with the upper arm horizontal and the lower arm moving forward in the vertical plane. Continue exercise with left arm.

Cable External Rotation

Muscle Group

Infraspinatus, teres minor, posterior deltoid

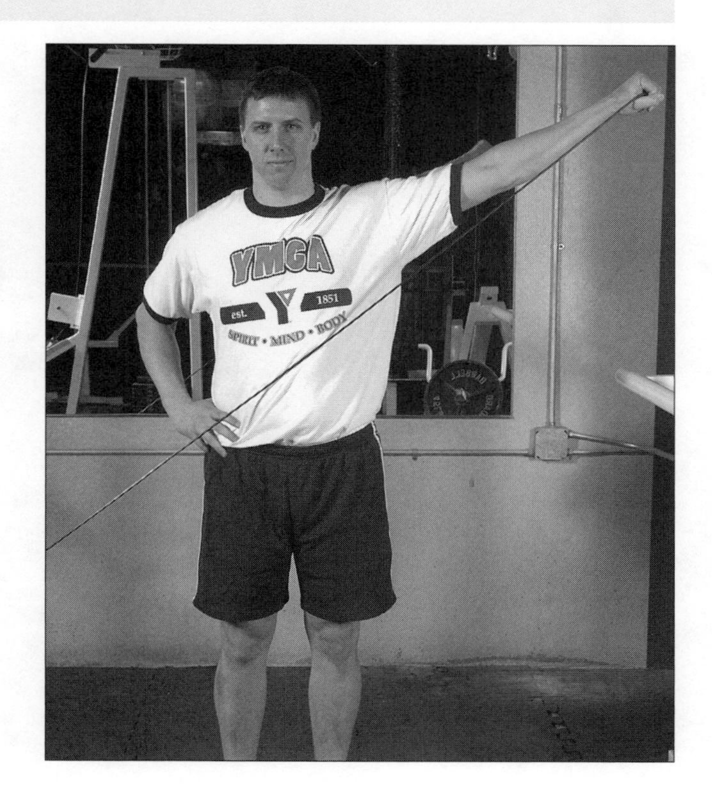

Stand with left side to cable resistance and grasp cable handle with right hand. With upper arm vertical against side, allow lower arm to rotate forward horizontal to floor. Slowly move lower arm backward as far as comfortable (external rotation). Pause, slowly return to starting position, and repeat. Continue exercise with left arm.

Note: Perform the same exercise with the upper arm horizontal and the lower arm moving backward in the vertical plane.

CHAPTER 6

Flexibility Training

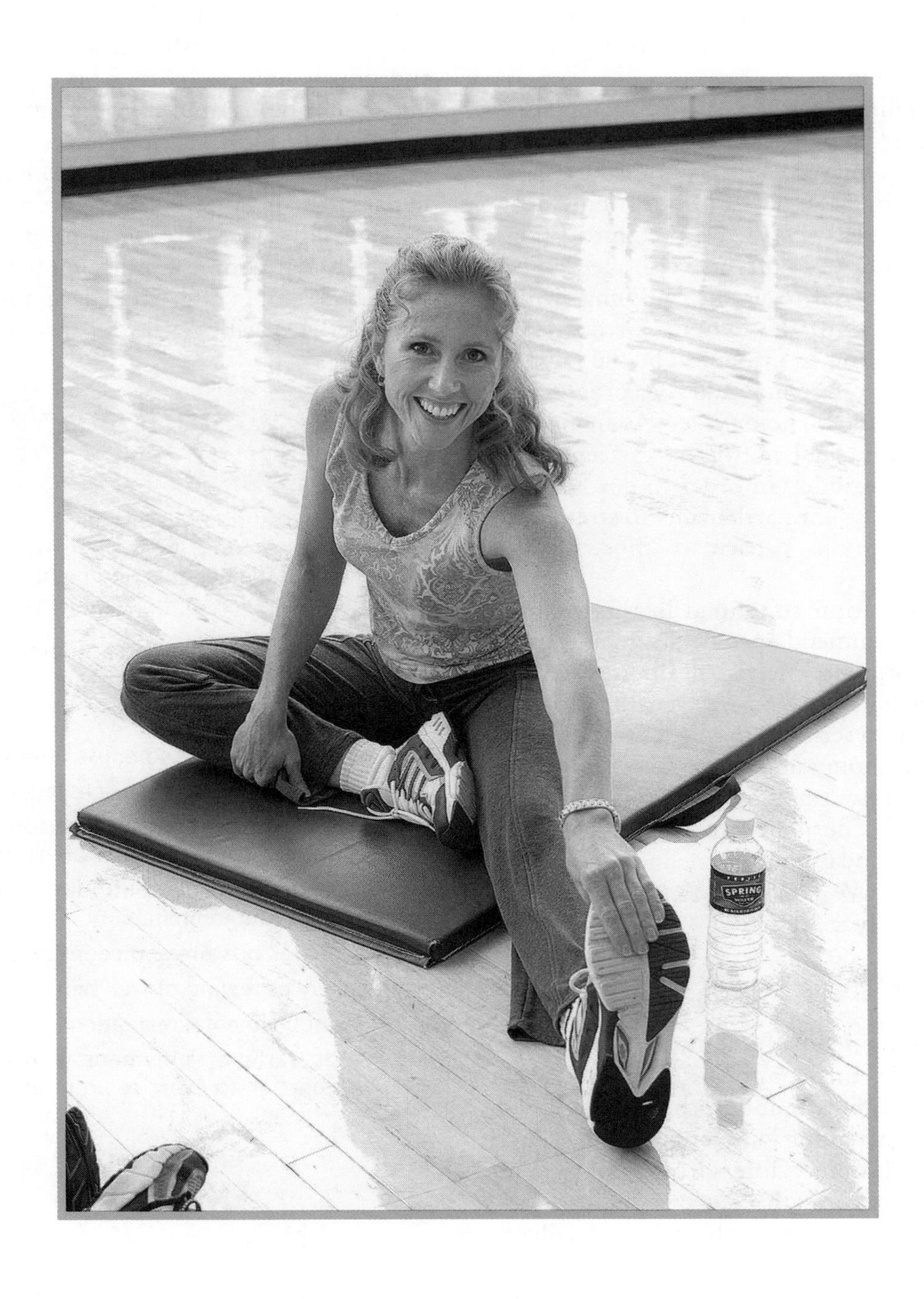

Flexibility is one of the three primary components of physical fitness, along with cardiorespiratory endurance and muscular strength and endurance. Flexibility allows a person to move the body in a greater range of motion. It also keeps muscles supple and responsive to the demands of daily activities, including leisure sports and exercise. Stretching to increase flexibility is a key component of a comprehensive personal training program.

Conditioning programs typically emphasize cardiovascular training and resistance training. Programs, equipment, and facilities do a good job of addressing the needs of most individuals in these two areas. However, the third fitness factor—flexibility—is often overlooked and is sometimes referred to as the "missing fitness link." Awareness of the benefits of flexibility training is growing, as evidenced by the increasing prevalence of stretching and yoga programs in fitness centers and on home video. As an instructor, you must understand the basic science and principles of flexibility in order to develop safe and effective ways for participants to stretch the major muscle groups, particularly those that are typically tight.

The information contained in this chapter helps you recommend specific stretching exercises and incorporate effective flexibility exercises in programs for members. We start by defining flexibility and describing the benefits. Then we discuss the anatomy and physiology and relate them to flexibility training. After reviewing the factors that affect flexibility, we talk about stretching techniques and training guidelines, along with teaching tips. We conclude the chapter with sample flexibility exercises.

DEFINING FLEXIBILITY

Flexibility is defined as the ability to move joints and use muscles through their full normal range of motion. Flexibility training is broadly accepted as a means of increasing joint mobility and reducing injuries. Flexibility differs from joint to joint and involves not only the muscles but also several other components of the musculoskeletal system.

There is no one way to assess an individual's total flexibility because flexibility at one joint does not validly predict the range of motion in another body area. The type of movement that a person typically performs often dictates the range of flexibility at that particular joint. For example, trained dancers might have much more flexibility in their lower extremities, whereas baseball pitchers might have more flexibility in the shoulder joint. Although research has shown that different stretching methods improve joint flexibility, inappropriate stretching can cause injury and impair joint stability. The goal of stretching should be to optimize joint mobility while maintaining joint stability. Recently, exercise researchers have promoted the concept of functional range of motion. This refers to developing the flexibility necessary for a specific activity or sport without compromising joint stability, and it can be useful in effectively designing exercises to meet the specific needs of participants.

Benefits of Flexibility Training

As a personal training instructor, you can be a valuable resource to members by educating them about the benefits of flexibility training. Following is a list of those benefits:

- Helps maintain or increase joint mobility
- Reduces muscle tension
- Helps prevent injuries
- Alleviates muscle soreness after exercise
- Delays the onset of muscle fatigue
- Contributes to enhanced performance in daily life, sports, or other physical activity
- Provides better equilibrium to maintain balance and joint stability
- Improves posture and coordination
- Enhances feeling of well-being
- Promotes mental relaxation
- Adds variety, enjoyment, and sense of satisfaction to exercise program

ANATOMY AND PHYSIOLOGY

To set up a flexibility program properly, you must understand the anatomy of joints and how physiology affects the development of flexibility.

Anatomy of a Joint

The nature of flexibility is complex and is influenced by many factors. Flexibility differs from joint to joint and involves not only the muscles but also several soft-tissue components of the musculoskeletal system at the joints. The properties of the soft tissues—the ligaments, tendons, cartilage, and muscles and their covering—are important in determining the contribution of each to the flexibility of a particular joint. Those tissues and their properties are as follows:

- **Ligaments.** Ligaments contain connective tissue fiber arranged in parallel lines packed closely together; they are inelastic and therefore do not stretch.
- **Tendons.** Like ligaments, tendons contain connective tissue fiber arranged in parallel lines packed closely together; they are inelastic and do not stretch.
- **Cartilage.** This tissue contains more elastic fibers to facilitate its shock-absorbing function.
- **Muscle and muscle fascia.** Muscles can be stretched to about 150 percent of their resting length. The fascia is a sheath that holds the muscle fibers together and it stretches.

Several physiological factors can limit an individual's functional range of motion around any particular joint. Those factors include

- skin, scar tissue, and excessive fat;
- the structure of the bone and type of joint;
- tight ligaments and tendons around the joint; and
- tight muscle tissue.

Physiology and Development of Flexibility

To teach flexibility exercises, you first must understand the physiological concepts of stretch reflex and reciprocal innervation.

Stretch reflex occurs when the motor receptors in the stretched muscle send a signal to the spinal cord, which sends a motor response back to generate a reflex action causing the muscle to contract against the stretch. This natural action protects the joint and muscles from injury, but it also can limit stretch effectiveness. The force of the reflex contraction is directly related to the force generated by the stretch. If a stretch is performed slowly and gently, the stretch reflex is minimal, if invoked at all. This provides an explanation of why slow, static stretches are the recommended technique to ensure safe and effective stretching. The components of the muscle tissue involved in the stretch reflex are these:

- **Muscle spindle.** This is a sensory motor receptor in the muscle that regulates changes in the length and tension of the muscle's fibers. It sends the signal to the spinal cord that invokes the stretch reflex.
- **Golgi tendon organ (GTO).** This is another sensory motor receptor, located in the muscle–tendon junction of a joint. When stimulated by excessive tension caused by a stretch or contraction, GTO receptors invoke an inhibitory reflex on the muscle, causing it to relax. This is called an *inverse stretch reflex*. The amount of force required to stimulate the GTO is much greater than the force required to stimulate the muscle spindles. A slow, long stretch will elicit a significant response from the GTO that causes the muscle to relax and stretch easily without injury.

Reciprocal innervation is the concept that when one set of muscles (agonists) contract, the opposing muscles (antagonists) relax. Muscles usually operate in pairs, so without this organization, coordinated muscular activity would be impossible. This phenomenon can be used to induce relaxation in the muscles you want to stretch by contracting the opposing muscle group.

FACTORS INFLUENCING FLEXIBILITY

You will find that the degree of flexibility in members with whom you work varies greatly. In addition to the physiological factors of the joint and muscle anatomy as previously discussed, several other factors influence flexibility. You must take all of these factors into consideration when prescribing flexibility exercises. Those factors include the following:

- **Age.** Muscle connective tissues naturally shorten with aging, as evidenced in the stiffness of older people. Contractility remains while elasticity is lost, resulting in tighter, stiffer muscles. Muscles must be regularly stretched to minimize this effect.

- **Gender.** Several studies have shown that females tend to be more flexible than males.
- **Exercise history.** It appears that active people tend to be more flexible than inactive people. Engaging in regular exercise can delay and even reverse the normal loss of flexibility caused by aging.
- **Temperature.** An increase in intramuscular temperature results in a decrease in intramuscular resistance, which translates into an increase in range of motion in associated joints. This points to the need to warm up before stretching.
- **Body type.** There is no indication that body type is a factor in determining one's flexibility.
- **Resistance training.** Proper strength training, in which exercises are performed through the full range of motion, probably enhances flexibility.

STRETCHING TECHNIQUES AND METHODS

Types of stretches commonly used are classified by the following three techniques—static, ballistic, and proprioceptive neuromuscular facilitation.

- **Static.** A low-force, high-duration stretch where the muscle is held at the greatest possible length for up to 30 seconds
- **Ballistic.** A high-force, short-duration stretch using rapid bouncing motions
- **Proprioceptive neuromuscular facilitation (PNF).** A static stretch of a muscle immediately after maximally contracting it; there are two types of PNF stretches:
    - **Contract–relax.** An isometric contraction of the muscle, followed by relaxing, then stretching to the point of limitation
    - **Contract–relax agonist contract.** An isometric contraction of the muscle, followed by relaxing, stretching to the point of limitation, then contracting the agonist muscle, followed by a stretch to the point of limitation.

The two most accepted techniques for improving flexibility are static and PNF stretching. Ballistic stretching was popular many years ago, but it is no longer recommended because it carries a greater risk of injury and is less effective than other techniques. Static and PNF stretching both operate on the premise that to increase flexibility and prevent injury, the muscle being stretched should be as relaxed as possible. Static stretching is probably the most widely used technique and is very safe and effective. This technique involves gradually stretching a muscle or muscle group to the point of limitation, then holding that position for 15 to 30 seconds.

PNF stretching techniques are also effective and safe for increasing flexibility. Developed in the 1950s as therapy for patients with paralysis and muscular diseases, they have been modified for use by fitness instructors and trainers. PNF techniques are based on the theory of reciprocal inhibition, which states that when the flexors of a joint (agonists) are voluntarily contracted, the extensors of that joint (antagonists) are automatically deactivated, and vice versa. The result is that after an isometric contraction of a selected muscle, there is a more profound reflexive relaxation in that muscle, thus facilitating a greater stretch.

The two methods for stretching are active and passive. Active stretching, in which the person's body movements cause the stretch, is most common. Passive stretching is usually performed with a towel, prop, or a partner who applies a stretch to a relaxed joint. Partner stretching requires close communication and an even and slow application of the stretch. Because there is the potential for injury if done incorrectly, its use is limited.

FLEXIBILITY TRAINING GUIDELINES

Few standard guidelines exist for prescribing the type, duration, and number of repetitions of any given stretching technique. Techniques continue to evolve, and ongoing research will continue to provide new information.

One principle underlying each of the flexibility techniques is the principle of specific adaptations to imposed demands (SAID). The SAID principle dictates that in order to increase flexibility, one must slowly and progressively stretch the muscle to the point of limitation, but not to the point of tearing.

Although a participant's fitness level, factors that limit flexibility, and goals should be considered when designing a safe and effective flexibility program, certain training guidelines should be followed.

- Prescribe exercises that will stretch all of the major muscle groups.
- Design a program that will assess and improve areas of inflexibility.
- Recommend daily stretching exercises.
- Suggest wearing clothing that will not constrict movement.
- Teach participants to do the following:
  - Warm up before stretching to increase the body temperature and range of motion.
  - Stretch opposing muscle groups equally.

Teaching Tips

You should make several decisions before you can effectively lead a flexibility training session, including what to teach, when to stretch, what the training program format should be, how to address safety concerns, and how to communicate the correct technique. Following are tips for teaching stretching exercises.

When do I stretch?

- If the goal is to *warm up*, incorporate gentle static stretches during the warm-up, being sure that each stretch is performed gradually and lasts no more than 10 seconds. Intersperse the stretches with rhythmic limbering movements, keeping in mind the purpose of a warm-up.
- If the goal is to *increase range of motion*, stretch right after the cardiorespiratory cool-down or after the muscle-strengthening section of the class. The muscles are still warm and are more likely to respond with an increase in flexibility.

For stretching-only workouts, perform a short warm-up of rhythmic limbering movements for all major muscle groups before stretching. Remember that all stretches are not appropriate for all people. Certain exercises should be modified or adjusted to correctly accommodate an individual's particular needs. Be especially aware of this when working with different populations, such as athletes, older adults, the inactive, youth, and pregnant women. Keep in mind that the following muscles are typically tight in the general population:

- Upper trapezius
- Shoulder protractors
- Trunk extensors
- Hip flexors
- Hamstrings
- Gastrocnemius

It is best to avoid stretching when the following situations are apparent:

- When the muscles are in the area of a recent fracture
- When there is evidence of a recent sprain or strain
- If osteoporosis is present or suspected (recommend a consultation with a physician)
- If pain occurs in the joint or muscle
- If the area is infected or inflamed

Explain each stretch and physically demonstrate the proper posture and positioning. Each stretch should begin gently and progress gradually. The sequence of exercises should work progressively through the entire body, targeting specific joints and muscle groups. Select exercises that will produce results with little risk of injury. Monitor participants for proper technique, form, and posture to ensure that they perform the stretches effectively and safely. If members have trouble with a stretch, gently guide them through the movement.

- Focus on the muscles involved in the stretch, minimizing the movement of other body parts.
- Hold stretches between 15 and 30 seconds. Research suggests that four sets of 15 to 20 seconds per stretch results in optimal gains (Taylor et al. 1990).
- Stretch to the limit of movement, not to the point of pain.
- Breathe slowly and rhythmically while holding the stretches.
- Stretch the muscles in various positions; stretching in different positions might enhance muscle relaxation and improve overall range of motion at the joint.
- Relax the target muscle before going into the stretch.
- Stretch after each vigorous workout to reduce the potential of delayed-onset muscle soreness and to encourage mind and body relaxation.
- Discontinue exercising in any position that causes unusual discomfort or pain. It might be necessary to correct technique or try another position or stretch variation for the target muscles.

SAMPLE FLEXIBILITY EXERCISES

The following are sample flexibility exercises. They are listed by areas of the body.

Neck

Neck stretch—Standing or sitting, tilt head to one side and relax the muscles along the side of the neck. Variation: Place hand on head, lift or tuck chin while tilting. ▼

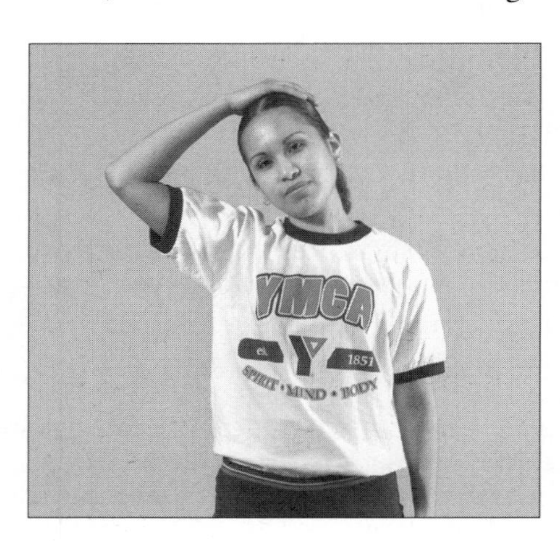

Shoulders and Arms

Triceps stretch—Standing with one arm held straight up over the head, bend the elbow so that the hand is behind head, hold elbow with opposite hand as you try to walk your fingers down your back. ▶

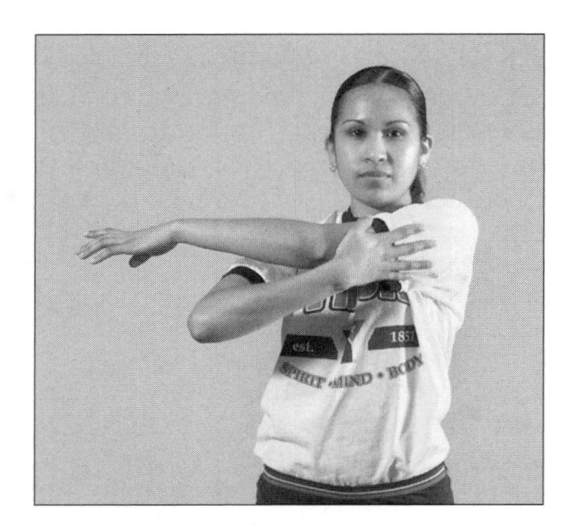

▲ Shoulder stretch—Standing, cross one arm in front of chest, hold elbow with opposite hand, and gently press shoulders down.

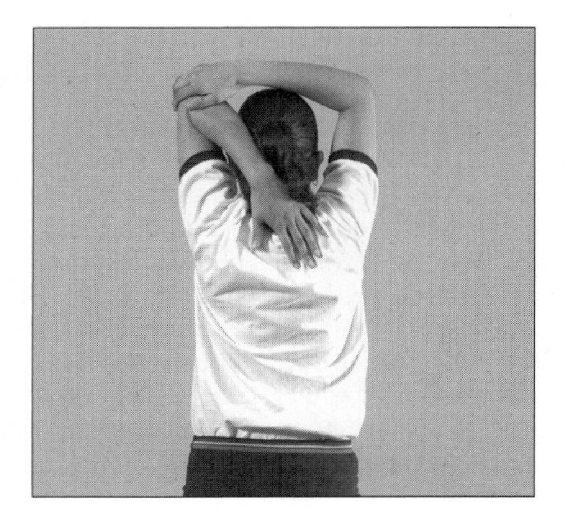

Torso

Pectoral stretch—Standing or sitting, place fingertips behind head and gently press elbows back to open the chest. ▶

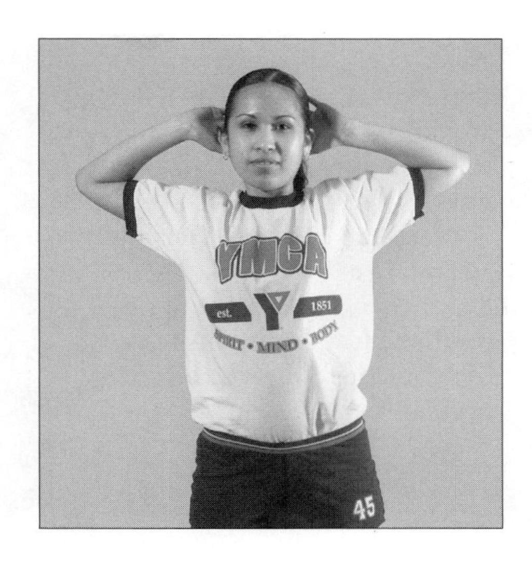

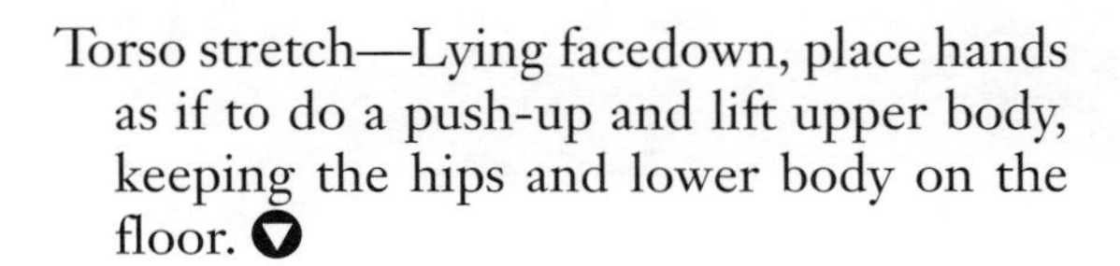

Torso stretch—Lying facedown, place hands as if to do a push-up and lift upper body, keeping the hips and lower body on the floor. ▼

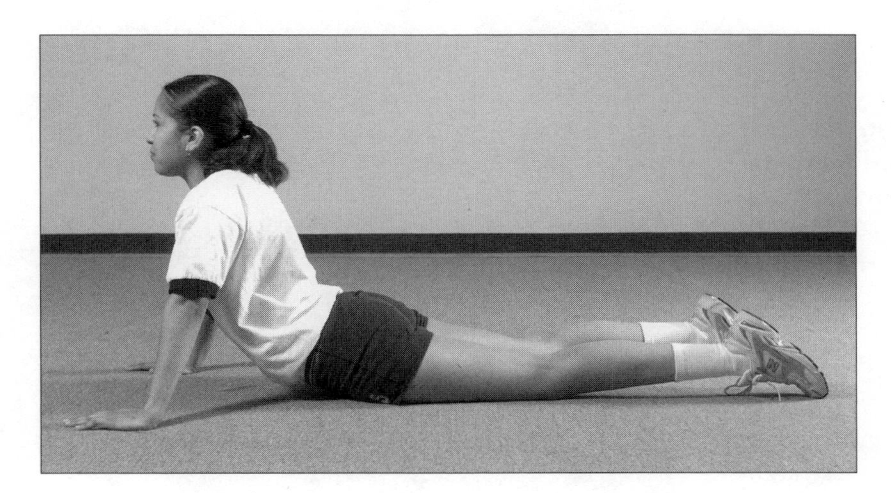

Obliques stretch—Lying on your back, tuck both legs into chest and slowly roll legs to side and rest on the floor. Extend arms out to sides, resting on floor for support. Repeat by rolling to the other side. ▶

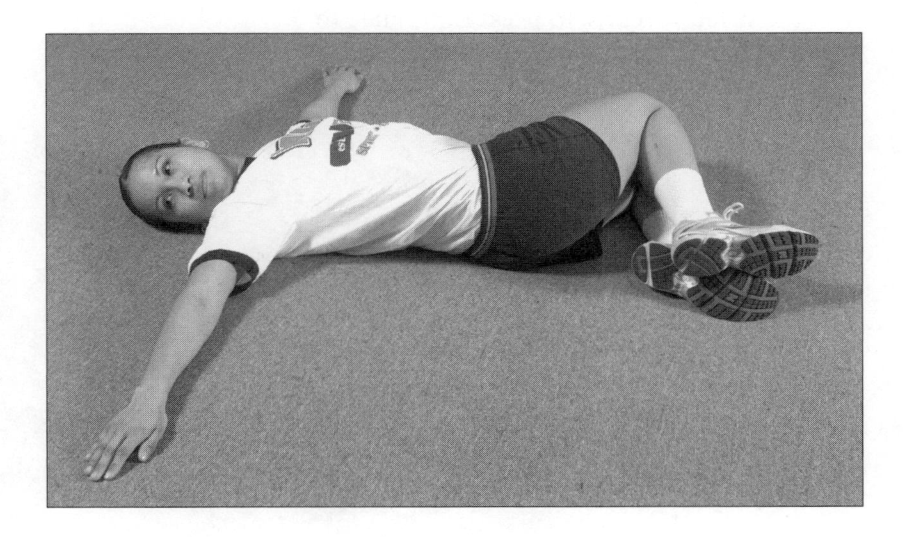

Low Back

Cat Stretch—Kneeling with hands and knees on floor, knees hip-width apart, and hands directly under shoulders, contract abdominals, tilt pelvis, and round the low back. Relax head, then release to neutral position. Caution: This is not recommended if wrist or knee problems are present.

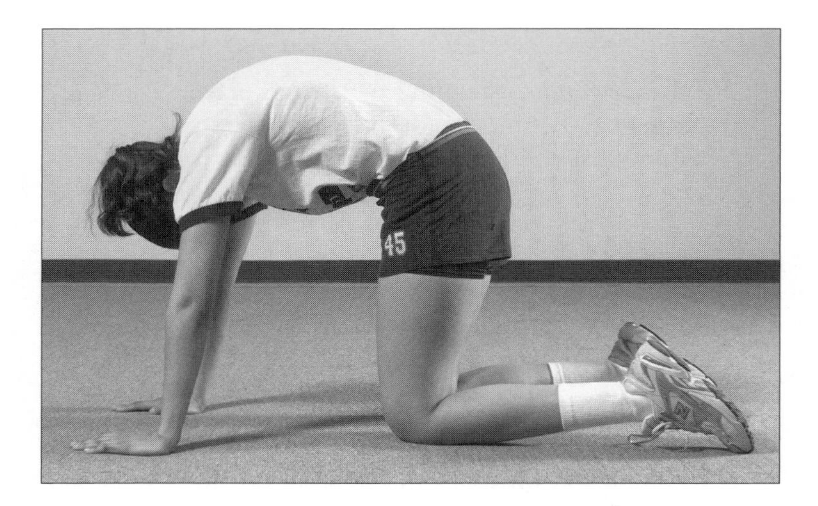

Low back stretch—Lying on your back, tuck your knees into chest, and grab behind thighs with hands. Pull thighs into chest, lifting tailbone off the floor.

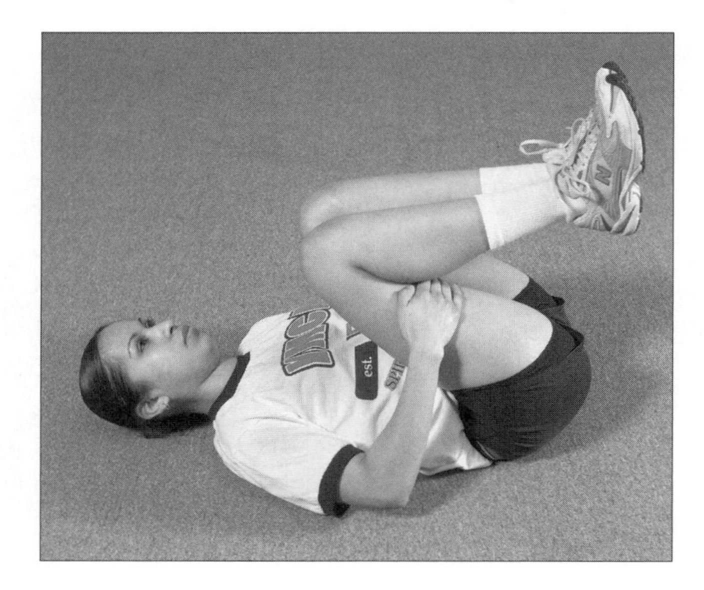

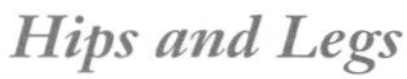

Hips and Legs

Hip abductor stretch—Sitting, flex right knee and cross right leg over straight left leg, placing right foot on floor. Use left forearm to press right knee to torso and turn torso to look over right shoulder.

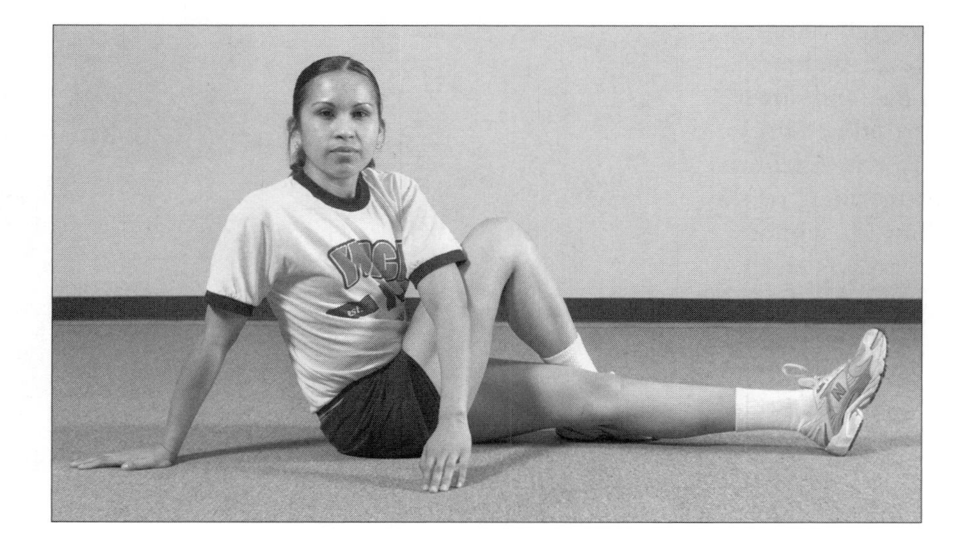

Hip adductors—Sitting with knees flexed and soles of shoes together, place hands on ankles and gently press knees toward floor, using elbows if needed. ▶

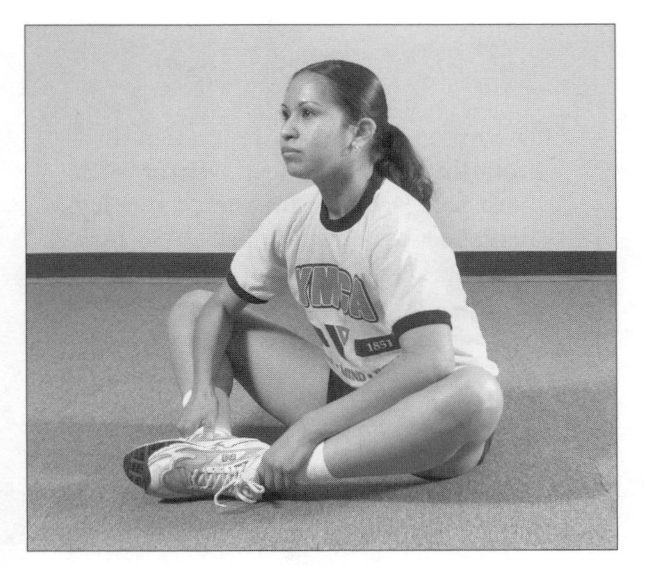

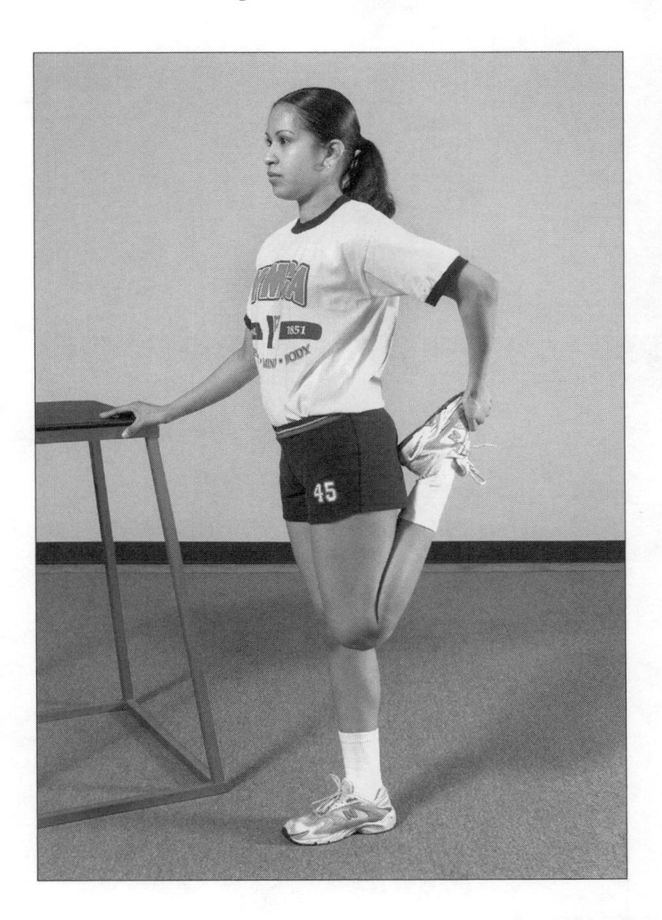

◀ Quadriceps stretch—Standing next to a wall or other support, place inside hand on the wall or other support to steady yourself, shift weight to the inside foot, and lift other foot to buttock. Grab foot with the outside hand and gently press heel toward buttock. Keep hips neutral, thighs parallel, and press hips forward and extend bent leg slightly.

Hamstring stretch—Lying on your back with both knees bent, feet flat on floor, tuck one leg to chest, then slowly straighten that leg, extending it toward the ceiling. ▶

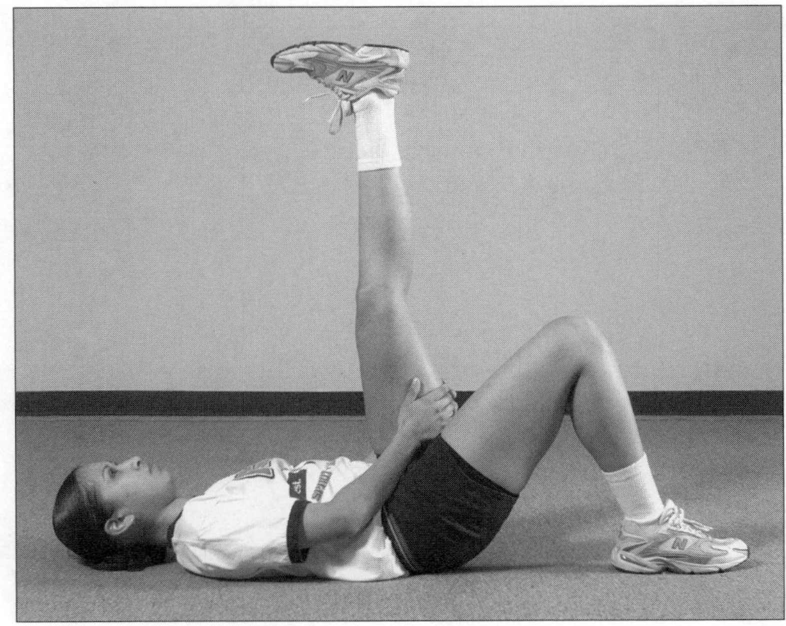

Gastrocnemius and soleus stretch—Standing in a stride position with both feet pointing forward, front leg bent, rear leg straight, press rear heel to floor. ▶

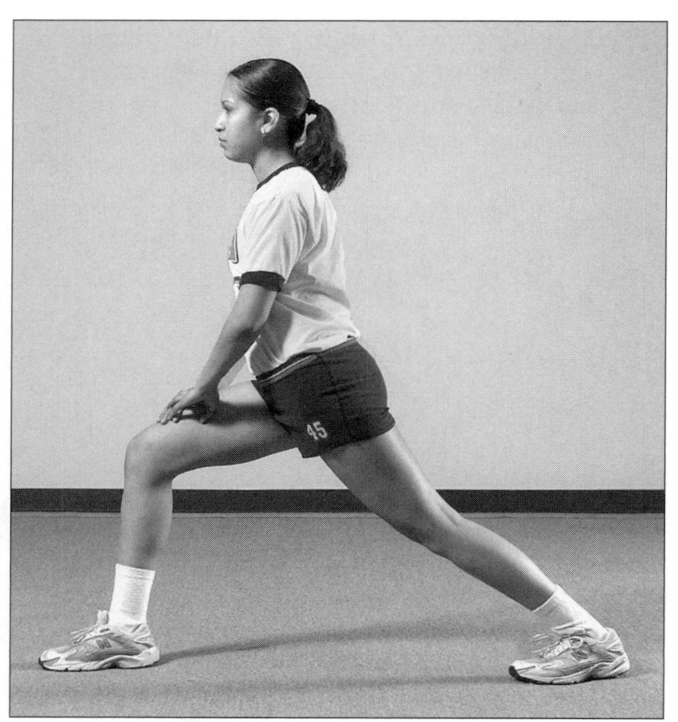

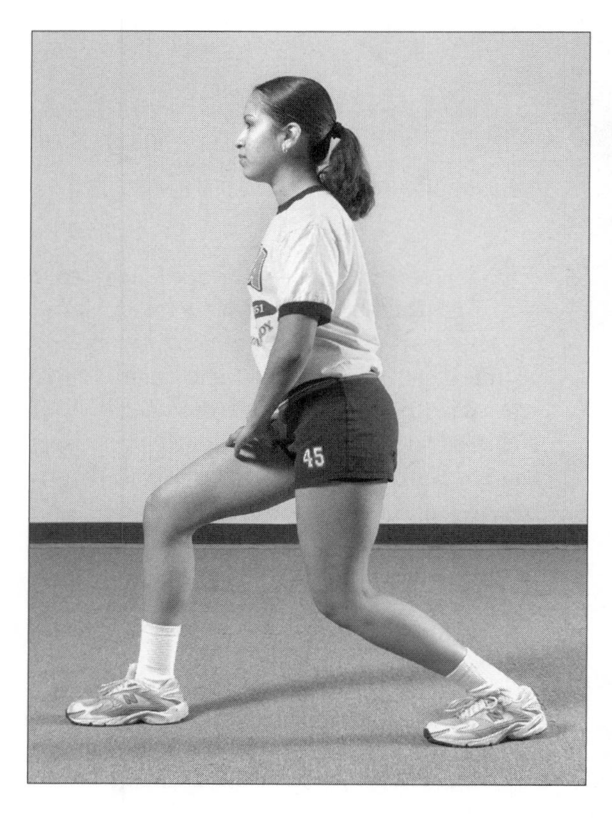

To stretch the soleus muscle, bend rear leg also, keeping heels on the floor. ▲

Hip flexor stretch—Standing in a forward lunge with the back heel raised and knee soft, tilt pelvis back (posterior tilt) and press hipbone of back leg forward. ▶

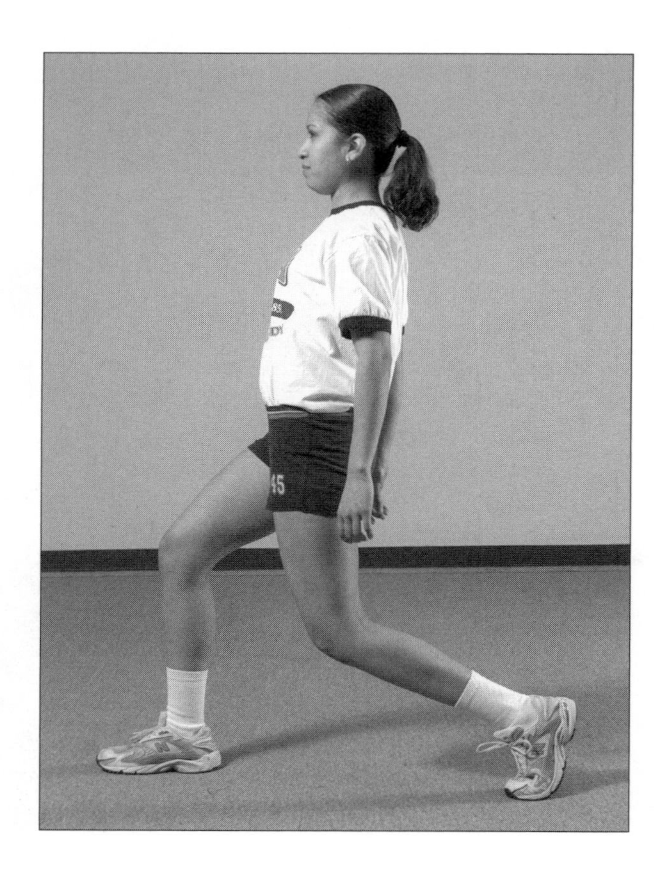

CHAPTER 7

Screening and Assessment

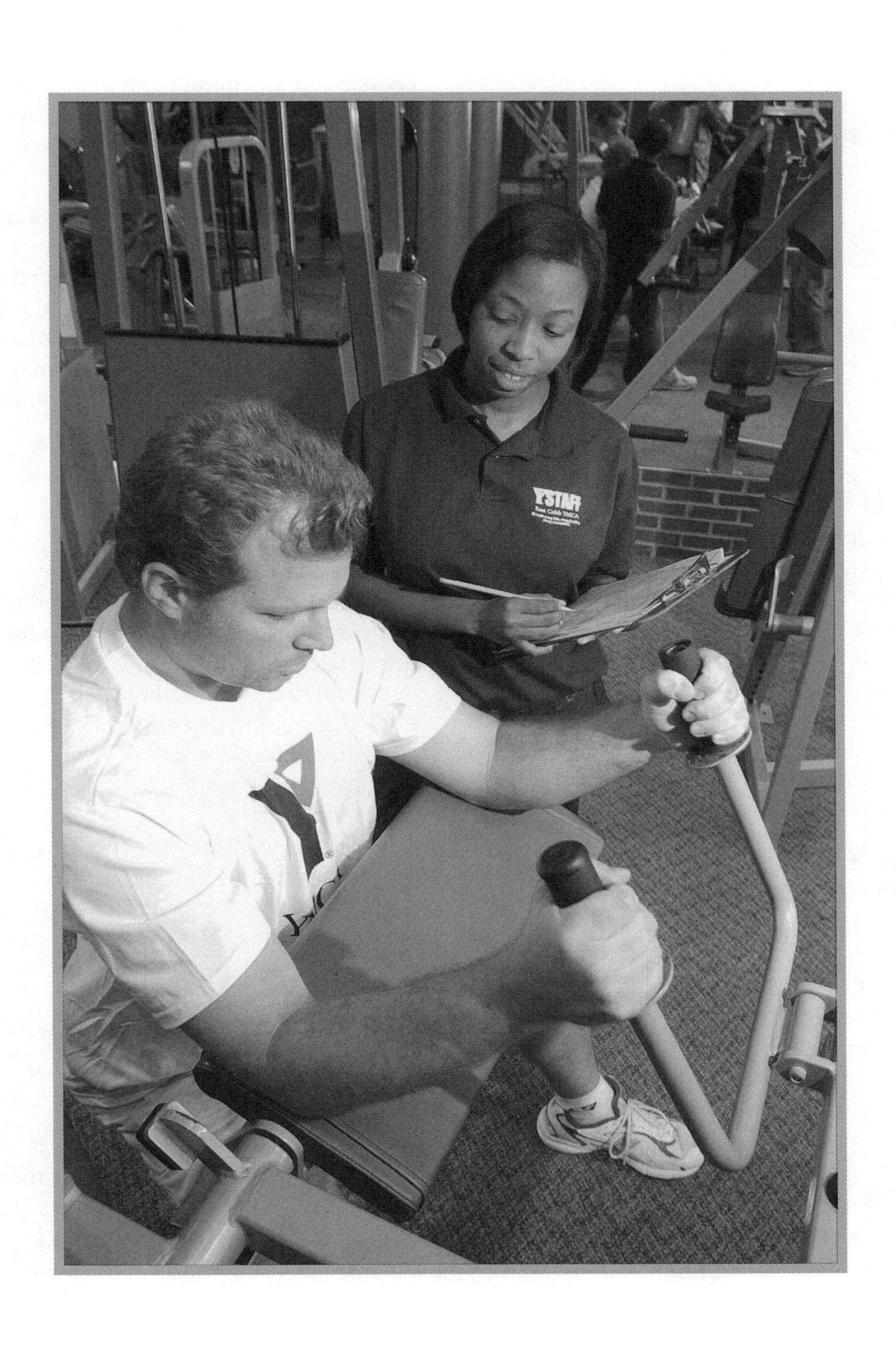

Personal training is by definition an individual activity that requires a personalized approach to help ensure safe and effective results. Health screening is the vital first step in developing a personal training program. It gives you essential information that will ensure safe and effective programming, and it also educates the participant about possible risks and realistic goals. Testing and assessing a participant using the YMCA of the USA's physical fitness test battery offers an opportunity to gather information related to the participant's current level of physical fitness. This information is essential in designing appropriate exercise programs and helping members develop exercise goals. Finally, an individual's exercise history must be taken into account when a personal training program is developed.

HEALTH SCREENING

The initial step for developing an individual exercise plan is screening for medical contraindications and coronary risk factors. The YMCA of the USA has established a series of forms and screening guidelines to help staff establish safe and effective programs for members. YMCA staff are strongly encouraged to administer the screening forms when participants begin a training program, and yearly thereafter. You should record, file, and use member forms when developing a personal exercise plan. The forms and their use are described in the following paragraphs, and copies of the forms are located in appendix B. They can be reproduced and used as needed for your YMCA personal training programs.

- **Health Screen Form (PAR-Q & You).** The PAR-Q is used to obtain general information about the participant's physical condition and to identify major risk factors. The YMCA of the USA recommends that all members and program participants complete this form before taking part in any activity. People with affirmative answers to the questions on the form should obtain medical clearance from a physician before being allowed to participate in YMCA fitness testing or exercise programs.
- **Medical Clearance Form.** This form is used by the participant's physician to report restrictions that should be placed on the participant during fitness testing or exercise programs. The physician should see both the form to be signed and the description of fitness testing and exercise programs. The description explains the general character of YMCA fitness testing and exercise programs and the risks associated with each.
- **Informed Consent for Fitness Testing.** This form ensures that the participant is aware of the risks involved in the fitness testing procedures. It documents that the description of the testing procedures has been read and that all questions concerning those procedures have been answered satisfactorily.
- **Informed Consent for Exercise Participation.** This form ensures that the participant is aware of the risks involved in exercise. It documents that the description of the exercise program has been read and all questions concerning the exercise program have been answered to the participant's satisfaction. It is recommended that each YMCA's legal counsel review this form to determine its effectiveness based on state laws.

The health screen form should be completed before a participant starts any program. The information obtained in these forms is valuable for educating participants about potential health and cardiorespiratory risk. These forms are not intended to be a substitute for a medical exam, but simply a means to obtain key health information. If a potential participant requires medical clearance before exercise participation, his or her physician must complete and sign the medical clearance form.

The informed consent forms are designed to notify participants of the inherent risks of fitness testing and exercise programs. Participants must read and sign them before fitness testing and participation in an exercise program.

PHYSICAL FITNESS ASSESSMENT

When members seek information about their fitness status, or when staff members feel it is appropriate, a physical fitness assessment can be administered to determine each participant's fitness level. The YMCA Fitness Testing and

Assessment protocol includes measurements in four key areas of physical fitness: cardiorespiratory endurance, body composition, flexibility, and muscular strength and endurance. Individual results are compared to tables of established norms that are age and gender specific and are used in a variety of ways:

- A fitness profile provides feedback to the participant on current strengths and weaknesses. After comparing the test results to norms, the person might be motivated to improve weak areas.
- Staff can use test results to help the participant set realistic short- and long-term goals and to assess progress over time. Setting goals and the subsequent reassessment can be effective motivational tools.
- Fitness test results can form the basis for exercise prescriptions. An appropriate exercise prescription ensures that participants start their program at the right level. A program that is too difficult or intense could cause injury or discouragement or both. And a program that starts at a level that is too low might not produce fitness benefits.

Although you might not be directly involved in performing fitness assessments, you should have a basic understanding of what the testing process is all about, which tests are generally conducted, how they are performed, and what test results will tell both participant and trainer. In the following section we briefly describe the standard YMCA of the USA fitness tests.

Cardiorespiratory Endurance

YMCAs might administer any of three kinds of cardiorespiratory tests: the cycle ergometer test, the bench step test, and the one-mile walking test. Details of these tests can be found in the *YMCA Fitness Testing and Assessment Manual* (cycle and bench step tests) and in the *YMCA Walk Reebok Instructor Manual* (one-mile walk test).

- **Cycle ergometer test.** This submaximal test in which the participant pedals a calibrated cycle ergometer at increasing workloads is designed to be safely administered by nonmedical personnel. Submaximal tests estimate aerobic capacity rather than actually measuring the maximum level. The person's heart rate response to the final workloads is used to estimate maximum capacity. An advantage to testing with the cycle is that the participant's body weight is supported by the machine, which makes the exercise easier on the body's joints than walking, jogging, running on the treadmill, or doing the bench step test. A disadvantage to the cycle ergometer test is that those unaccustomed to cycling might rapidly fatigue their thigh muscles. This could result in an elevated heart rate and the onset of fatigue due to the newness of activity, reducing the accuracy of the test results.
- **Bench step test.** The three-minute bench step test is also a safe submaximal test of cardiorespiratory fitness. The test, developed by Kasch and Boyer (1968), requires stepping in an established cadence up and down on a bench. The recovery heart rate from the test is used to determine the level of fitness. Although the bench step test is easy to administer, especially to a group, participants must carry their body weight up and down with each step. People who are overweight or those with joint problems might experience pain associated with the repetitive jarring of the up-and-down motion and might have difficulty completing the test.
- **One-mile walking test.** Fitness walking tests are a safe, easy way to assess cardiorespiratory fitness. The participant walks one mile as fast as possible and then takes his or her heart rate at the end of the test. The time in which the walk is completed and the heart rate are used to determine the fitness-level rating. The YMCA of the USA uses the one-mile walking test developed by The Cooper Institute for Aerobics Research. See the *YMCA Walk Reebok Instructor Manual* for more information on this test.

Body Composition

Body composition refers to lean body weight plus fat weight, which together make up total body weight. Fat weight is calculated by multiplying the total body weight by the percentage of body fat. The percentage of body fat is estimated from skinfold measurements. The *YMCA Fitness Testing and Assessment Manual* describes how to take these measurements.

Flexibility

No general test accurately reflects total-body flexibility. However, because of the incidence of low back pain and disability among the general population, the YMCA of the USA uses the trunk-flexion sit-and-reach test to measure the flexibility of the hip and back along with the elasticity of the hamstring muscle group (at the back of the upper leg).

Muscular Strength and Endurance

The bench press and the one-minute timed half-sit-up tests assess muscular strength and endurance. The latter is particularly important because it assesses abdominal strength and endurance, and the fitness status of abdominal muscles is related to correct posture and alignment of the pelvis. Weak abdominal muscles do not adequately support the pelvis, which can cause low back discomfort.

Test results can be summarized on a fitness profile summary sheet for each participant. Values recorded on this form can be quickly scanned to determine strengths and weaknesses.

For a detailed explanation of these assessments, refer to the *YMCA Fitness Testing and Assessment Manual*, available from the YMCA Program Store. The YMCA of the USA strongly recommends that certified YMCA Fitness Testing and Assessment Specialists perform these assessments. To be trained and certified to administer the test battery, staff must attend a YMCA Fitness Testing and Assessment Specialist certification course. This 40-hour training is available at selected YMCA of the USA Program Schools and other training sites across the country. Refer to the current YMCA of the USA Training Course Catalog or contact the YMCA of the USA for specific dates, locations, and the name of a contact person.

CONSULTATION AND DEVELOPMENT OF TRAINING GOALS

After the health screening and fitness assessment have been completed, discuss the results and the implications for a training program with the participant. Although it is important to address all of the fitness parameters (body composition, muscular strength, cardiorespiratory endurance, and joint flexibility), each person might have specific training objectives.

For example, some participants might want to lose weight, and others might want to gain weight. Some might be more concerned with muscular strength, while others are more concerned with cardiorespiratory endurance. Some might prefer upper-body conditioning, and others might prefer lower-body conditioning. Some might be more interested in physical appearance, while others are more interested in improved sports performance.

In addition to training objectives, the participant's exercise preferences and time constraints should be carefully considered when designing the fitness program. For example, some might prefer free weights, and others might prefer machines for strength training. Some might schedule 90-minute training sessions, and others might schedule 30-minute training sessions. Staff should be sensitive to these needs. A well-designed program will be of no benefit if it doesn't fit into the member's schedule.

EXERCISE HISTORY

Another factor that you should consider before designing a personal training program is the participant's previous exercise experience. People who have never exercised need a gradual introduction to training. Also, caution is recommended when training former athletes who have not exercised for several years; they may be inclined to train more intensely than they should. At the other extreme, endurance exercise enthusiasts who already train extensively might need to be guided into a more balanced program of physical activity. Flexibility and strength training are especially useful for endurance athletes to reduce their risk of overuse injuries. A sample Exercise History Form is included in figure 7.1.

Exercise History Form

1. Name ______________________________ Date ______________
2. Address ____
3. Phone number (home) ________________________
4. Age __________ Sex: M ______ F ______
5. Height _____________
6. Occupation: Physical ______ Nonphysical ______
7. Do you currently exercise: Yes ______ No ______

   If you answered yes; how long have you been exercising? __________________

   Briefly describe your program: ______________________________

   ____

   ____

8. Rate yourself on a scale of 1 to 5 (1 indicating the lowest value and 5 the highest) circling the number that applies most closely:

a. Daily stress level:	1	2	3	4	5
b. Competitive personality (pertaining to physical activity)	1	2	3	4	5
c. Aerobic (endurance) fitness level:	1	2	3	4	5
d. Muscular (strength) level:	1	2	3	4	5
e. Flexibility level:	1	2	3	4	5

9. Check the description below that most closely describes your diet:

   _____ High fat, high sodium, low carbohydrate

   _____ Low fat, low sodium, high carbohydrate

   _____ Moderate fat, moderate sodium, moderate carbohydrate

   _____ Other: Briefly describe your typical dietary habits: __________________

   ____

   ____

10. Are you on a calorie-restrictive diet?

    Yes _____ No _____

11. Based on your lifestyle, how much time can you comfortably allocate per workout session? Check the answer that most closely applies:

    _____ 45 minutes or less _____ 45 to 60 minutes _____ 60 to 90 minutes

12. Briefly describe the goal(s) you have set for your exercise program:

    ____

    ____

    ____

Figure 7.1 Exercise history form.

CHAPTER 8

Designing Individual Exercise Programs

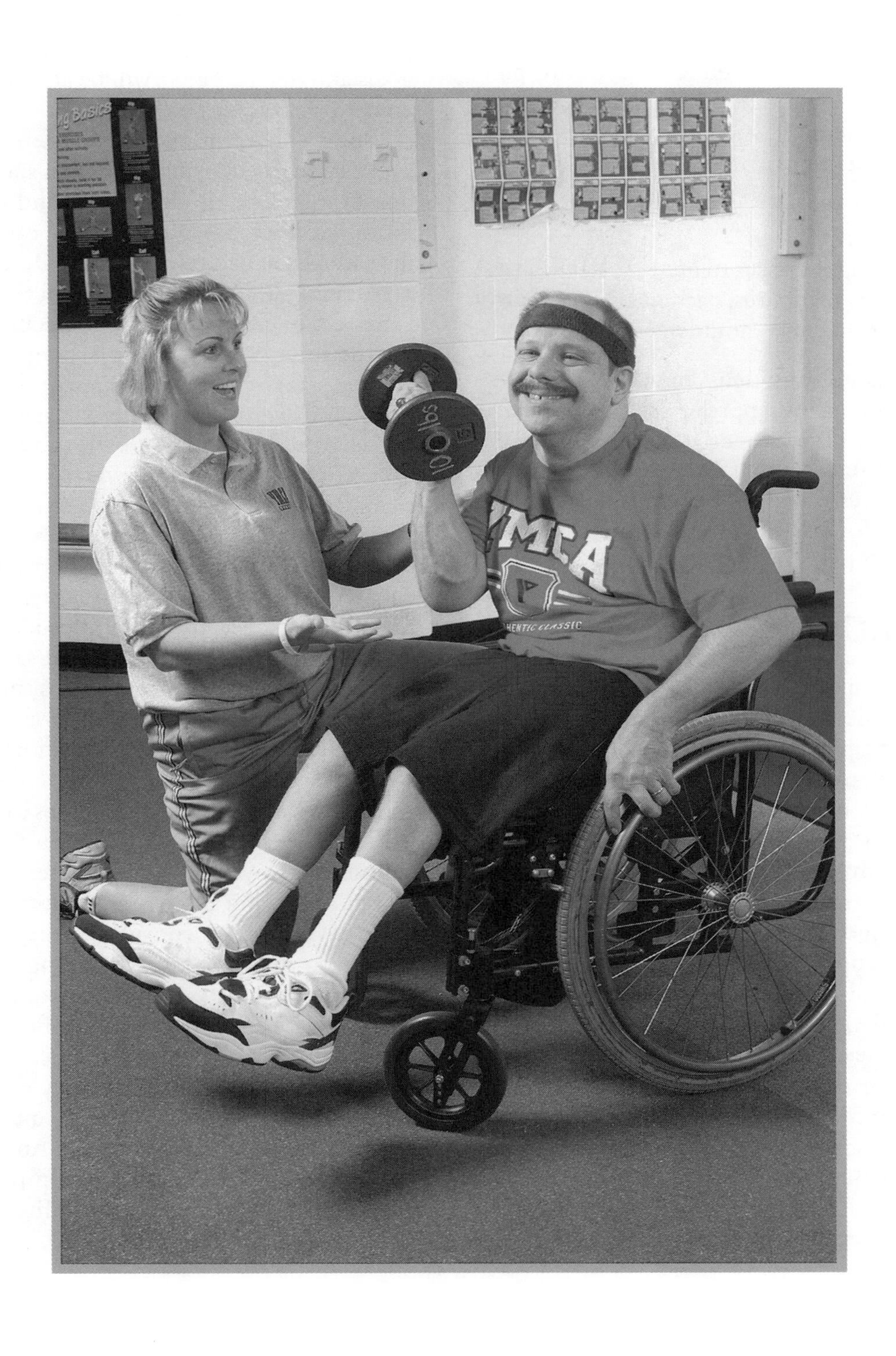

As a personal training instructor, you have the unique opportunity to develop individualized exercise programs to meet the fitness needs of YMCA members. In developing programs that best meet members' expectations in a safe and effective manner, you should keep participants' distinctive goals, interests, health and fitness status, age, and motivation in mind.

A comprehensive personal training program includes the following three components:

- Aerobic exercise to enhance cardiorespiratory endurance, typically by means of sustained large-muscle activity (such as walking, running, swimming, cycling, stair climbing, or rowing)
- Strength training exercise to develop the major muscle groups
- Stretching exercises to increase flexibility in the major joint structures, particularly the injury-prone hip, trunk, and shoulder areas

In this chapter we discuss how to design exercise programs using appropriate guidelines, as well as how to implement these programs and to modify them so that the member's fitness progresses over time. We conclude with recommendations for orienting new participants and working with participants effectively.

PROGRAM DESIGN

Every fitness program should include comprehensive physical conditioning based on sound exercise principles, individual goals, and personal training preferences. This approach reduces the risk of injury, increases the rate of compliance, and facilitates the desired fitness results. Previous chapters of this book have presented information on health screening, fitness assessment, and training components of cardiorespiratory fitness, muscular strength and endurance, and flexibility. This chapter discusses how these components can be combined to provide a comprehensive exercise program for each of your participants. There are four steps for designing a comprehensive exercise prescription. The first three are to screen for health, assess physical fitness, and select the exercise mode for each specific training component (cardiorespiratory, strength, and flexibility). The fourth step is to quantify the intensity, frequency, and duration of each workout based on the person's capabilities and goals.

Guidelines for Exercise Programming

Health screening and physical fitness assessments provide the personal trainer with information on each member he or she works with. The trainer then uses that information to design an exercise program that will meet each member's needs and goals and that he or she will be able to follow and enjoy for a long time.

Once you have assessed a person's fitness capacity, learned his or her health status through questionnaires and clearances, and determined his or her interests and goals, you can provide an individualized exercise program. To be effective, a program should be based on all three of these factors. You can then develop specific guidelines for the intensity, duration, frequency, type, and progression of exercise—the integral components of a sound exercise program. Because the reasons for exercising can vary greatly among people at different fitness levels, the need for precision in recommending exercise also varies. Whereas competitive athletes and people limited by disease might need careful and precise programs, average, apparently healthy adults rarely need precision, and a generalized program is usually adequate. The important point is that the same training principles apply to everyone. Most people select activities that they enjoy or that provide social and recreational interaction. Modifications are usually associated with the absence or presence of medical contraindications, types of activities to be avoided, the initial level of fitness, the intensity of participation, and the rate of improvement expected.

The following discussion focuses on the five primary factors to consider in developing fitness programs for apparently healthy adults: frequency, intensity, duration, mode of activity, and rate of progression. These five factors are discussed for the three primary components of physical fitness: cardiorespiratory conditioning, muscle strength and endurance, and flexibility. This information is based on the American College of Sports Medicine's position paper on the recommended quantity and quality of exercise training for healthy adults (1998).

Cardiorespiratory Conditioning

1. Frequency of training: 3 to 5 days per week.

2. Intensity: 55/65 to 90 percent of maximal heart rate. Exercise of low and moderate intensity provides important health benefits and results in increased levels of fitness in people who are sedentary or at low fitness levels. Higher intensity of exercise is appropriate as training progresses and fitness level increases.

3. Duration of training: 20 to 60 minutes of continuous aerobic activity. The length of time spent exercising aerobically depends on the relative intensity of the activity. For example, low-intensity activities should be conducted for a longer time, particularly early in a training program.

4. Mode of activity: An appropriate activity for developing cardiorespiratory fitness is one that uses the large muscle groups, can be maintained at submaximal levels continuously, and is rhythmical. Examples are walking, jogging, running, bicycling, swimming, aerobic dancing, machine-based stair climbing, rowing, or cross-country skiing. Activities such as walking, jogging, or cycling are particularly good activities for a beginner's exercise program.

5. Rate of progression: Because of the body's ability to adapt to the stresses placed on it (referred to as the *training effect*), people are able to gradually increase the total amount of work they can do over time. With cardiorespiratory exercise, the workload can be increased by increasing the intensity of the exercise, the duration of the exercise, or by a combination of the two. The most significant training effects are typically observed during the first six to eight weeks of an exercise program. A person's exercise prescription can be adjusted as they become more fit. The extent of the adjustment depends on the person involved and his or her performance during exercise sessions.

Muscle Strength and Endurance

1. Frequency of training: A minimum of two days per week.

2. Intensity: Moderate-intensity resistance training sufficient to develop and maintain lean body tissue.

3. Duration of training: 1 set of 8 to 12 repetitions of each exercise.

4. Mode of activity: 8 to 10 exercises that train the major muscle groups.

5. Rate of progression: In general, when 12 repetitions of an exercise can be completed with the proper form and technique, the resistance can be increased by 5 percent or less. This may not be practical in all circumstances, and each case must be evaluated individually.

Flexibility

1. Frequency of training: A minimum of two or three days per week.

2. Intensity: To a position of mild discomfort.

3. Duration of training: 10 to 30 seconds for each stretch.

4. Mode of activity: Stretching should include appropriate static and dynamic techniques with an emphasis on the low back and hamstring area because of the prevalence of low back pain.

5. Rate of progression: Gradually increase the time of each stretch by 2 to 6 seconds.

See table 8.1 for a sample training outline.

Developing an Appropriate Exercise Program

A variety of exercise programs can produce desired fitness results for any given member. Successful programs can vary considerably in terms of mode, frequency, intensity, and duration. In addition, some people will achieve greater results than others, and some achieve results more quickly. For these reasons, it is important to tailor each exercise program to the individual.

Members who have been relatively sedentary for years should be counseled to progress slowly. They should begin exercising at a level that they can successfully complete and then gradually increase the amount of work they perform. This slow progression not only reduces the potential for injury, it also ensures appropriate adaptations in previously unused or underused muscles. On the other hand, active people might progress more rapidly and are ready for greater physical challenges. As a skilled personal trainer, monitor how participants are adapting to an exercise

Table 8.1 Sample Training Outline

Warm-up activity	5 minutes
Cardiorespiratory exercise Examples	20 min—choose one or cross-train Running Swimming Cycling Stair climbing Rowing Walking Cross-country skiing Basketball Racquetball Group aerobics
Strength exercise Examples	20 min—all major muscle groups Leg extension (quadriceps) Leg curl (hamstrings) Chest cross (chest) Pullover (upper back) Lateral raise (shoulders) Arm extension (triceps) Arm curl (biceps) Trunk extension (low back) Trunk flexion (abdominals) Neck extension (neck extensors) Neck flexion (neck flexors)
Flexibility and cool-down activity	15 min

Reprinted, by permission, from the *YMCA Exercise Instructor Manual*, © YMCA of the USA, 1995, Human Kinetics.

routine and make necessary and appropriate adjustments to their prescriptions. With periodic adjustments as appropriate, you will give each member a prescription for a lifetime of health and fitness.

PROGRAM IMPLEMENTATION, PROGRESSION, AND REDESIGN

The first step in implementing a program is conducting an orientation with the member. This step is essential to the development of the personal trainer to member relationship, as well as the safety and success of the program. Unless there is a contraindication, the initial program should be followed for four to eight weeks. This allows the participant time to establish a familiar exercise routine, to develop a degree of training consistency, and to obtain observable results from the fitness program.

Record individual programs on a form like the one shown in figure 8.1, a workout card, or a log book for each participant. Examples of workout cards are included at the end of the chapter (see figures 8.2 to 8.4 on pages 166-168. Once the program is established on paper, implement it in a persistent and progressive manner.

PROGRESSION RATE AND PROGRAM REDESIGN

Because the human body tends to adapt to a given exercise program, the training protocol should change periodically. The rate of progression in any exercise program depends on many factors, including the participant's initial fitness and health status, age, motivation, and the frequency and intensity of training. Many beginning exercisers will make greater measurable gains during the first three to six months of an exercise program than current exercisers will, relatively speaking. The following three progression stages in an exercise program is based on the American College of Sports Medicine's guidelines (1995):

1. **Initial conditioning stage.** This stage typically lasts four to six weeks. The ACSM recommends that the intensity, duration, and frequency of exercise sessions be at the low end of the training ranges during this stage, to minimize muscle soreness, injury, discomfort, and discouragement. Gradual progression is urged to help ensure that members feel successful in modifying their lifestyles.

2. **Improvement conditioning stage.** This stage usually lasts 12 to 20 weeks, with a more rapid rate of progression. Intensity, duration, and frequency all should be gradually increased to at least the middle of the recommended training ranges. Discuss with the member the possibility of retesting all fitness components about three months after the program starts, to help members maintain interest and motivation. Fitness objectives can be altered after the retesting session to help members aim for higher goals or to maintain goals already attained.

3. **Maintenance conditioning stage.** Once the desired level of fitness is reached, the maintenance stage of an exercise program is reached. This stage usually begins five to six months after the start of training and can last a lifetime. To ensure compliance, the program should be enjoyable, fit into the member's daily schedule, meet his or her personal needs and goals, and be adaptable to changes in location.

Numerous research studies have shown that people must regularly engage in physical activity in order to maintain fitness benefits. Stopping exercise training results in a rapid decrease in both cardiorespiratory and muscular conditioning. However, people can maintain physical fitness even if they work out less, as long as they maintain the intensity. It takes a lot of work to achieve desirable fitness levels, but once the habit is established, maintaining fitness is a bit easier. Recognize, however, that many members need continual help in maintaining the motivation that will enable them to continue to enjoy the fitness benefits that they have worked so hard to attain.

Recommended First-Session Guidelines

The first session with new members is critical to making them feel comfortable with you and in the training environment. When teaching members their new training programs, cover the basic information about each piece of equipment or each exercise.

- **Explain the equipment.** Demonstrate correct positioning on the equipment (either cardio or strength) and how to operate the machine.
- **Demonstrate the exercise.** Point out proper form and technique.
- **Adjust the equipment.** Ask the member to position himself or herself on the equipment, then make necessary adjustments for size. Explain that this will help the member use proper technique and improve safety. Write down all of the adjustments on the member's workout card.
- **Watch the member perform the exercise.** Ask the member to attempt a trial exercise slowly and with little resistance, providing oral cues about form, body alignment, and exercise technique. Cover the following points:

  Major muscle group used

  Proper starting position

  Description of movement

  Breathing

  Speed of movement

  Proper grip for strength exercises
- **Set the starting level.** Cardiorespiratory conditioning should begin at a pace and duration that the member can comfortably handle. Use caution and don't ask him or her to attempt too much too soon. As a general guideline for strength training, start members with the heaviest weight they can lift for 8 to 12 repetitions with good technique and form. Document the weight on the member's workout card. Beginners should use a resistance that allows them to perform 12 repetitions.
- **Discuss the progression.** Explain that the member should perform at the starting level and gradually progress in intensity and duration. For example, strength exercise should progress to where 12 repetitions can be accomplished comfortably; then the weight can be increased by 5 percent.
- **Answer questions.** Ask if the member has questions. Review the notes on the workout card. Review equipment adjustments.
- **Set a schedule.** Discuss the days of the week and times that the member will work out. New exercisers generally need to set a specific schedule, which helps them adhere to a routine in the beginning stages of an exercise program.

The YMCA Exercise Program Design Form

Warm-Up

Purpose: To gradually elevate the heart rate and increase body temperature by engaging in 5–10 minutes of low-intensity activity.

Cardiorespiratory Fitness

Purpose: To improve one's cardiorespiratory system by continuous, rhythmic, and vigorous exercise for 20–30 minutes, 3 times a week.

Frequency: Days a week of exercise: Mon. Tues. Wed. Thurs. Fri. Sat. Sun.

Intensity: % of heart rate: Max. HR – Age × 55% = Low end of training HR range

_______ – _______ × _______ = _______________

Intensity: % of heart rate: Max. HR – Age × 90% = Upper end of training HR range

_______ – _______ × _______ = _______________

Duration—No. of minutes per session: 10–20 20–30 30–45

Mode—select activity: _______________________________

Cool-Down

Purpose: To gradually decrease the heart rate by slowing the intensity and pace of the activity for 5–10 minutes.

Muscle Strength and Endurance

Purpose: To develop muscular strength and endurance using various calisthenics and weight training exercises for 10–20 minutes.

Exercises:

Muscle: _______________ Exercise: _______________

Resistance: _______________ Repetitions: _______________

Muscle: _______________ Exercise: _______________

Resistance: _______________ Repetitions: _______________

Muscle: _______________ Exercise: _______________

Resistance: _______________ Repetitions: _______________

Muscle: _______________ Exercise: _______________

Resistance: _______________ Repetitions: _______________

Muscle: _______________ Exercise: _______________

Resistance: _______________ Repetitions: _______________

Muscle: _______________ Exercise: _______________

Resistance: _______________ Repetitions: _______________

Flexibility:

Purpose: To stretch the major muscles and joints using static stretching techniques for 5–10 minutes.

Exercises: _______________________________

____

____

Figure 8.1 Sample program form.

Reprinted, by permission, from *YMCA Strength Training,* © YMCA of the USA, 1994, Human Kinetics.

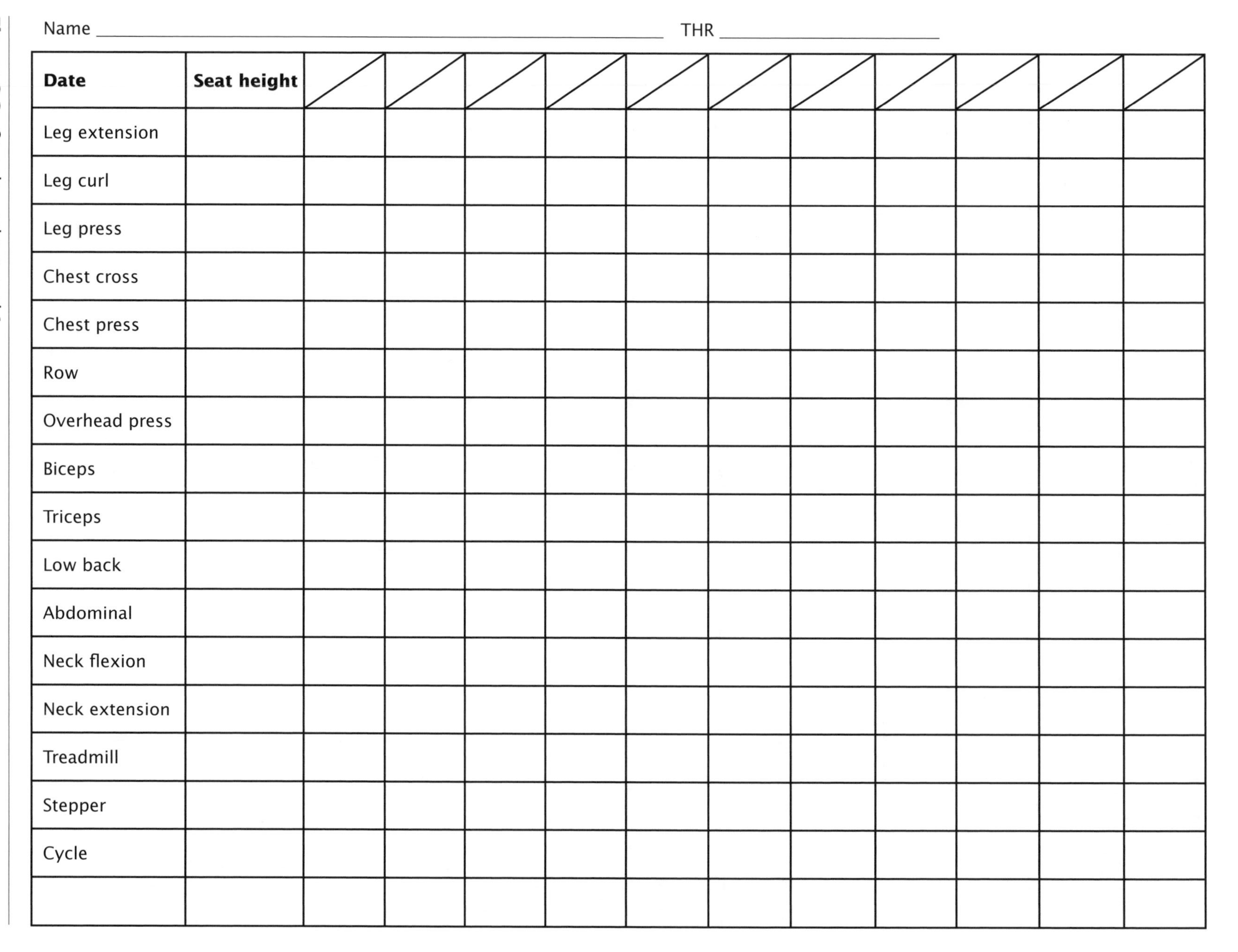

Name ______________________ THR ______________________

Date	**Seat height**											
Leg extension												
Leg curl												
Leg press												
Chest cross												
Chest press												
Row												
Overhead press												
Biceps												
Triceps												
Low back												
Abdominal												
Neck flexion												
Neck extension												
Treadmill												
Stepper												
Cycle												

Figure 8.2 Sample workout card 1.

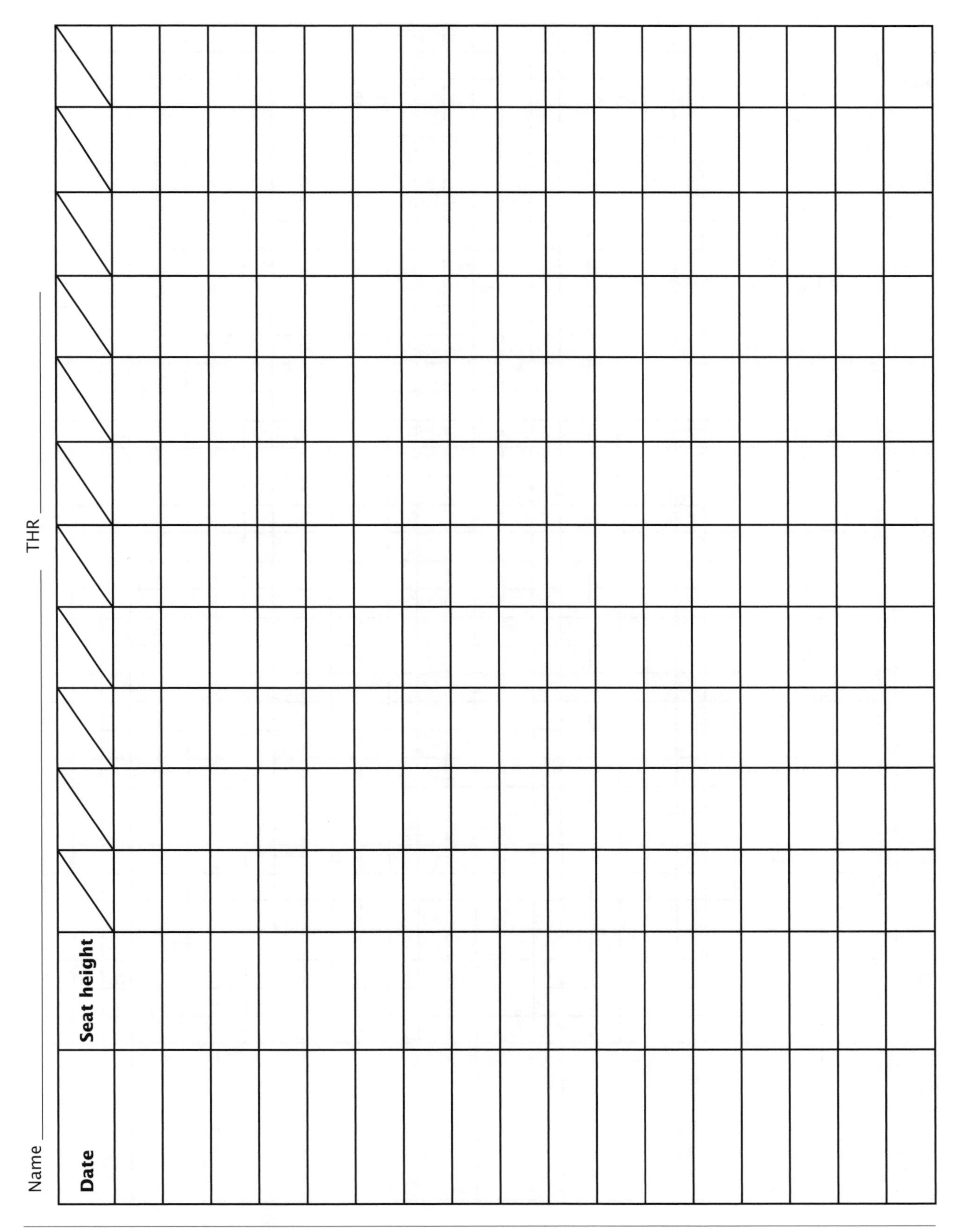

Figure 8.3 Sample workout card 2.

Name ______________________________

Date	**SET**	**WGT**	**REP**	**SET**	**WGT**	**REP**	**SET**	**WGT**	**REP**	**SET**	**WGT**	**REP**	**SET**	**WGT**	**REP**	**SET**	**WGT**	**REP**	**SET**	**WGT**	**REP**	**SET**	**WGT**	**REP**	**SET**	**WGT**	**REP**	**SET**	**WGT**	**REP**	**SET**	**WGT**	**REP**	**SET**	**WGT**	**REP**

Figure 8.4 Sample workout card 3.

CHAPTER 9

Nutrition

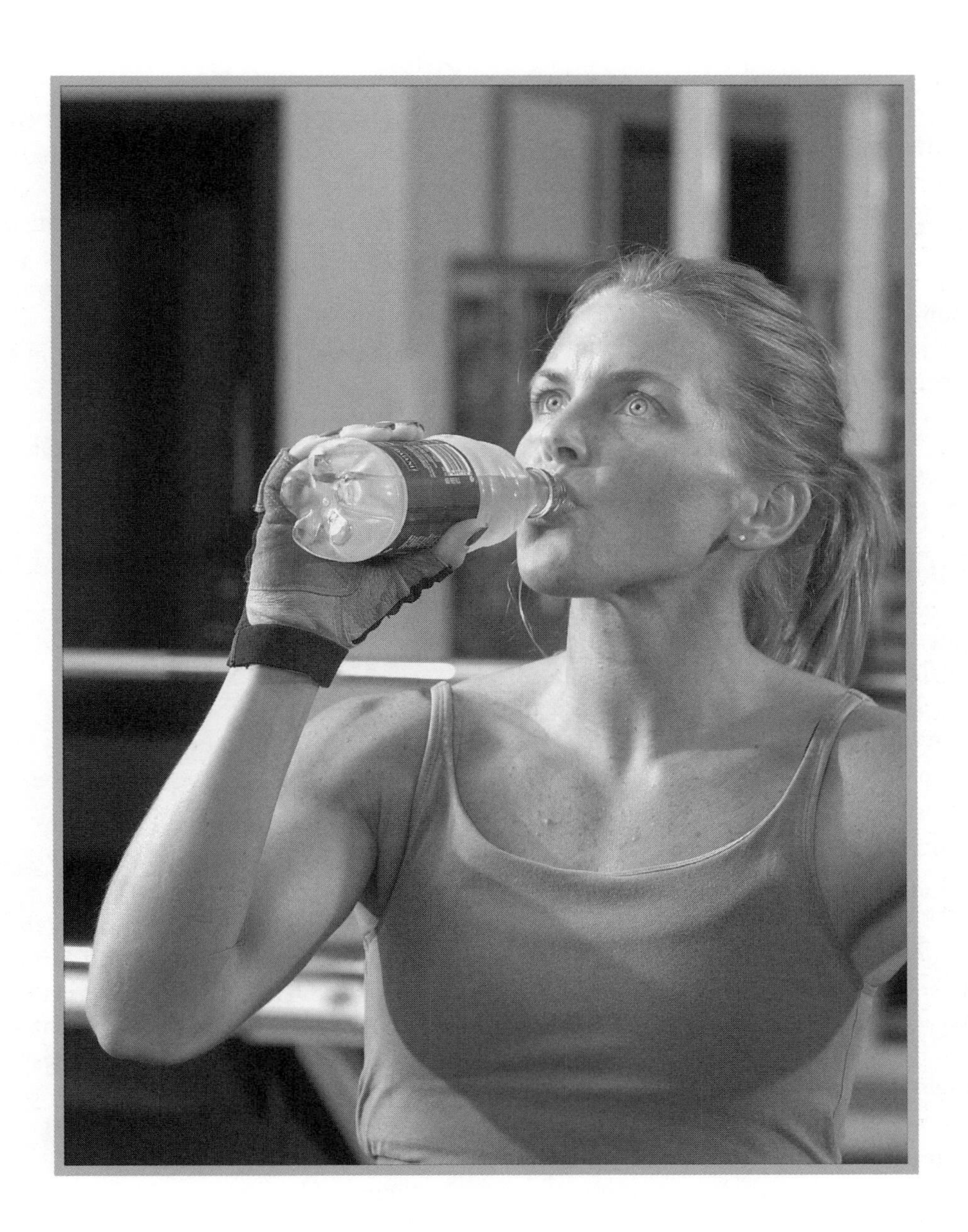

From chapter 2 of *Personal Training Manual*, National Exercise Trainers Association (NETA), 2001.

The study of nutrition involves complex theories and diverse issues. It is vital that fitness professionals understand basic nutrition principles. Our dietary habits affect our overall health and exercise performance. According to a 1991 American Dietetic Association survey of American eating habits, only 28 percent of those surveyed rated themselves knowledgeable of basic food guidelines.

In recent years, the science of sports nutrition has dramatically altered what and how athletes eat. The emphasis is on the application of sound nutrition principles such as promoting the consumption of ample carbohydrates for fuel, sufficient protein to build and repair muscle tissue, and plenty of water. Restrictive dietary habits are not recommended. Eating regular, well-balanced meals of nutrient-dense, low-fat foods, getting regular exercise, and maintaining reasonable body weight can substantially influence health and longevity.

TERMINOLOGY

Antioxidant Vitamins: substances that attach to harmful metabolic products (free radicals) and are thought to reduce the risk of developing cardiovascular disease and cancer. Beta-carotene, vitamins E and C are touted as antioxidants.

Calorie: a measure of energy, also called kilocalorie.

Macronutrient: the three food categories (fats, carbohydrates, and proteins) that supply energy.

Percent Daily Value (%DV): each macronutrient, sodium and cholesterol listed on a nutrition label is expressed as a percentage of the total daily calorie intake that a serving supplies based on a 2000 calorie daily caloric intake.

Recommended Daily Allowance (RDA): these are recommended daily values for most vitamins and minerals that were developed by the National Research Council of the Academy of Sciences. The RDA's are thought to be adequate to promote good nutrition in the majority of healthy people.

Weight Bearing Exercise: represents any exercise that requires a person to bear his or her own body weight during the exercise activity (i.e., walking, running, cross-country skiing, resistance training).

DIETARY GUIDELINES

One of the promotion strategies designed to encourage Americans to eat a healthful diet is the *Dietary Guidelines* developed by the Department of Health and Human Services and the U.S. Department of Agriculture (USDA). These guidelines were first published in 1980 and are revised every 5 years based on developments in scientific research. They apply to healthy Americans ages two years and up. The 2005 *Dietary Guidelines* identifies 41 key recommmendations, of which 23 are for the general public and 18 for special populations. They are grouped into nine general topics:

- Adequate nutrients within calorie needs
- Weight management
- Physical activity
- Food groups to encourage
- Fats
- Carbohydrates
- Sodium and potassium
- Alcoholic beverages
- Food safety

FOOD GUIDE PYRAMID

A more recent promotion strategy introduced by the Department of Health and Human Services and the USDA in August 1992 is the *Food Guide Pyramid.* (Note: The most recent version was released in April 2005.) It is a visual tool that encourages Americans to choose a wide variety of foods, in recommended servings and serving sizes to get the required nutrients. (See figure 9.1 on pages 172-173.)

ESSENTIAL NUTRIENTS

Essential nutrients are those necessary for body functions that are not synthesized in the body. They include carbohydrates, protein, fat, vitamins, minerals, and water.

Carbohydrates

- Provide approximately 4 calories per gram
- USDA recommends that carbohydrates represent 55-60% total caloric intake
- Most readily available source of energy—most important nutrient in energy production

All carbohydrates must be converted into their simplest form, glucose. Glucose is the only form of carbohydrate the body can use as a fuel source. Any glucose not used immediately is stored in the liver and skeletal muscles in the form of glycogen. Excess glucose can also be converted into fatty acids and stored as adipose tissue (body fat). Fat cannot be converted back to glucose and can only be utilized for energy as fatty acids.

Substantial reduction of dietary carbohydrates may result in significant weight loss, but is primarily from loss of lean muscle mass and fluid. If carbohydrates are unavailable or in very limited supply, protein can be used for energy. When protein is used as a fuel source the body must eliminate excessive quantities of fluid to complete the metabolic process. This loss of fluid can result in a dramatic loss of body weight but is temporary and can be very unhealthy. Weight is regained rapidly once "normal" eating is resumed whereas lean muscle tissue may not be regained leaving the person at a higher level of body fat than before carbohydrate restriction.

Carbohydrates are subdivided into three main types of sugars differentiated by their chemical structure. *Monosaccharides* (glucose, galactose, and fructose) are the simplest, consisting of a single saccharide molecule. *Disaccharides* (sucrose, lactose, and maltose) consist of two saccharide molecules linked together. *Polysaccharides* (starch and cellulose) consist of a long chain of many saccharide molecules. Polysaccharides are generally associated with the term *complex carbohydrates*. They require energy to digest, entering the blood stream more gradually than simple sugars and can be found in cereals, potatoes, rice, pasta, and bread.

Carbohydrates can be divided into two categories: simple carbohydrates and complex carbohydrates. *Simple carbohydrates* are generally associated with a low-nutrient density and include honey, corn syrup, and refined sugars such as table sugar. *Complex carbohydrates* are those carbohydrate sources that are nutrient dense, such as whole grains, vegetables, and fruits. They are typically high in essential vitamins and minerals, contain longer chain sugars (polysaccharides) and contain dietary fiber (fiber is discussed on page 176). The USDA recommends that 55-60% of the total number of calories consumed be in the form of carbohydrates. Only 10% of the total number of calories consumed should be in the form of simple carbohydrates.

Protein

- Provides approximately 4 calories per gram
- USDA recommends that protein represent approximately 10-15% of the total caloric intake
- Adult requirement–0.8 grams of protein per kilogram of body weight (infants to about 14 years old require more protein than adults)

Protein supplies the body with amino acids. Amino acids are absorbed and used primarily to build new and rebuild damaged body proteins such as hair, skin, muscles, cartilage, hemoglobin, enzymes, hormones, and various proteins in the blood. Unused amino acids are stored as body fat. The waste products from fat conversion must be excreted in the urine, requiring additional work for the kidneys. While protein provides the basic building blocks for body tissues, research has not shown that mega-doses of protein (amino acids) will increase muscle tissue growth during training or contribute significantly to energy needs.

Protein quality counts. There are 20 required amino acids found in the human body. Eight to ten are considered essential. *Essential amino acids* must be ingested as part of one's regular diet because the body cannot manufacture them. The other required amino acids can be constructed from other substances. Amino acids can be combined in innumerable ways to form thousands of different proteins. High-quality or *complete proteins* contain all the amino acids, including the essential amino acids. Complete proteins include foods from the meat, fish, poultry, eggs, and dairy products. Lower quality or *incomplete proteins* are found in vegetables, fruit, legumes,

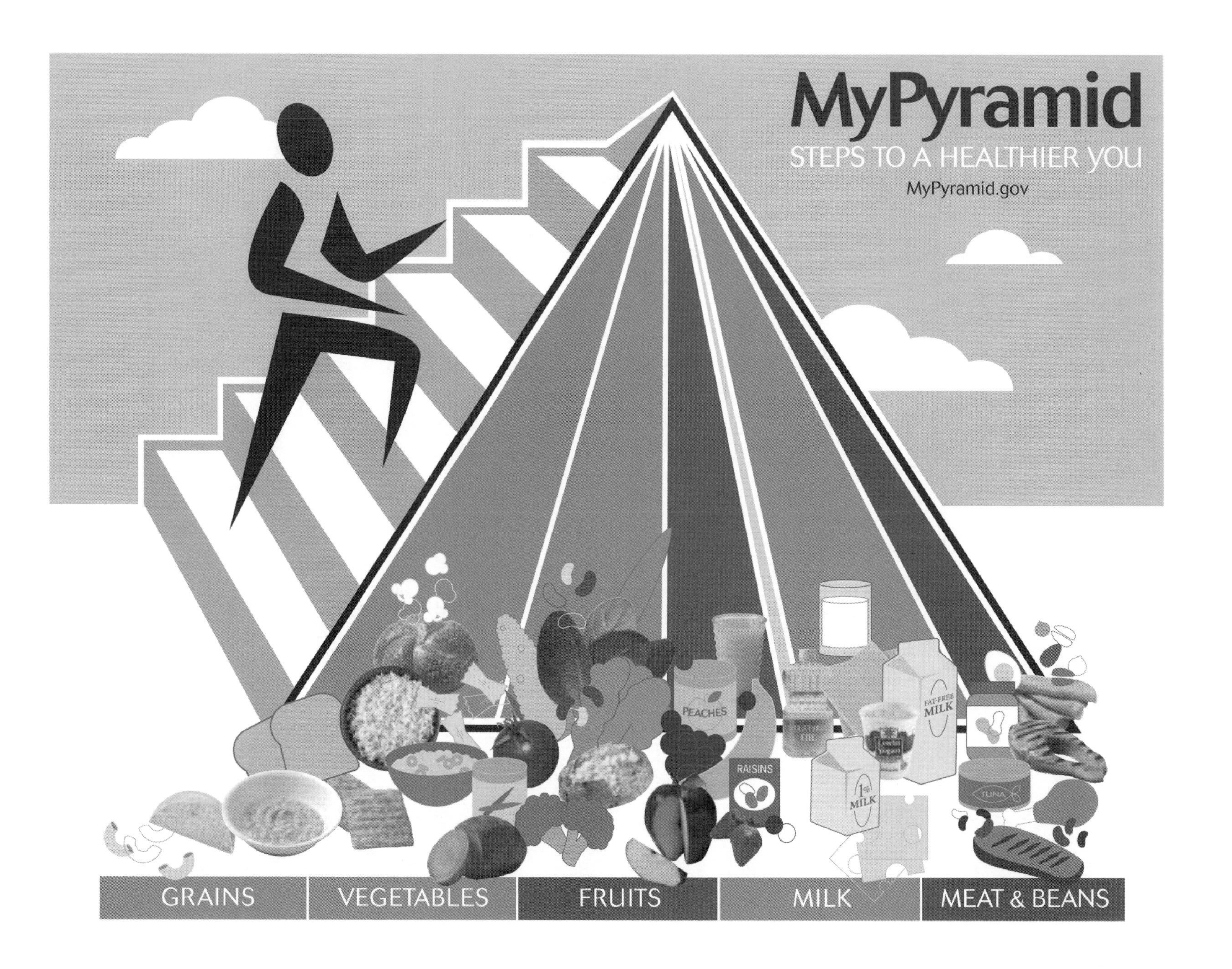

MyPyramid
STEPS TO A HEALTHIER YOU
MyPyramid.gov
PEACHES
RAISINS
FAT-FREE MILK
1% MILK
TUNA
GRAINS
VEGETABLES
FRUITS
MILK
MEAT & BEANS

GRAINS *Make half your grains whole*	VEGETABLES *Vary your veggies*	FRUITS *Focus on fruits*	MILK *Get your calcium-rich foods*	MEAT & BEANS *Go lean with protein*
Eat at least 3 oz. of whole-grain cereals, breads, crackers, rice, or pasta every day 1 oz. is about 1 slice of bread, about 1 cup of breakfast cereal, or ½ cup of cooked rice, cereal, or pasta	Eat more dark-green veggies like broccoli, spinach, and other dark leafy greens Eat more orange vegetables like carrots and sweetpotatoes Eat more dry beans and peas like pinto beans, kidney beans, and lentils	Eat a variety of fruit Choose fresh, frozen, canned, or dried fruit Go easy on fruit juices	Go low-fat or fat-free when you choose milk, yogurt, and other milk products If you don't or can't consume milk, choose lactose-free products or other calcium sources such as fortified foods and beverages	Choose low-fat or lean meats and poultry Bake it, broil it, or grill it Vary your protein routine—choose more fish, beans, peas, nuts, and seeds
For a 2,000-calorie diet, you need the amounts below from each food group. To find the amounts that are right for you, go to MyPyramid.gov.				
Eat 6 oz. every day	Eat 2½ cups every day	Eat 2 cups every day	Get 3 cups every day; for kids aged 2 to 8, it's 2	Eat 5½ oz. every day

Find your balance between food and physical activity	**Know the limits on fats, sugars, and salt (sodium)**
▪ Be sure to stay within your daily calorie needs ▪ Be physically active for at least 30 minutes most days of the week. ▪ About 60 minutes a day of physical activity may be needed to prevent weight gain. ▪ For sustaining weight loss, at least 60 to 90 minutes a day of physical activity may be required. ▪ Children and teenagers should be physically active for 60 minutes every day, or most days.	▪ Make most of your fat sources from fish, nuts, and vegetable oils. ▪ Limit solid fats like butter, margarine, shortening, and lard, as well as foods that contain these. ▪ Check the Nutrition Facts label to keep saturated fats, *trans* fats, and sodium low. ▪ Choose food and beverages low in added sugars. Added sugars contribute calories with few, if any, nutrients.

Figure 9.1 The Food Guide Pyramid.
Courtesy of the United States Department of Agriculture.

and grains. They are incomplete because they are missing one or more of the (essential) amino acids. Combining complete and incomplete protein foods works well to form a complete protein. Grains, seeds, and legumes teamed up with any plant protein forms a complete protein source (see table 9.1). For example, dry beans, peas, lentils, and peanuts eaten with any whole grain food provides a quality protein, Tofu is made from coagulated soymilk. Although it is not from an animal source, tofu provides a complete protein source. It is a high quality alternative to animal protein, is low in saturated fats, low in calories, and is cholesterol free.

Research has yet to define a specific amount of protein needed by sports-active people. Individuals who may require more protein than the current RDA include athletes, intense exercisers, and dieters who consume insufficient calories.

Fat

- Provides approximately 9 calories per gram
- USDA recommends that fats represent 30% or less of total caloric intake (10% saturated fats, 10% monounsaturated fats, and 10% polyunsaturated fats)
- Linoleic acid is the only essential fatty acid that must be ingested because the body cannot manufacture it

Fats provide more than twice the energy as the same amount of protein or carbohydrates. They are important in energy production, temperature regulation, distribution of vitamins A, D, E and K, and protect vital internal organs.

During digestion, dietary fats are broken down into fatty acids and glycerol, forming triglycerides. *Triglycerides* are three molecules of fatty acids plus (+) one molecule of glycerol. Any fatty acids not used as energy are transported in the blood as *lipoproteins* and stored as triglycerides in the *adipose tissue* (fat cells). Stored adipose tissue, or fat, can be used to provide energy. Triglycerides are divided into saturated and unsaturated fats.

Saturated fatty acids generally come from animal products and are solid at room temperature. The vegetable oil from palm kernel, coconut, palm, and cocoa oils also contain large proportions of saturated fat. Consuming saturated fat which are generally associated with high cholesterol content (discussed on page 177) also stimulates the liver to produce excess cholesterol.

Unsaturated fatty acids are further divided into mono- and polyunsaturated fats and are usually liquid at room temperature. Unsaturated fatty acids are generally associated with plant sources but fish and chicken also contain unsaturated fats. Healthy sources are canola, olive, and fish oils. It is heart-wise to cook with mono- or polyunsaturated fats versus saturated fats.

Vitamins

- Thiamin
- Niacin
- Folic Acid
- Pantothenic Acid
- Riboflavin
- Biotin
- Vitamin K
- Vitamin A

Table 9.1 Protein Teams

Animal and grain proteins	Animal and legume proteins	Legume and grain proteins
Milk and cereal	Cheese and bean stew	Baked beans and brown bread
Cheese sandwich	Milk and rice pudding	Blackeyed peas and rice
Tuna and rice casserole	Ham and split pea soup	Beans and cornbread
Macaroni and cheese		Peanut butter sandwich
Cheese pizza		Beans and pasta

- Vitamin B-6
- Vitamin B-12
- Vitamin C
- Vitamin D
- Vitamin E

Vitamins are organic substances essential to the normal function of the human body. They help control the growth of body tissues, production and release of energy, and *(antioxidant vitamins)* may be effective in decreasing the risk for developing cardiovascular disease and certain forms of cancer. The human body only requires small amounts, and there is no evidence that vitamins taken in excess of the USDA Recommended Daily Allowance (RDA) of any vitamin will enhance performance. However, vitamin deficiencies can impair physical performance and health. Special care must be taken to not consume excessive amounts of *fat-soluble (A, D, K and E) vitamins* that are stored in the body fat. Excess vitamin A and D can retard growth and permanently damage organs. Excess *water-soluble vitamins*, such as the Band C vitamins, are excreted in the urine. Taking vitamin supplements will not alleviate stress, supply energy, or make up for lost sleep and missed meals but may be helpful in maintaining overall health.

Minerals

- Calcium
- Magnesium
- Potassium
- Chromium
- Fluoride
- Iron
- Molybdenum
- Zinc
- Chloride
- Phosphorous
- Sodium
- Copper
- Iodine
- Manganese
- Selenium

Minerals are inorganic chemical elements that must be present for the maintenance of health. They are important for body structures and for controlling body processes, but do not supply calories. Except for iron, minerals are not used up in the body, but are excreted after carrying out their respective functions. This is why mineral losses must be replaced regularly. Four of the minerals that are found in the largest quantities are calcium, iron, magnesium, and potassium. These minerals serve important roles:

Calcium is the most abundant mineral in the body, and is critical for strengthening teeth and bones. About 99 percent of the body's calcium is found in the skeleton. Calcium is essential for cell function, muscle contraction, blood clotting, and the transmission of nerve impulses from nerve endings to muscle fibers. Vitamin D is important in promoting calcium absorption. Most milk is fortified with vitamin D. Milk, shellfish, dark green vegetables, and nuts are excellent sources of calcium. A lifelong calcium-rich diet combined with weight-bearing exercise can help reduce the risk of osteoporosis. Osteoporosis affects primarily older, postmenopausal women; however, it can also affect young female athletes who have irregular menstrual periods or have stopped menstruating altogether. Both groups of women have inadequate estrogen production, which helps maintain bone density. The National Institute for Health (NIH) recommends 800-1500 mg of calcium per day. Pregnant, lactating, and postmenopausal women need to consume calcium at the 1200-1500 mg levels. Men and children under 10 years of age require approximately 800 mg/day.

Iron is essential in the formation of certain enzymes and is the core element in hemoglobin, which is the oxygen-carrying structure of the red blood cell. People with diets low in iron may develop a blood disorder called anemia. Anemia is a condition that reduces the blood's hemoglobin concentration. It is often categorized by fatigue, general sluggishness, and loss of appetite. Red meat, eggs, spinach, and prunes are excellent sources of iron. Consuming vitamin C with meals increases the body's ability to absorb iron. The recommended intake of iron for postmenopausal women and men is 10 mg/day and 15 mg/day for females in their childbearing years.

Magnesium is required for teeth and bone formation, muscle contraction, transmission of nerve impulses, and activation of many enzymes. Nuts, seafood, whole grains, and leafy green vegetables are good sources of magnesium.

Potassium is a mineral that, in combination with sodium and calcium, maintains normal heart rhythm, regulates the body's water balance, aids in muscle contraction, and conducts nerve impulses. Citrus fruits, bananas, vegetables, and milk provide good sources of potassium. Sodium is found in table salt and is commonly found in high levels in canned, pre-packaged foods and baked goods.

Water

Proper hydration is essential for energy production because water is the medium in which all metabolic reactions take place. It accounts for about 60% of the body weight. Fluids regulate body temperature and carry nutrients to cells, aid in digestion and excretion of waste products, and are necessary for all chemical reactions within the body. Most adults need at least 10 (8-ounce) glasses of water per day. Athletes and people living in hot climates require considerably more. Beverages and foods containing caffeine should be limited because caffeine acts as a diuretic, forcing excessive amounts of water to be excreted.

For exercisers, one of the most important functions of water is its cooling capacity. During exercise, heat is generated within the body as a by-product of the working muscle. Heat must be removed to maintain normal body temperature. If heat builds up, body temperature rises and performance suffers. The body loses water in the form of sweat, urine, feces, and exhaled water vapors. The amount lost as sweat depends on physical activity and the external temperature. The amount lost as urine depends on fluid intake. Sweat evaporates from the skin as the body cools down. Heavy sweating significantly reduces the body's water content. Water should be consumed before, during, and after exercise. Exercisers who sweat heavily should drink at least two cups (16 ounces) of water for each pound lost during exercise to rehydrate. (See table 9.2.) Dark gold urine may indicate a water deficiency, assuming no influence from medications.

Fiber

Dietary fiber aids in proper digestion. It consists of the indigestible components of plants, and includes certain types of polysaccharides, cellulose, hemicelluloses, gums, and pectin. Humans do not possess the necessary enzymes to digest fiber; instead, they pass through the digestive system in the same form as they were ingested rendering fiber unusable as energy. It is recommended that people consume 20-35 grams of fiber per day to help prevent cancers of the digestive system, hemorrhoids, constipation, and diverticular diseases. The easiest way to increase fiber content in the diet is to increase consumption of unrefined carbohydrates such as whole-grain breads, cereals, root vegetables, yams, potatoes, and fruits.

Cholesterol

Cholesterol is a major constituent of cell structure. It is involved in the formation of hormones and bile salts, and transports fats from the bloodstream to tissues throughout the body. Although animal (saturated) fats are associated with high levels of cholesterol, cholesterol and fats are not the same thing. Cholesterol is a fat-like substance found in the lean and fat parts of meat, fat in dairy products and the skin of poultry. Egg yolks, liver,

Table 9.2 Water Intake

Before exercise	During exercise	After exercise
16 ounces up to 2 hours before	As much as possible (as tolerated) as often as possible	At least 16 ounces for each pound of body weight lost
Another 4–8 ounces 5–10 minutes before	At least 8–10 ounces every 15–20 minutes	As much as possible until urine is pale yellow and you are urinating every 2–4 hours

and other organ meats are loaded with vitamins and minerals but are also high in cholesterol. In the human body cholesterol is found in the blood, brain, nervous system and cell structure. Sex hormones and cortisone are made from cholesterol. The body normally synthesizes about 1000 mg of cholesterol each day.

The body produces low-density lipoprotein cholesterol (LDL-C) and high-density lipoprotein cholesterol (HDL-C). These fat and protein (lipoprotein) molecules distribute cholesterol throughout the body. HDL-C and LDL-C comprise the majority of what is called "total cholesterol." Researchers believe the desirable cholesterol level for American adults is below 200 milligrams per deciliter (mg/dl) of blood. Epidemiological surveys indicate that the risk for heart attack at cholesterol levels of 250 mg/dl is twice that of 200 mg/dl, and at least four times as high with a level of 300 mg/dl. However, the single most important factor in determining risk for heart disease is the ratio of HDL and total cholesterol. (See table 9.3 for cholesterol ranges.)

LDL-C carries cholesterol into the system leaving fatty residues along the arterial walls. HDL-C carries cholesterol out of the vascular system and transports it to the liver to be eliminated. Therefore, LDL-C is known as *bad* cholesterol and HDL-C is known as *good* cholesterol. Genetics or a diet high in saturated fat also contributes to high cholesterol levels. Elevated cholesterol levels, especially LDL-C, indicate a higher risk of developing heart disease. The National Cholesterol Education Program recently classified total blood cholesterol levels for American adults as shown in table 9.3.

Alcohol

Technically, alcohol is not a nutrient because it does not contribute to cellular growth, maintenance, or repair. Alcohol is more like a drug, but it provides 7 calories of energy per gram. Alcohol acts as a depressant to the central nervous system. Even at low levels, alcohol can slow reaction times, and impair balance and coordination. Alcohol decreases the liver's output of glucose and dehydrates the body. The stomach absorbs about 20 percent of the alcohol ingested; the remainder is absorbed in the intestines. Alcohol is water soluble and is diluted by the body's water content. Organs that have a higher water content and rich blood supply, like the brain, receive the highest initial alcohol concentration. Alcohol affects all the body's cells, but the extent depends on the blood–alcohol concentration. Alcohol is converted into fat when the caloric intake from carbohydrates, protein, and fats exceed daily need.

Food Labeling

Nutrition Panels

The new nutrition labeling requirements issued by the Food and Drug Administration (FDA) and the USDA's Food Safety and Inspection Service became effective May 8, 1994. By law, a revised list of nutrients must appear on the nutrition panel of all processed and packaged foods. The revisions include percentages of calories from fat, saturated fat, cholesterol, sodium, carbohydrates, protein, sodium, vitamin A, vitamin C, calcium, and iron. Thiamin, riboflavin, and niacin levels are no longer required because deficiencies in these vitamins are not considered a significant public health problem.

Percent Daily Value (%DV)

Macronutrients, cholesterol, and sodium are also expressed as a percent of the Daily Value (%DV). The %DV is based on a 2000-calorie diet (except when noted) and is intended to help consumers understand the role of individual

Table 9.3 National Cholesterol Education Program (NCEP) Guidelines

	Total cholesterol (mg/dl)	LDL (mg/dl)	HDL (mg/dl)	Triglycerides (mg/dl)
Normal–desirable	≤ 200	≤ 130	≥ 45 (> 60 ideal)	≤ 200
Borderline	200–239	130–159	36–44	200–399
Unhealthy	≥ 240	≥ 160	≤ 35	≥ 400

foods in the total daily caloric intake. However, not all people require 2,000 calories per day; some require more, others less. The factors that predict calorie requirements are body size, age, height, weight, activity level, and metabolism. (See figure 9.2.)

Example:

According to the food label (see figure 9.2) 13 grams of fat represents 20% of the recommended fat for a person consuming 2000 calories per day.

USDA recommends fat intake be less than or equal to 30% of total caloric intake

- 30% of 2000 calories = 600 calories
- 13 grams of fat = 9 calories/gram × 13 calories = 117 calories
- 117 ÷ 600 = 19.5% = rounded up to 20%

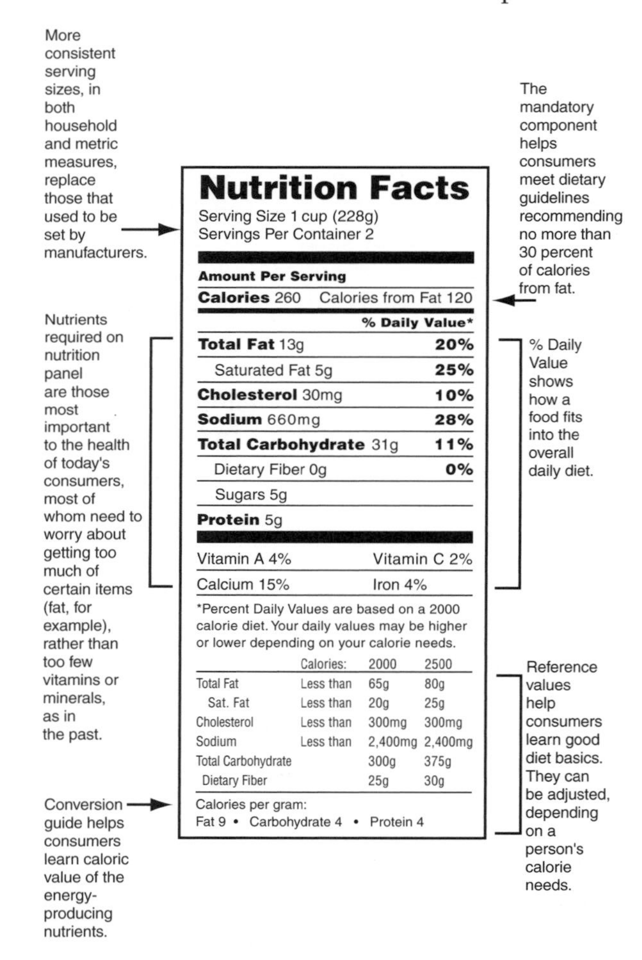

Nutrition Facts
Serving Size 1 cup (228g)
Servings Per Container 2

Amount Per Serving
Calories 260 Calories from Fat 120

	% Daily Value*
Total Fat 13g	20%
Saturated Fat 5g	25%
Cholesterol 30mg	10%
Sodium 660mg	28%
Total Carbohydrate 31g	11%
Dietary Fiber 0g	0%
Sugars 5g	
Protein 5g	

Vitamin A 4% Vitamin C 2%
Calcium 15% Iron 4%

*Percent Daily Values are based on a 2000 calorie diet. Your daily values may be higher or lower depending on your calorie needs.

	Calories:	2000	2500
Total Fat	Less than	65g	80g
Sat. Fat	Less than	20g	25g
Cholesterol	Less than	300mg	300mg
Sodium	Less than	2,400mg	2,400mg
Total Carbohydrate		300g	375g
Dietary Fiber		25g	30g

Calories per gram:
Fat 9 • Carbohydrate 4 • Protein 4

Figure 9.2 Sample nutrition food label.
Reprinted, by permission, from National Exercise Trainers Association (NETA), 2001, *Personal trainer manual* (Minneapolis, MN: NETA), 29.

Serving sizes are expressed in both metric and household measurements. They are more uniform across product lines and the nutritional qualities of similar products more easily comparable.

Common Serving Sizes

Breads, Cereals, Rice and Pasta

- 1 slice of bread
- 1/2 cup cooked rice or pasta
- 1/2 cup cooked cereal
- 1 ounce ready-to-eat cereal

Fruits

- 1 medium sized piece of fruit
- 1 melon wedge
- 3/4 cup juice
- 1/2 cup canned fruit
- 1/4 cup dried fruit

Vegetables

- 1/2 cup chopped raw or cooked vegetables
- 1 cup leafy raw vegetables

Meat, Poultry, Fish, Legumes, and Nuts

- 1-1/2 to 3 ounces cooked lean meat, poultry, or fish
- 1-1/2 cups cooked beans
- 3 eggs = 2-3 ounces of cooked lean meat, poultry, or fish
- 6 tablespoons peanut butter = 2-3 ounces of cooked lean meat, poultry, or fish

Dairy Products

- 1 cup milk or yogurt
- 1-1/2 to 2 ounces of cheese

Nutritional Claims

Many nutritional claims are false. For example, "light" vegetable oil is merely light in color, and "light" cheesecake light in texture. With new labeling, any term used to describe a particular food's nutrient content has a universal meaning. The list of acceptable claims includes such descriptions as "free," "low," "light or lite," "less," and "high." There are regulations prescribing which nutrient content claims are allowed and in what circumstances they can be used.

Only under certain circumstances can claims link a nutrient or a food to the risks of disease. The January 6, 1993, issue of the Federal Register permits the following nutrient-health relationships:

- Calcium and reduced risk of osteoporosis
- Dietary fiber and reduced risk of certain cancers
- Sodium and increased risk of hypertension
- Dietary saturated fat and cholesterol, and increased risk of coronary heart disease
- Dietary fat and increased risk of certain cancers

These regulations allow information on food labels that can help educate the public about recognized diet–disease relationships. Authorized claims must meet requirements to prevent label information that would be false or misleading. The FDA and USDA have begun a multi-year labeling education campaign designed to increase consumer knowledge and to help consumers make accurate and sound dietary choices.

Serving Percentages

The new labeling system does not require listing percentage of nutrients per serving, but lists percentages of daily values based on a 2,000-calorie diet. To calculate the percentage of nutrients per serving, the grams per serving are converted to calories. Proteins and carbohydrates have four calories per gram, and fat has nine calories per gram. The following formula calculates the total percent- age of protein, carbohydrates, or fat per serving.

1. (Total grams of specific nutrient) multiplied by (number of calories per gram for that nutrient) = calories of nutrient
2. Divide (calories of nutrient) by (total calories per serving) = percent of nutrient/serving

Example:

1 serving of wheat 'n cheddar snack crackers
Total calories = 200
Fat grams = 10
Formula:

1. (10 grams of fat) × (9 calories/gram) = 90 calories of Fat
2. 90 calories ÷ 200 total calories = 45%
   Fat = 45% of serving

Weight Management

Weight management can apply to weight gain, weight loss or weight maintenance. The same principles apply to all weight management goals. Balancing calories consumed and calories expended during exercise activity to meet the desired goal and the application of behavior modification techniques are the main strategies in achieving a healthy weight.

Dieting

Americans spend billions of dollars on weight loss programs and diet products each year. The media continues to inundate the public with confusing and contradictory information about diets and weight loss. Despite the emphasis on being thin Americans are even fatter after a decade of "low-fat" hype. The high-protein, low-carbohydrate diet has made a dubious comeback. It's hard to get down to the truth. Most restrictive diets promote weight loss but less than 95% promote the maintenance of that weight loss. Fitness professionals must be diligent in providing clients with safe, healthy nutritional information.

According to the Dietary Guidelines and the Food Guide Pyramid, consuming a balanced diet high in complex carbohydrates and moderate in protein may be the most effective way to manage weight. Balancing calories consumed and calories expended during daily activity is the most important factor in weight management. Evidence suggests that it is healthier to maintain a small weight loss, rather than repeatedly take off and put on weight (yo-yo dieting).

Most experts recommend a gradual weight loss of 1/2 to 2 pounds per week. This can be achieved with a moderate decrease in calories consumed (less than or equal to 500 calories) and moderate increase in physical activity (approximately 500 calories). This method may provide gradual, healthy weight loss. One pound of fat is about 3,500 calories. Reducing daily calorie intake by 250 calories and expending 250 calories exercising would result in a loss of approximately one pound per week. However, severe caloric restriction and over exercising may reduce metabolism, making weight loss more difficult.

Behavior modification strategies, another important component in weight management, involve making short- and long-term changes in lifestyle patterns. Along with achieving caloric balance through diet and exercise, some other behavior modification strategies include: keeping a food/ mood/activity journal; setting reasonable behavior and weight loss/gain goals; planning meals and snacks (if you fail to plan, you plan to fail); seeking a support network; developing a healthy reward system; avoid negative self talk and committing to life-long maintenance.

Eating Disorders

Eating disorders are characterized by severe imbalances in eating and food-related behaviors. Symptoms can range from self-imposed starvation to episodes of binge eating. Binge eating, which is characterized by eating unusually large amounts of food in a short period of time, accompanied by feelings of anxiety and loss of control, may be present in any of the three medically recognized eating disorders: anorexia nervosa, bulimia nervosa, and binge-eating disorder (BED). They also understand that not everyone fits into a neat little diagnostic category as some patients may exhibit major symptoms of anorexia, bulimia, or BED but do not meet specific diagnostic criteria. Each disease has its own characteristics and has its origin in psychological issues, which need to be addressed as well as the eating disorder behaviors. Individuals with eating disorders frequently suffer from depression, anxiety, and chemical abuse.

Anorexia Nervosa (AN)

AN is characterized by self-starvation and is present in only about 1 percent of the population. It is most prevalent in cultures where food is abundant and thinness is the cultural ideal. Individuals who are at the highest risk of developing anorexia nervosa are females (especially Caucasian and Asian), who are from an upper-level socioeconomic status, who demonstrate a marked preoccupation with thinness, who constantly discuss food and body image, and who may be seriously involved in activities requiring a low body weight (i.e., gymnastics, ballet, diving, modeling, and running).

In the United States most anorexics are female, in their mid-teens, from a middle-class, well-educated family. Anorexics tend to be highly competitive and strive for perfection. The "perfect body" is the ultimate goal, and in their minds, they can never become too thin. Weight loss becomes an obsession, losing control becomes a great fear, and self-imposed starvation takes over. Exercise is often used in conjunction with caloric restriction to enhance weight loss. Many anorexics may also abuse laxatives.

Anorexia is very difficult to treat and should be dealt with by qualified professionals. A study from the Renfrew Center in Philadelphia, a treatment center for anorexics and bulimics, reported that females with eating disorders often begin dieting much earlier than their peers (average age 15). The prognosis for treatment is fairly good with early intervention; however, if left untreated, it is associated with early death.

Characteristics of Anorexia Nervosa—Summarized from *Diagnostics and Statistical Manual (DSM IV)* of the American Psychiatric Association:

- A refusal to maintain body weight at or above a minimally normal weight for age and height
- Intense fear of becoming fat or gaining weight
- Distorted body image
- Undue influence of body shape and size on self evaluation
- Denial of seriousness of the current low body weight
- Absence of menstrual cycle for at least 3 consecutive cycles in post pubescent females
- Two types: restrictive (no binge or purge behaviors) and binge-eating/purging

Symptoms of Anorexia Nervosa may include:

- Dramatic weight loss, including muscle tissue
- Dry skin, which is sometimes tinged yellow from an accumulation of stored vitamin A
- Growth of fine body hair
- Intolerance to cold
- Lowered blood pressure and basal metabolism
- Anemia
- Various hormonal changes
- Retarded bone growth

- Amenorrhea (temporary cessation of the menstrual cycle)

Bulimia Nervosa (BN)

BN is characterized by cycles of binge eating and compensatory purge behaviors. Purge behaviors include self-induced vomiting, abuse of diuretics, laxatives or enemas, fasting and excessive exercise. According to the American Psychiatric Association exercise may be considered excessive when it interferes with important activities, is done at inappropriate times or in inappropriate places, or when the individual exercises despite injury or medical complications. Bulimia nervosa may be exacerbated by our cultural obsession with thinness. The obsession with body image and weight gain have an unhealthy correlation with the bulimic's self worth and self-esteem. Bulimics have a morbid fear of fatness. Many fear they won't be able to stop binge eating voluntarily. Most bulimics report feeling depressed after a binge episode, even though the binge eating may have resulted from depression. Ninety percent of bulimics are white females, ranging from 15 to 30 years of age. They may be of normal weight or slightly underweight; however, many remain extremely thin. There are very few reports of male bulimia. Bulimics may eat as much as 6000 calories in one sitting, and spend as much as $50 per day on food. During binges, the bulimic may have low self-esteem or feel out of control, guilty, and shameful. To control fluctuations in body weight, purging may follow binge eating. This cycle may produce a variety of health complications with potentially life-threatening consequences.

Over 40 percent of bulimics report menstrual irregularities or amenorrhea (lack of menses), especially those with low body weight (less than 92 percent of ideal body weight). The effect of amenorrhea on the bone density of young female athletes is of great concern. It is estimated that 60 percent of competitive female runners are amenorrheic. Bone density of the lumbar spine is lower among amenorrheic athletes, and tibial and metatarsal stress fractures are also more common.

Binge eating can cause dilation and possible rupture of the gastrointestinal tract due to excessive food intake within a short period of time. Vomiting after binging may damage tooth enamel and upset the body's electrolyte balance. Repeated use of syrup of ipecac to induce vomiting can cause myocardial abnormalities. Abuse of laxatives by bulimics may promote a sense of purging, but seldom prevents the absorption of calories.

Characteristics of Bulimia Nervosa—Summarized from *Diagnostics and Statistical Manual (DSM IV)* of the American Psychiatric Association:

- Recurrent episodes of binge eating which are characterized by:
  - Eating unusually large amounts (more that most people would eat in the same period of time) of high calorie, otherwise forbidden foods, within a short period of time (about 2 hours)
  - A sense of loss of control and intense anxiety over binge eating behaviors
  - Recurrent use of unhealthy purge behaviors including
  - Binge and purge behaviors occur at least twice a week and continue for at least 3 months
  - Self-evaluation is highly influenced by body shape, size, and weight

Binge-Eating Disorder (BED)

BED, also commonly known as compulsive overeating, is the most common yet most recently recognized eating disorder. It represents about 25-30% of the individuals seeking treatment in a clinic-based weight management program. BED is similar to bulimia nervosa except that individuals with BED do not use the compensatory purge behaviors. Individuals with BED are almost always overweight.

Binges may be triggered by stressful situations, eating even small amounts of "forbidden" foods or negative moods. The binges bring on feelings of shame and self-loathing, which only seem to keep the negative cycle in motion.

Characteristics of Binge-Eating Disorder—Summarized from *Diagnostics and Statistical Manual, (DSM IV)* of the American Psychiatric Association:

- Recurrent episodes of binge eating which is characterized by:
  - Eating unusually large amounts (more that most people would eat in the same

period of time) of high calorie, otherwise forbidden foods, within a short period of time (about 2 hours)
  - A sense of loss of control and intense anxiety over binge eating behaviors
- Binge episodes are associated with 3 or more of the following:
  1. Eating rapidly
  2. Eating until uncomfortably full
  3. Eating large amounts of food when not physically hungry
  4. Eating alone to avoid embarrassment
  5. Feeling disgusted, depressed, and guilty about overeating
- Marked anxiety about binge eating
- Binges occur at least two days a week for six months, on average
- There is no use of compensatory purge behaviors

Professional Ethics

It is of utmost importance that fitness professionals refer an individual that is suspected of having an eating disorder to a qualified medical/ psychiatric professional. Fitness professionals must be careful not to overstep professional, ethical boundaries. We can, however, communicate genuine concern and provide individuals with a list of community resources. Peer support and encouragement are very important when guiding those with eating disorders to seek treatment. The following signs that may indicate a client has an eating disorder are from an article written by Dr. Peter D. Vask, titled *"Spotting the Problem Exerciser"*:

- A need to exercise excessively
- Frequent, wide fluctuations in weight (5-10 pounds or more)
- Fatigue, muscle cramping, lack of stamina
- Irritability or significant mood shifts, especially depression and frustration with performance
- Frequent complaints about weight that appear groundless
- Edema or fluid retention (unrelated to menstrual periods) of face, hands, or ankles
- Complaints of abdominal bloating or stomach pain that resembles heartburn
- Questions about laxatives, diuretics, or thyroid medication and their relationship to weight loss
- Reports of needing extensive dental work or having more cavities

Resources

For more eating disorders information and resources in your local area contact:

EDAP
(Eating Disorders Awareness & Prevention, Inc.)
603 Stewart Ave. Suite 803
Seattle, WA 98101
Phone: (206) 382-3587
FAX: (206) 829-8501
Toll-free information and referral hotline: (800) 931-2237
Web Site: *www.edap.org*

Academy for Eating Disorders
672:6 Old Mclean Village Drive
McLean, VA 22101
Phone: (703) 556-9222
FAX: (703) 556-8729
Web Address: *www.acadeatdis.org*

CHAPTER 10

Motivating Your Participants

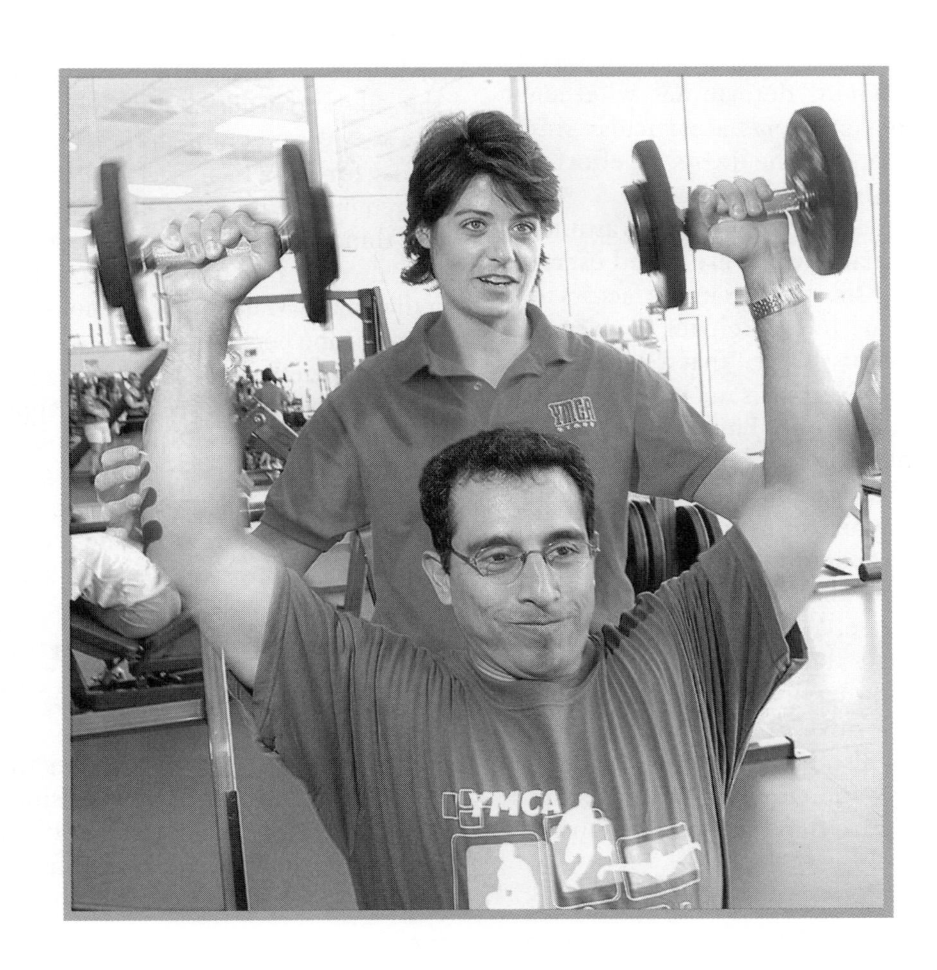

Every personal training instructor is confronted with the challenge of motivating participants to stick with the program. Just as the people with whom you work have a wide range of biological fitness levels and abilities, they also have a wide range of psychological outlooks on exercise. The more sensitive you are to factors that motivate exercisers to stay committed to a program, the easier it will be for you to identify participants who are more likely to drop out.

Motivation is a broad term that describes a variety of behaviors. In general it refers to the direction or intensity of a person's behavior. Direction of behavior determines whether a person approaches or avoids a particular situation. Intensity relates to the degree of effort put forth to accomplish a certain behavior.

Exercise scientists who study people's attitudes, beliefs, and personality traits are called exercise or sport psychologists. They examine factors that influence decisions to participate in exercise. Most exercise scientists agree that a psychological prescription for exercise is not quite as easy to write as a physiological one. This chapter presents the basic elements of psychological exercise prescriptions geared toward motivating participants to stick with their programs. Some elements to take into account include participants' needs and various factors that influence participants' decisions to exercise. You can help participants by guiding them as they set goals, providing a supportive training environment, and keeping the atmosphere positive. In addition to helping yourself, you will also help members if you are aware of your motivation for becoming a personal trainer and are aware that you are a role model for participants.

IDENTIFYING PARTICIPANTS' NEEDS

People are motivated to fulfill their needs. If you understand what your participants need and you are able to help them fulfill these needs, you possess the key to their motivation (Martens et al. 1981, 49).

How can you help fulfill participants' needs if you don't know what they are? Take the time to get to know your participants. Talk with them about their fitness goals, jobs, interests, and so on. These conversations give you opportunities to learn what they like and dislike about their exercise routines. Always ask for comments in a manner that makes it easy for them to answer. For example, say, "Tell me your favorite thing about your workout and one thing that you would like to see changed." You can also use this time to encourage participants individually. Many sport psychologists believe that one-on-one encouragement to keep exercising is much more effective than encouragement directed at an entire group. You can even approach this job more formally. After a while, you can conduct a short, written survey asking for participants' suggestions. Read the comments carefully and amend your program to address the responses that aren't as positive as you'd like.

FACTORS INFLUENCING DECISIONS TO EXERCISE

Listed in table 10.1 are variables that have been found to influence people's decisions to exercise. The main categories of exercise determinants are biological, psychological, and situational.

Table 10.1 Factors Influencing Decisions to Exercise

Biological traits of the exerciser	Psychological traits of the exerciser	Situational factors
Body weight	Attitudes	Support from family and friends
Fitness level	Beliefs	Job status
Health status	Personality traits	Recreational habits
		Location of exercise facility
		Facility atmosphere

These factors do not operate in isolation within a person. A continual, complex interaction between these and other variables is always at work influencing decisions. Let's discuss each factor briefly and examine how you can influence it while leading your participants.

Biological

It's been shown that a participant who has more biological advantages initially (for example, is close to ideal body weight, has a greater genetic capacity to become physically fit and hence sees training benefits occurring faster, or is less predisposed to coronary heart disease) is much more motivated to begin and continue an exercise program. Unfortunately, a person who is undermotivated, overweight, and less fit is less likely to begin training and more likely to quit once he or she gets started. You need to be aware, then, that participants who might benefit most from a personal training program are also the very people most likely to drop out.

Psychological

An exercise psychologist looks at three areas when studying the psychological traits of an exerciser: attitudes, beliefs, and personality traits.

- **Attitudes.** A person's attitude is how he or she feels or thinks about something. Participants will begin training with a variety of attitudes about exercise formed from past experiences as well as expectations for the new program. Although attitudes can predict the likelihood of initial involvement in exercise and the type of program selected, the fact that a person thinks of exercise as a positive experience is no guarantee that he or she will stay with the program (Dishman 1984, 420-435).
- **Beliefs.** What a person believes about the health benefits of exercising affects his or her participation in and commitment to a program. Some people believe strongly that exercise will produce many health-related benefits, whereas others believe just as strongly that exercise will do very little for them. Participants who enter your program with a particular health problem or a belief that exercise is an ounce of prevention against future health problems will probably be more motivated to stay.
- **Personality traits.** Personality traits are those complex characteristics that distinguish one person from another. One of the most studied personality traits in terms of exercise adherence is self-motivation. A self-motivated person is one who is reinforced more by his or her own ideas and goals than by those of others. Self-motivated people have much higher success rates in staying with exercise programs. These people seem to be better suited to overlook factors such as their physical appearance, the exercise room, and the convenience of the location that other participants might use as excuses not to exercise.

Situational

Because biological and psychological traits are very personal factors, as an instructor your ability to alter these influences on motivation is limited. Because situational factors are often environmental, you have a better chance of altering them in hopes of increasing your participants' motivation to exercise regularly. The training setting, its location and accessibility, and the atmosphere in which you conduct it are a few of the situational factors you can control, at least to some degree.

HELPING PARTICIPANTS SET GOALS

Helping people establish realistic exercise goals is important to motivation. Many participants drop out because they expect to become fit immediately, and they are disappointed when this does not happen. You must warn participants, in a positive manner, of the various pressures that might tempt them to drop out (hard work, discomfort, time commitment). Keep encouraging participants to make each appointment and exercise a habit. Helping participants set realistic goals is one way to reinforce the exercise habit.

Short-term and long-term goals provide participants with objectives to work toward, and the goal-setting process is an effective means of eliciting commitment to the program. Discussing goals with participants gives you an opportunity to help them modify unrealistic goals. For example, a participant has set a goal of losing 20 pounds after eight weeks of training. However, you know that exercising alone will not accomplish this goal and that 2 pounds per week ($2 \times 8 = 16$) is a recommended and safe rate of weight loss. Therefore, you must explain the amount of weight loss the participant can expect from her or his program. The participant must understand that diet and exercise together is the best approach to attaining and maintaining weight loss. A more appropriate short-term goal would be to lose 1 to 2 pounds a week by exercising regularly and reducing caloric intake. At this rate, a safer, more desirable long-term goal of losing 10 to 15 pounds in two months could be accomplished. When planning goals with participants, take into account their physical ability, their expressed commitment, and their previous ability to accomplish goals.

PROVIDING A SUPPORTIVE TRAINING ENVIRONMENT

A supportive training environment might provide the most powerful positive reinforcement. People generally like to exercise where they are known by name, treated with respect, and instructed in a professional manner. A user-friendly facility is clean, spacious, and well lit. It has plenty of professional staff and educational materials. Specific member services might include quality equipment, easy-to-read instructional charts, spray bottles and towels at exercise stations, a convenient workout card system, easy room access, smooth traffic flow, cold-water dispensers, and a systematic participant orientation program.

Physical features of the exercise facility, such as its size, furnishings, lighting and ventilation, and temperature, contribute to participants' perceptions of how enjoyable the workout environment is. Although budgetary constraints or the facility design might limit your options, try to provide your participants with the best that is available.

- **Size of the facility.** The amount of space participants have to move around in affects their perception of the experience. Participants need to feel that there is enough room to freely perform movements and exercises without interfering with other exercisers. Mirrors add to the attractiveness of an exercise facility and make it appear larger. Many participants also enjoy the visual feedback as they work out. Mirrors should be high quality so that they maintain an accurate reflection over time.
- **Furnishings.** The decor of the workout facility should be both professional and attractive. You can hang posters, fill bulletin boards with exercise tips, post educational materials on training-related topics, and display information participants bring to share. Always keep the workout area clean and free of safety hazards such as dirt, clothing on the floor, or water tracked in on participants' shoes.
- **Lighting and ventilation.** Exercise facilities need to be well lit and well ventilated. Bright lighting will help participants feel positive and ready to work out. Windows are a welcome addition to any exercise facility. Ceiling fans or large floor fans, if you have space for them, circulate the air.
- **Facility temperature.** Facilities within a building or complex are typically controlled by a central thermostat. Pay attention to the temperature of the workout facility. The YMCA recommends a temperature of 68 to 72 degrees Fahrenheit in exercise facilities.

CREATING A POSITIVE EXERCISE ATMOSPHERE

The atmosphere in which personal training sessions are conducted affect participants' motivation. Try to create a comfortable, *noncompetitive* atmosphere in which participants will enjoy working out. Encourage participants to work out at their own pace and to have fun. As a leader you can facilitate this type of environment by always being positive and giving participants encouragement, feedback, and positive reinforcement. Try to be in an uplifting mood and to express confidence. If you establish a positive and helpful rapport with participants, they will be understanding and positive toward you in return.

Being a Positive Communicator

An effective motivator is first an effective communicator. When talking with participants, keep these points in mind:

- Don't treat participants as inferior or naive. Speak to them in the same way you want to be spoken to.
- If you ask participants for suggestions, do not ignore what they say; use their suggestions, when appropriate, to show that you are listening.
- Always be positive or provide constructive feedback. No one should be embarrassed by trying to perform a movement, only to be told point-blank that it is being done poorly.
- Don't become defensive when participants criticize you. Listen and try to turn the conversation into a positive situation for everyone involved. Asking a clarifying question can help get at the cause for the criticism.

In addition to communicating with participants, work toward communicating effectively with your colleagues.

Providing Encouragement

Encouragement is essential not only for new personal training participants, but also for regular exercisers. For those just starting out, their feelings of insecurity and inadequacy can be offset by encouragement from you, which helps them develop confidence and competence. For regular exercisers, your encouragement might be their main source of motivation to continue training, particularly when they experience progress plateaus or lose interest in the activity. Encouragement comes in many forms, including greeting participants by name, inviting them to try new exercises, and showing enthusiasm for their training program and progress.

Giving Feedback

Your feedback should provide specific information about the exerciser's performance and progress. Feedback should always be honest and be given constructively. Although participants need to know precisely what they are doing properly and improperly in order to improve their performance, the way in which you address participants' mistakes can affect their attitude toward training. For example, if you say, "Don't you remember you're not supposed to let your elbows come out on triceps press-downs?" it could be taken as personal criticism. Saying "You will get better results if you keep your elbows against your sides during triceps press-downs" instead is both more precise and more positive. The same logic applies when you comment on participants' progress. Saying "You haven't increased your workout weight at all in three weeks" is probably less effective than saying "Your training over the past three weeks indicates that you should increase your weight loads by 2.5 pounds next workout."

It is essential that you give participants feedback about their performance and progress clearly, concisely, and objectively. Remember that you can provide relevant feedback through periodic fitness evaluations as well as observation. Evaluations could include assessments of body measurements, body composition, muscle strength, joint flexibility, resting heart rate, and resting blood pressure.

Another important source of feedback for participants is their workout charts or exercise logbooks that contain written records of each training session. Self-recording has been shown to be a very effective means of motivation, particularly when reviewed regularly by concerned personal trainers.

Using Positive Reinforcement

Positive reinforcement refers to anything that maintains or increases a particular behavior. In terms of exercise adherence, positive reinforcement might include compliments on appearance, praise for performance, and rewards and incentives. Although compliments are almost always welcomed, they are not always meaningful. For example, simply saying "Good job" or "You're looking good" might become so routine that it has little impact. Praise is more effective when it provides specific information. That way the exerciser knows you actually observed the behavior that prompted your comment. Here are examples of specific positive reinforcement: "Good job. You're performing every repetition in a slow and controlled manner." "You're looking good. The back and shoulder exercises you added have improved your posture."

Rewards and incentives are most meaningful when they are based on personal goals and abilities. The performance criteria should be challenging, yet attainable with appropriate effort. For example, an undermuscled participant might be motivated to train regularly if you make the award of a T-shirt contingent upon adding three pounds of lean (muscle) weight.

Checking Your Mood

Common sense tells us that the mood you bring into the session affects participants. An effective instructor leaves his or her troubles outside of the exercise facility and enters with an uplifting spirit. This is the mark of a professional. Encourage participants to do the same to help them get the most out of the session. Remind them that this is one hour of the day in which they can relax and do something beneficial for their minds and bodies.

Displaying Confidence

The level of self-confidence an instructor displays can influence some participants' motivation to stick with the program. Your self-confidence comes across through both your words and your actions. Verbal confidence usually takes the form of clear instructions, positive comments from systematic observations, and an assured tone of voice as you ask and answer questions. Nonverbal confidence is usually displayed by body language, appropriate and effective use of the hands to assist and direct, and pleasant facial expressions. Being well prepared to teach can only boost your level of self-confidence.

EXAMINING YOUR OWN MOTIVATION

Besides considering what you can do as an instructor to motivate your participants, you should also occasionally think about what motivates you to be a personal training instructor. The factors might include prestige, teaching experience, personal enjoyment, or salary.

Take the time to identify your reasons for wanting to be a personal trainer. As you identify key factors that motivate you to be an instructor, ask yourself how they affect, positively or negatively, your leadership.

BEING A ROLE MODEL

Whether you like it or not, being a personal training instructor makes you a role model in the eyes of many participants. To many participants, the stereotypical instructor is physically fit, at proper body weight, and skilled at performing movements and exercises. The stereotype might also extend to a picture of someone who doesn't smoke, drink alcoholic beverages in excess, eat junk food, or indulge in any other "unhealthy" behaviors.

How you perceive yourself as a role model depends on your own philosophy. There are many professional variations of a good role model. You should take time to identify your beliefs and attitudes so that you are ready to articulate them if the subject comes up with participants or with other instructors. Your participants' perceptions of you as a role model can be motivating or not-so-motivating factors for them. For example, participants who expect you to be in top shape and at your ideal body weight might question the benefit of your program if you are neither.

Personal training instructors who display positive attitudes and demonstrate that they value exercise typically influence their participants to do the same. A friendly, courteous, and respectful staff is the key to friendly, courteous, and respectful members who enjoy their exercise experiences. The three most desired instructor qualities are (1) knowledge of exercise science, (2) good teaching skills, and (3) enthusiasm. Because knowledgeable instructors who communicate effectively and enthusiastically play a major role in motivating members, it is in everyone's best interest for you as an instructor to demonstrate these important characteristics.

CHAPTER 11

Communication and Teaching Techniques

Amy Jones, M.Ed.

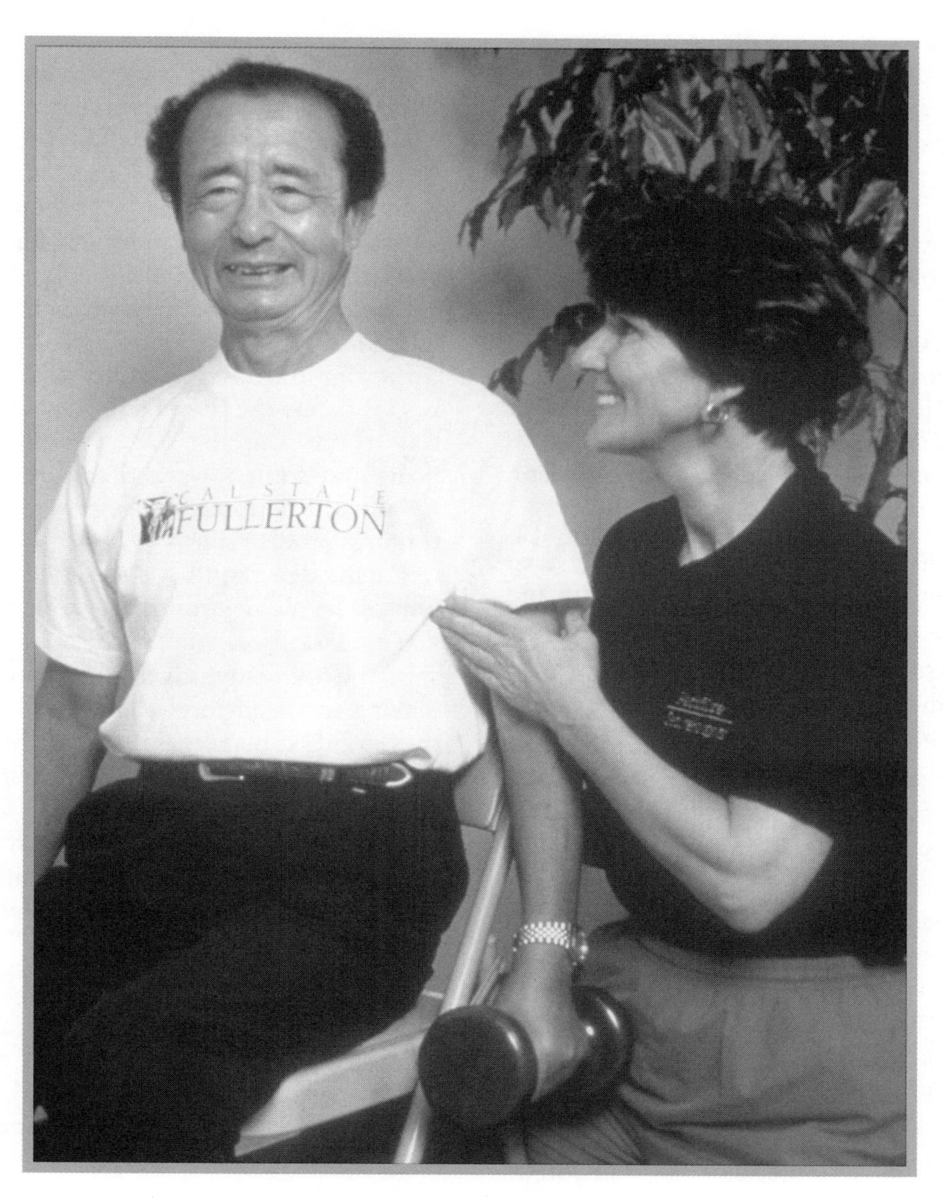

Amy Jones, M.Ed., L.P.C., is a licensed psychotherapist and leads the organizational capability practice for The Feld Group, a firm specializing in Information Technology transformation in Fortune 500 companies. In addition to working with executive teams in leading organization change and transformation efforts, much of her time is spent coaching and training executives in interpersonal communication, leadership development, and organizational effectiveness. She was formerly the director of programs for the Cooper Fitness Center in Dallas, Texas, for 12 years, served on the American Council on Exercise Board of Directors, and was a technical advisor to the National Aerobic Championship.

A personal trainer's relationship to a client is clearly the helping relationship of educator to student. Helping relationships differ from most other kinds of relationships encountered in daily routines. Most ordinary experiences are dialogues in which both individuals seek personal enhancement or the mutual exchange of ideas or information. In the helping relationship, one person temporarily sets aside personal needs to help another person. The focus of the relationship is on the client's needs and on goals that will lead to new behavior. Simply put, helping is enabling another person to change. Instead of encouraging dependence, the purpose of helping is to enable the client to take more control and become self-sufficient. Helping is an active process of advising, informing, correcting, and directing.

There are many kinds of helping relationships. Because there is usually a fee for service in personal training, you can be classified as a structured, professional helper, like social workers, teachers, school counselors, and legal advisors. In contrast to this professional level are unstructured levels of helping such as friendships and family relationships. Your role is complex, as you will function as a teacher, coach, advisor, supporter, counselor, and negotiator.

Teacher: Explaining to clients what they need to know and must do (e.g., outlining and explaining an aerobic exercise program).

Coach: Training clients in desired skills (e.g., coaching during a free-weight workout).

Advisor: Telling clients the wisest course of action (e.g., warning about potential dangers associated with nutritional supplements containing ephedra).

Supporter: Encouraging clients as they work on specific lifestyle changes (e.g., providing emotional support for a client who has stopped smoking).

Counselor: Helping clients sort through personal problems (e.g., listening to a client's frustrations regarding problems at work).

Negotiator: Bargaining with clients to reach an acceptable agreement (e.g., negotiating an exercise contract with a client for a period of travel).

These roles are described only in a general sense. You should be acutely aware of your limitations and must not exceed the professional parameters of offering advice or counseling about personal problems. You can obviously listen and offer support, but you should know when to refer clients to other qualified professionals.

STAGES OF THE PERSONAL TRAINER/ CLIENT RELATIONSHIP

There will be distinct stages in your relationships with clients and they form a general model or framework for the divisions and related skills of the helping relationship (figure 11.1). They may not always occur in this exact sequence, nor are all stages always present. Their length also may vary from client to client. Generally, the initial contact between the personal trainer and client is made in the **rapport** stage. The process of gathering information after the relationship has begun forms the investigation stage. This gives way to the planning stage in which the client's goals and steps toward them are mapped out. Finally, the action stage begins when the actual training process starts.

Each stage requires specific skills and techniques. In the beginning, for example, attentive listening skills can build the working relationship; the following stages require more decision-making and behavioral-change skills. Developing these skills can increase your effectiveness as a personal trainer. Because the personal trainer/ client relationship is dynamic and ever-changing, these stages and skills overlap and may not occur in the exact order given. The specific stages and required skills are outlined as follows:

Stage 1: Rapport—interpersonal communication skills

Stage 2: Investigation—information gathering skills

Stage 3: Planning—problem-solving or decision-making skills

Stage 4: Action—behavioral change skills (e.g., feedback, contracting, modeling)

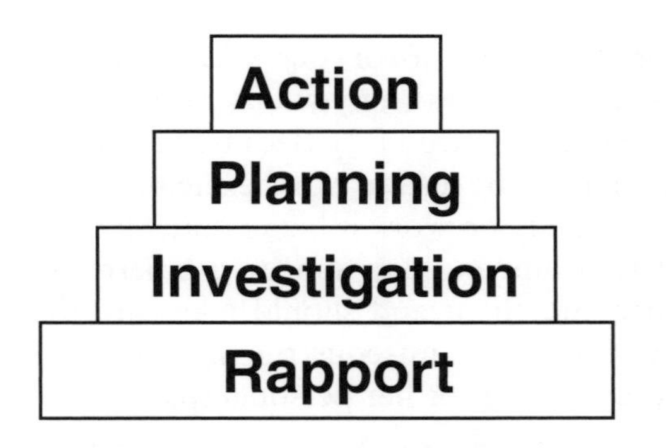

Figure 11.1 Stages of the personal trainer/client relationship.

The **rapport** stage is the foundation for the entire relationship between you and your client. Rapport means a relationship of mutual trust, harmony, or emotional affinity. Establishing it entails building a certain level of comfort or shared understanding into a relationship. The rapport stage begins at first contact. Whether in person or on the telephone, the client is check-ing out" the personal trainer and answering the question, "Can this person help me?" Confidence or trust in your skills must be established early because only then will the client be willing to receive guidance.

According to Rogers et al. (1967), people in the helping profession need to communicate three basic attributes or qualities for the helping relationship to be successful. These three primary qualities are (1) **empathy,** (2) warmth, and (3) genuineness. The importance of these qualities has been demonstrated repeatedly in research by Truax and Carkuff (1967) and others. They are the foundation for a successful helping relationship and are key factors during the rapport stage.

Empathy is the ability to experience another person's world as if it were one's own. It is understanding the client's point of view or where the client is "coming from." The empathetic personal trainer will be able to respond appropriately to the client's covert feelings and verbal messages by communicating perceptions to the client. The absence of empathy may lead the client to think the trainer does not understand what they are experiencing and, therefore, will block the entire helping process.

Warmth is an unconditional positive regard or respect for another person regardless of their individuality and uniqueness. It bridges professional distance through friendliness and consideration regardless of a "liking" for another person. Warmth is about caring and understanding rather than judging and impersonalizing. This quality will convey a climate that communicates safety and acceptance to a client, even when they are making mistakes.

Genuineness can be defined as authenticity or being honest and open without putting up a front. It is a state in which the helper's words and actions are congruent. For example, when you greet a client with "I'm glad to see you're here today," your body language must be consistent with the words of welcome. Genuineness is the ability to relate to people without hiding behind a clipboard or white coat. It is not necessarily being fully self-revealing, but rather being committed to a responsible honesty with others.

Empathy, warmth, and genuineness are paramount in establishing trust in a working relationship. At first glance, they may seem simplistic because they are the outgrowth of ordinary effective human qualities. However, relevant research and cumulative experience points out the necessity for continuous monitoring of the timing and amount of conditions that facilitate the development of these qualities.

Interpersonal communication skills are the primary skills needed to establish rapport and thereby build a relationship. They are not only important during the rapport stage, but are necessary throughout the relationship. Interpersonal communication skills can be broadly categorized as nonverbal and verbal. The nonverbal category includes such behaviors as attending and perceiving nonverbal and verbal messages. The verbal category includes paraphrasing, reflecting, and clarifying. Many of these skills are natural for anyone genuinely involved in helping another person, but specific communication skills can be learned, practiced, and continuously mastered.

Nonverbal Behaviors

Listening is the primary nonverbal communication skill. It is a complex concept and is not the same as hearing, which is the perception of sound through the ear. Listening obviously involves the physiology of hearing, but also is a more complex psychological procedure of involvement with the other person that includes skills in attending, perceiving verbal and nonverbal messages, and even verbal responding. All of these skills overlap and are difficult to treat separately.

Attending

Attending behaviors are exhibited by the listener to put the speaker at ease and entail being attentive or giving physical attention to them. Instead of interrupting, the listener gives nonverbal acknowledgments during the conversation through posture, eye contact, and gestures. Verbal responses also are a form of attending. The listener may say, "Yes, I see," to encourage the speaker to continue.

Effective attending can build trust and can work wonders in human relationships. Conversely, nonattentive behavior can be devastating. For example, when you are speaking to someone who appears bored and whose eyes are continually distracted to other things, you may feel ignored and not encouraged to continue the conversation. The trainer interested in developing good attending behaviors or skills needs to be aware of the following:

1. **Posture:** When you and your client are seated, specific postures can communicate your interest. To show involvement, face the client squarely at eye level and lean toward them in a relaxed manner. Avoid expressing defensiveness by maintaining an open position with arms and legs uncrossed. This posture says, "I am interested in you and am ready to listen." Research has shown that these postural behaviors demonstrate to the client the traits of empathy, warmth, and genuineness.

2. **Positioning:** Position yourself at an appropriate distance from the client to demonstrate a respect for his or her personal space. Hall (1966) describes an 18-inch (46 cm) or less distance between two people as "intimate space," an 18-inch to 4-foot (46 cm to 1.2 m) distance as "personal space," a 4-foot to 12-foot (1.2 to 3.7 m) distance as "social distance," and beyond 12 feet (3.7 m) as "public distance." Most normal conversation will occur in the personal space. However, the very nature of your working relationship demands at times that you enter the client's intimate space (figure 11.2). Because of this intimate positioning, be sensitive to the client, particularly when hands-on work is being done. Early in the relationship you may want to ask permission to touch the client and should take care that the client does not misconstrue your touching or presence in his or her personal space.

3. **Mirroring:** Another technique you can use to establish rapport is mimicking or **mirroring.** Mirroring may be either conscious or unconscious, but its purpose is to establish rapport with another person. The technique of mirroring involves sensitively matching the posture and gestures of the other person, and may include matching voice tone and tempo and breathing patterns. These techniques often occur naturally as people interact.

4. **Eye Contact:** Eye contact is a key vehicle for indicating interest in a person. Good eye

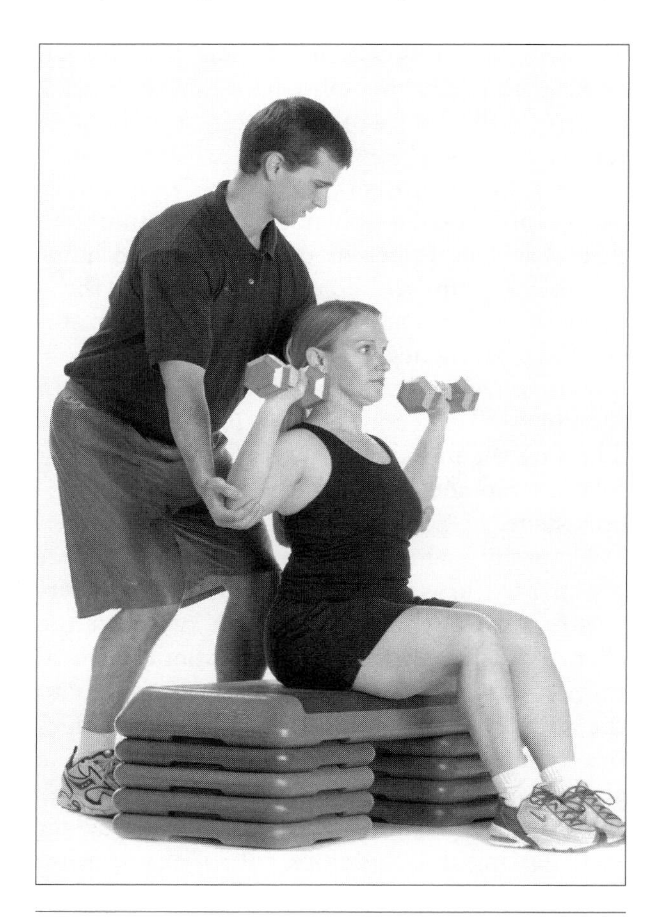

Figure 11.2 Trainer working in a client's intimate space.

contact is not a fixed stare but rather a relaxed focus on the client's eyes, face, and body gestures. It enables the client to feel safe and comfortable and conveys your interest at the same time.

5. **Gestures:** Appropriate body movement is essential in attending. Try to use relaxed motions instead of appearing rigid and unmoving. Nervous mannerisms such as playing with objects, jingling pocket change, waving to others, and drumming fingers should be avoided.

6. **Environment:** Since much of the personal training process takes place in a gym that is usually full of talking people, blaring music, and clanging weights, a quiet place is preferable for effective communication. Pleasant surroundings facilitate conversation, so initial sessions should be conducted in a nondistracting environment. To give someone your undivided attention when distractions are present is difficult. Distractions may consist of a blaring TV or radio, a ringing telephone, people stopping by to talk, uncomfortable room temperature, and inappropriate lighting. Another type of distraction is seating arrangement. Sitting behind a desk not only puts up a physical barrier, but can be an interpersonal barrier as well. Attempts should be made to limit environmental distractions so that the client's thoughts are not interrupted and effective communication can take place.

Perceiving Nonverbal Messages

The saying "actions speak louder than words" is especially true in communications. Mehrabian (1972) determined that 93% of communication is nonverbal, leaving only 7% for actual content of spoken words. A person's expressions, gestures, posture, and other actions provide a constant source of information. Therefore, improving your interpretation of body language is a valuable communication skill. Nonverbal messages are usually a means of expressing emotions. We search someone's face to determine feelings of anger, sadness, or disgust. Nonverbal messages tend to be more reliable than verbal messages and are essential to understanding many of the most important things others are trying to communicate to us (table 11.1).

Although voice intonation is verbal and explained in more detail later, it is appropriate to mention it as a nonverbal behavior. The sound of the voice communicates beyond the specific words. The words spoken may be fast, slow, high-pitched, loud, or whispered. The voice tells much about the mood of the speaker. For example, some people may speak very rapidly or at a high pitch when they are nervous or fearful.

General appearance also is a nonverbal cue. The way in which a person grooms and dresses is a statement to others. One aspect of interpreting body language is noting discrepancies between verbal and nonverbal messages. It is easy to note incongruence in a person who says he is not angry while slamming his fist on the table. When you note a difference between words and nonverbal behavior, it may be helpful to search for the meaning of both. Body language can have multitudes

Table 11.1 Examples of Nonverbal Cues

Feature	Nonverbal Cues
Head	Nodding, cocked to side, thrown back, motioning a direction
Facial	Frowning, grimacing, animated, expression distracted
Eyes	Squinting, wide open, closed, winking, blinking, rolling, teary
Mouth	Smiling, pursed lips, lip licking, lip biting, open, closed
Skin	Blushing, paleness, perspiration, rashes
Body	Relaxed, rigid, stooped shoulders, posture leaning forward, leaning backward, chest extended out
Hands/arms	Fidgeting, tapping, laced fingers, fisted, pointing, touching, crossed arms
Feet/legs	Foot tapping, legs crossed, legs open, knee knocking

of meanings and should be interpreted in context. A single gesture does not stand alone, but should be seen in relationship to other body movements and related to a person's words.

Misunderstandings often occur when listening only to words or observing only body language. Clarify the accuracy of your interpretation with the client.

Perceiving Verbal Messages

To understand verbal messages, you must be able to recognize both the apparent and the underlying content. The apparent or cognitive content is composed of the actual words and facts of the message. Cognitive messages are more easily recognized because they are stated and usually involve talking about things, people, or events and may include one or more themes or topics. The underlying or affective content is composed of emotions, attitudes, and behaviors. Affective messages are communicated both verbally and nonverbally and are more difficult to perceive and interpret. The client may not even be aware of their own feelings and might be surprised when you reveal your perceptions of what they are saying. Generally, emotions can be grouped into four major categories—sadness, anger, fear, and happiness—and a feeling from one category may often cover up a feeling from another. Discriminating between cognitive and affective messages will allow you to respond appropriately to the client. Many cognitive themes may be communicated at once, but hearing the emotional message will help you to establish priorities for cognitive topics. It seems listeners will often respond to the most recent verbal theme instead of the most important one. To illustrate, a client says to a personal trainer in their first meeting, "There is so much going on right now. I have gained 25 pounds since starting school. I'm about to flunk chemistry and if I do, my dad said he would take me out of school. I can't concentrate and I'm not sleeping at night. It seems I just keep gaining weight." In this situation, it is necessary for the personal trainer to listen to the whole message and prioritize the cognitive themes. It may be helpful for this client to learn some stress reduction techniques from a qualified professional even before being put on a weight-control and exercise program.

Verbal Behaviors

Verbal responses are a form of listening and they demonstrate to the client an understanding of what he or she is saying and feeling. Appropriate responses will encourage the client to continue talking and will allow for more exploration. The following are commonly used verbal responses:

- Minimal encouragers—brief words or phrases that allow the client to continue speaking. These verbal prods let him or her know that you are following what is being said. Examples of minimal encouragers are "Mmmhmmm," "I see," "Yes," and "Go on."
- Paraphrasing—a response that concisely restates the essence of the speaker's content. For example:

  Client: I didn't sleep well and don't feel like working out.

  Personal Trainer: You're tired today.
- Probing—an attempt to gain more information. Statements such as, "I'm wondering about . . ." and "Let's talk about that" will help reveal more information.
- Reflecting—restating feelings and/or content in a way that demonstrates understanding. You can reflect stated or implied feelings, nonverbal observation, specific content, and even what has been omitted. Examples of reflecting are: "You're feeling uncomfortable about starting an exercise program," and "Sounds like you are angry at your husband for insisting that you come today."
- Clarifying—an attempt to understand what the client is saying. "I'm confused about . . ." and "Could you please explain that again?" are examples of clarifying statements.
- Informing—sharing factual information, as when you explain the pros and cons of a particular piece of exercise equipment.
- Confronting—providing the client with mild or strong feedback about what is really going on. Confrontations are more easily heard when communicated with "I" messages such as "I feel you really don't want to be here today." Another example of confronting is "It seems to me you say . . . and yet you do . . . "

- Questioning—asking for a response. Questions may be closed or open. Closed questions direct the client to give a short response such as "yes" or "no." Open questions provide space for them to explore their own thoughts without being hemmed in. "What's on your mind today?" is an example of an open question.
- Summarizing—recapping what has been communicated and highlighting major themes. Effective summarizing can tie loose strands of a conversation together at its conclusion. A summary might begin with "Let's recap what we've discussed so far."

As mentioned earlier, the way in which we speak is often more important than what we actually say. An effective communicator is aware of the quality of delivery of the message. The elements of voice in delivery are intensity, pitch, and pace. The intensity, or force, is an important factor in delivery. Some personal trainers speak so softly that they cannot be heard, while others speak with such volume that they become annoying. Delivery should be loud enough to be heard, while reserving a range to emphasize important points. When working in the weight room, you may find an unusual amount of interference from others talking, background music, and weights clanging. This situation provides you with a challenge to determine an effective intensity for your voice. Decreasing voice volume in a noisy situation can actually increase the attentiveness of the other person. For example, instead of shouting to a client in a noisy gym, you can experiment with lowering your voice volume to encourage him or her to listen more intently. This technique also will reduce vocal stress.

Pitch is the general level of the voice on the musical scale. Everyone has a characteristic pitch. Some speak in a singsong fashion while others speak in a monotone. Some people may end their sentences with an upward inflection while others end with a downward inflection. A noticeable rise in pitch level may decrease effective delivery because it usually denotes incompleteness of thought or indecisiveness. Experienced personal trainers cultivate a wide range of pitch, which they use effectively during delivery.

Rate means the speed of the utterance, or the number of words spoken per minute. Most people speak at the rate of 115 to 150 words per minute. Variations in rate depend upon such factors as the importance of the material, the desire for emphasis, and the mood of the content. Speaking too quickly reduces clarity and can be confusing for those listening. Even though speaking at a slower rate allows others time to absorb what is being said, speaking too slowly may bore the listener. Pausing gives people time to think about what is being said and can accentuate important information.

The rapport stage, which begins at first contact, is critical to establishing a good working relationship between the personal trainer and client. Sometimes a level of comfort may be quickly established, while at other times more time and energy may have to be expended to win a client's trust. Interpersonal communication skills can be learned and mastered. Merely reading about these skills does not necessarily improve application to everyday situations; they must be continuously practiced. Even though the rapport stage is presented as the first stage, there is really no end to it. The primary qualities (empathy, warmth, and genuineness) and the interpersonal communication skills are important and valuable throughout the entire personal trainer/client relationship.

INVESTIGATION STAGE

The goal of the investigation stage is to gather information about your client's present fitness level, personal goals, and physical and psychological limitations. This may begin in the initial interview, when the client is encouraged to talk about desires and expectations for training. Health history and lifestyle questionnaires can yield a wealth of information. Additional data can be gathered from fitness assessments. Historically, health history and lifestyle questionnaire forms are filled out by the individual client. However, you are encouraged to ask these questions orally. This method requires more time, but it can be valuable in establishing rapport. In addition, clients will probably reveal more about themselves when they observe your interest. At a minimum, you and your client should discuss his or her written responses to the questionnaire. During the discussion you can probe, question, and clarify to gain more information. After all the information is gathered, you and your client can begin planning by setting goals and making decisions about how to achieve them.

PLANNING STAGE

Up to this point, most of your time with your client has been spent building rapport and gathering appropriate information regarding lifestyle behaviors and current fitness level. In the planning stage, the personal trainer and client begin setting goals according to the client's needs and desires. Because there are usually several ways to reach any goal, you must make use of decision-making skills to determine the best course of action. The outcome will be more effective if the process is done together than if you dictate to the client what to do each step of the way.

Decision-making occurs frequently as we go about our daily activities; we must constantly decide how we will spend our time, money, and energy during any given day. Many of these decisions are second nature for us, so we do not consider the process we go through in determining what is best in a particular situation. Even though there are many decision-making models, the basic process for the personal trainer/client relationship consists of the following steps:

1. Setting goals
2. Generating alternatives
3. Exploring the alternatives
4. Making the decision
5. Formulating a plan
6. Evaluating the implementation

Setting Goals

Clients will seldom approach you with neatly stated goals. They are usually expressed in vague statements, such as, "I want to be in better shape," or "I want to lose some weight." It is your responsibility to translate these general aims into precise goals.

Effective goals must be SMART, which means they are

Specific—The goals must specifically tell what is to be accomplished. They must be easily understood and unambiguous.

Measurable—The goals must be measurable so there is no question of attainment. Examples of measurement would be percent body fat, number of pounds, or a specific fun run.

Attainable—The goals must be attainable, not too difficult or too easy. Easy goals do not motivate and overly difficult ones may frustrate.

Relevant—The goals must be relevant or pertinent to the particular interest, needs, and abilities of your client.

Time-bound—The goals must be time-bound with specific deadlines for completion.

It is difficult to know when a client has obtained a goal that is expressed in terms such as "I want to get in better shape." However, both parties would know when the goal is attained if it is stated as, "I want to be able to walk three miles in 45 minutes by March 31st," or "I'd like to drop 20 pounds by the end of the year." According to Dick, Carey, and Carey (2000), one method of clarifying a broad goal is to follow these steps:

1. Write the goal down.
2. Write down things the client can do to demonstrate they have achieved the goal (e.g., lose 20 pounds, drop to 12% body fat, fit into a size 10 dress they have not worn in three years).
3. Sort through the statements and pick out the ones that best represent the original goal.
4. Rewrite the original goal to include your new statements or make smaller goals.

Express the goals in terms of client actions rather than personal trainer actions. A goal stated as, "the trainer will get me in shape," does not give the client ownership of or responsibility for the goal. The goals must also be attainable. It would not be attainable for a nonrunner client to say, "I want to run a 10K next week." Attainable goals will help ensure the client's success. Finally, setting both short- and long-range goals will be helpful. For example, a female client who is 30% body fat may have a long-range goal of reaching 20% body fat in six months.

The short-range goal might be to reach 27% in the next six weeks. Setting a time line, or date of completion, often creates a sense of urgency for both the client and the personal trainer and can be effective in overcoming client procrastination. You also can help the beginner client create behavioral goals that will remove intimidating evaluation procedures like body-fat tests, tape measures, and weight scales. For example, a behavioral goal can be stated as, "I want to exercise three times per week, for 30 minutes of aerobic training, 20 minutes of strength training, and 10 minutes of stretching, for 12 consecutive weeks starting January 1st." In this example, the personal trainer and client are establishing positive lifestyle changes rather than strictly emphasizing physiological changes.

Generating Alternatives

This step in the decision-making process involves proposing all possible alternatives for reaching the goal. This brainstorming process gives the client more choices. For example, a client might define his or her goal as, "I want to get my thighs stronger for the upcoming ski season." In exploring alternatives to reach this goal, you and your client might generate the following:

a. I could increase my thigh strength by riding the stationary cycle.
b. I could increase my thigh strength by performing squats with free weights.
c. I could increase my thigh strength by climbing stairs.
d. I could increase my thigh strength by stepping up and down on a bench.

The client now has several viable options for obtaining their goal.

Exploring Alternatives

After brainstorming the list of options, the next step is to weigh or rank them. Evaluate the alternatives for implementation realities and hypothesized consequences. Some options may immediately be thrown out because they are impractical, making it easier for the client to prioritize the remaining alternatives. From the previous example, a client may discard option b because of its relative inconvenience. With your help, he or she may then rank the rest of the alternatives according to interest, availability, and time.

Making the Decision

You and the client now decide on one or more of the alternatives. Choose the most effective strategy or a combination of the options for this person at this time. For example, our skier may choose to train for skiing by doing squats with free-weights at the gym at least two days a week. In addition, he or she can climb stairs at home when there is no time to get to the gym.

Formulating a Plan

At this point you and the client determine a specific sequence of action that likely will result in the accomplishment of the goals. Formulating an action plan includes determining who needs to do what, when, where, what materials are required, and so forth. This step is further developed as exercise programming, which is covered in chapters 8 and 10.

Evaluating the Implementation

This step measures accomplishment in relation to the predetermined goals and may occur in a formal setting where the client's fitness level is reassessed. The evaluation process may also occur informally during the training sessions as both client and trainer report progress. Either way, together you determine the accomplishment and, if necessary, a new set of action steps.

ACTION STAGE

Once rapport has been established, information has been gathered, and goals have been set, the action stage, or actual training, begins. You coach the client toward his or her goals. As a teacher or tutor, you may use many methods of education.

In a broad sense, personal training is similar to an individual approach to direct instruction, which is essentially active learning. It consists of the personal trainer explaining a new concept or skill to the client. Afterward, the client demonstrates understanding by practicing under the personal trainer's direction, while the trainer encourages him or her to continue to practice until the skills become natural. The climate of direct instruction is task-oriented and is high in expectations. The client will be more motivated to learn in areas they find interesting and may actively resist learning in areas they do not. You can increase motivation by teaching information that meets the needs and desires of the client. Once an area of interest is discovered, you can use a variety of teaching techniques to help the client feel successful with learning. According to Wlodkowski (1998), an initial small success can lead to greater confidence in the learning process, improved self-esteem, and increased motivation to learn new things. Your selection of techniques will depend upon your style and that of the client. What works well for one client may not work for another. Having a variety of teaching techniques is essential to the success of the trainer/client relationship.

Multisensory Input

Clients gather information through their senses (visual, auditory, kinesthetic, smell, taste) and this creates a pathway for information to be received and processed. Pathways often overlap with clients showing a "preference" for gathering information in one pathway over others. Approximately 60% of the population prefers a primary visual pathway, while 20% accesses information auditorily and another 20% prefers to kinesthetically receive data. Even though a client may enjoy charts and pictures because he or she prefers to gather information visually, the client is still able to gather information verbally, although it is not their dominant pathway.

You can identify which pathway the client prefers by observing actions during learning situations and by listening for clues in language (table 11.2). For example, a personal trainer is discussing basic anatomy with a client using an anatomy chart on the wall. The visual learner may focus directly on the chart and may walk right up to it while the trainer is talking. The auditory learner may ignore the chart and focus directly on the trainer's words. The kinesthetic learner may touch the chart or touch and move the corresponding muscles as the trainer describes them. If you can identify the learning pathway that the client prefers, you can match your words and behaviors to that preference (see table 11.2). This not only enhances learning, but it also allows you to maintain rapport with your client.

"Tell, Show, Do"
I hear and I forget
I see and I remember
I do and I understand
—Confucius

This proverb is at the heart of day-to-day personal training. As early as the 1930s, John Dewey advocated "learning by doing." Probably the most effective systematic method of teaching a skill is by explanation, demonstration, and execution, also known as "tell, show, do." It involves observing how something is done correctly and then performing it under the supervision of an instructor (figure 11.3). The instructor provides an auditory, visual, and kinesthetic learning experience, thus stimulating all learning pathways.

Table 11.2 Learning Pathways

	Visual	Auditory	Kinesthetic
Participant actions	Watches intently Prefers reading	Listens carefully Prefers hearing	Touches or holds Prefers to be spotted
Participant statements	"Oh, I see." "Let me see that again."	"Yeah, I hear you." "Say that one more time."	"I feel that." "This does not feel right."
Strategy	Demonstrations	Question and answer	Hands-on supervision

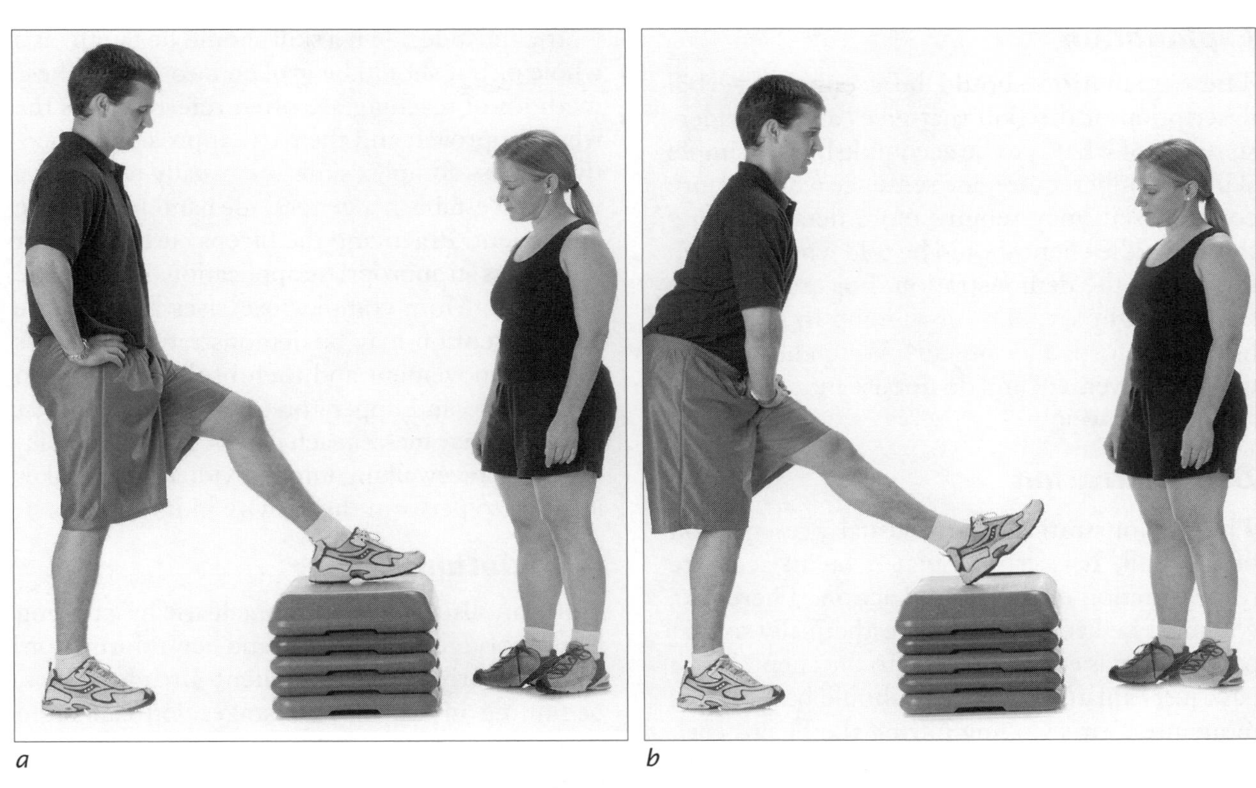

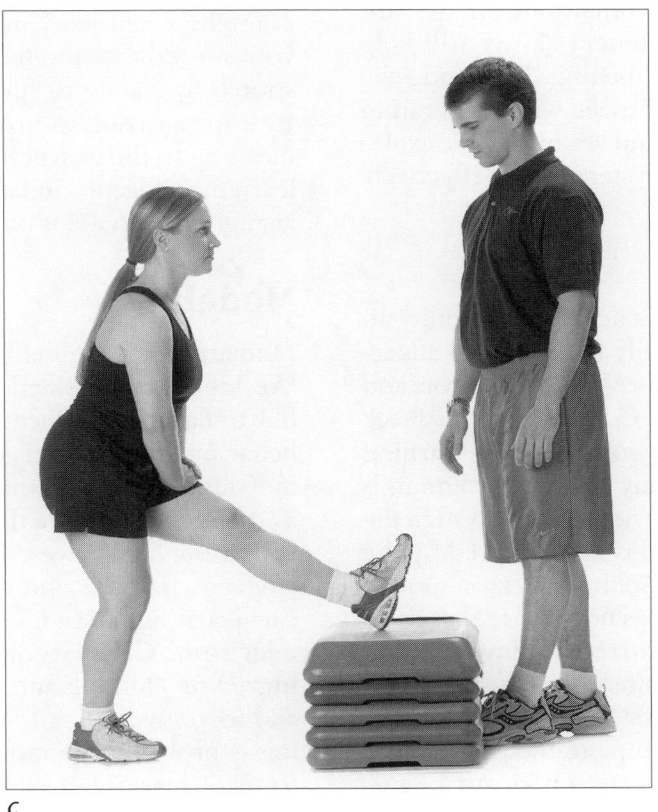

Figure 11.3 "Tell, show, do."

Explanation

The explanation should be a concise verbal description of the skill that gives a clear understanding of what is to be accomplished. A simple skill may only require one sentence while a more complex skill may require more detail. During this time, the client should be told what to watch for during the demonstration. For example, the trainer might say, "I'm now going to show you how to perform a biceps curl. Watch how I control the movement and do not use momentum to help lift the weight."

Demonstration

The demonstration is the visual presentation of the skill. It is critical that it be an accurate representation of the desired action. Therefore, you must be keenly aware kinesthetically so that proper form is communicated to the client. If you have just explained that there should be no use of momentum or swinging during the biceps curl, then you must perform the curl with complete control without using momentum for the lift. Demonstrating the movement slowly will help the client see what is happening. Repeating the demonstration at normal speed while reiterating the main points also will aid learning. The explanation and demonstration steps can be effectively combined to save time.

Performance

The performance is the client's opportunity to practice the skill. Carefully monitor and supervise the client's performance to correct errors and encourage proper form. Constructive feedback and more practice time complete the learning loop. The problem in many teaching programs is that all the above steps are not followed. Often the explanation or "tell" step is not followed by the "show" and "do" steps. Telling a person exactly how to perform a skill does not ensure that he or she will be able to do it correctly. Simply telling a client to "stretch the hamstrings after you jog" does not ensure that he or she will perform the stretch effectively. To complete the process, the client should be shown how to perform a hamstring stretch properly, and then given an opportunity to practice it while you coach proper form and execution.

You must decide if a skill should be taught as a whole or if it should be broken into parts. These methods of teaching are often referred to as the whole approach and the parts approach, respectively. Less complex skills are usually taught as a whole to establish a general idea and feel for the movement. Practicing the biceps curl from start to finish is an appropriate application of the whole approach. More complex exercises that require much attention may be demonstrated by you as a whole movement and then broken down into lower torso and upper-torso movements so that the client may master each part of the skill. Breaking down racewalking into individual parts makes it easier to perform the activity in its entirety.

Association

you can also help the client learn by creating links or bridges between old and new information. By discovering what the client already knows, beginning in the rapport stage, you can build on preexisting knowledge. Each client will have unique personal experiences to draw from. For example, when working with a client who skis, you can redirect the feet during a standing calf stretch by cueing to "point both skis downhill." By using an association, you allow clients to place meaning to the instruction, and, ultimately, they learn more deeply and are more likely to make a lasting improvement on performance.

Modeling

Humans want to identify with other humans. We look at others and imitate traits we would like to have. The concept of emulating another's behavior or attitudes is called modeling and the individual demonstrating the behavior is known as the model. We see many examples of modeling in our daily lives. Children adopt parent's language patterns and nonverbal cues and they can learn aggressive behavior from watching television. Celebrity models have a profound impact on clothing and dress, hair styles, music, and food. According to Bandura (1977), modeling is probably the most efficient and effective form of learning a new behavior. This places both enormous opportunity and responsibility on the personal trainer. Two forms of modeling are identified by Good and Brophy (1999). The first is simply imitation, or "monkey see, monkey do." The observer adopts the behavior of the model. The second is more complex because the observer must infer attitudes, values, beliefs, or personality characteristics as a result of watching the model. The observer draws his or her own conclusions and, over time, may change a behavior. This is a common occurrence in the personal trainer/client relationship. As a result of observing your dedication to a healthy and fit lifestyle, the client may choose a healthier alternative to the regular Friday afternoon happy hour. In this form of modeling, people often communicate attitudes unconsciously and are unaware of the effects. Students constantly observe a teacher's approach to a subject, studying the teacher's attitudes and beliefs. They watch the way the teacher interacts with other students and colleagues and the student may then make inferences regarding the learning process. The way in which a teacher responds to a student's question can affect the learning climate. The response, "I don't know . . . let's find out," models enthusiasm for learning and makes not knowing the answer acceptable. This form of modeling is both subtle and powerful.

There are several factors that influence modeling. The first is the state of the learner. The more uncertain a learner is, the more significant the effects of the model will be. Therefore, a client is more susceptible to the effects of your modeling at the beginning of the relationship. A second factor that influences modeling is the status of the model in the eyes of the learner. Students are more likely to adopt the behaviors of a teacher they like and respect than of one they do not.

You cannot escape being a model. However, you can decide what kind of model you will be. Who a personal trainer is and what he or she does sends loud and clear messages to the client about what is important and how the program is really supposed to work. In other words, the way you behave is just as important as what you say. The personal trainer who advocates doing what he or she is unwilling to do will more than likely be unconvincing. For example, it is fruitless for a personal trainer to tell clients that steroids are bad for their health when it is known that the trainer uses steroids. "Do as I say, not as I do" has no place in the personal trainer/client relationship. The client views you as an expert and will generally believe everything that you say and do with regard to fitness. Therefore, it is critical that you be aware of your influence. Be competent and wise in fitness matters and obtain at least a level of fitness that corresponds to the level of teaching. Going beyond mere competence is even more desirable.

Contracting

Contracting finds its roots in the behavioral theory of reinforcement that says rewarded behavior tends to be repeated. Contracting systematically arranges the rewards so that the probability of the desired response is increased. Most behavioral **contracts** are verbal or written agreements between two or more people and consist of two primary parts (figure 11.4). The first part is specifying the behavior to be achieved. The second part is stating specific reinforcements that will reward the desired behavior. It may take the form of, "If you will do ___________, I will do _________." A contract does not necessarily require involving other people. It is possible to make an agreement with oneself by preparing a self-contract (figure 11.5).

All helping relationships have implied contracts or understandings that both people will have responsibilities to carry out. Verbal or informal contracts are used when there is little chance of a misunderstanding of the conditions. The written contract is used to prevent those misunderstandings and to add impact by having the client sign to indicate a commitment.

Several features are necessary for an effective contract. The terms should be explicitly stated so that the expectations are clearly understood by all parties. An example of an unclear contract statement is, "I agree to lose some weight so I may do something I enjoy." A more clearly stated contract term might be, "I will lose 5 pounds and then I'll be permitted to buy that new dress." Many contracts fail because of impossible terms, so they should be feasible and reasonable. "I will lose 50 pounds this month so I can buy that new dress," is an unreasonable goal. "I will lose 1 to 2 pounds a week for the next two months," is a more reasonable goal. Composing the contract in positive rather than negative terms will encourage a more favorable attitude toward the contract. "If

I, the undersigned, agree to the following conditions, which I will follow to the best of my ability.

From ________ to ________, for a period of one week, I will choose to eat at meal time only.

From ________ to ________, for a period of one week, I will eat foods recommended by the American Heart Association and the American Dietetic Association.

At the end of the week, as a reward for fulfilling the above conditions, I will attend a movie or other social function with my husband.

Date ______________________________

Signature of wife ______________________________

I, the undersigned, agree to take my wife to a movie when the above conditions are met.

Date ______________________________

Signature of husband ______________________________

Figure 11.4 Example of a contract between two people.

I will walk in my target zone a minimum of _______ minutes _______ times per week.

I will record my progress in my personal log.

The following people will help me reach my goal:

Person Method

Person	Method
1. ________________	1. ________________
2. ________________	2. ________________
3. ________________	3. ________________
4. ________________	4. ________________

I will reward myself for adhering to the above for _______ weeks with the following:

____

____

____

I will begin the program _______ and will reevaluate it on _______.
(date) (date)

Figure 11.5 Example of a personal exercise contract.

you do not quit smoking, I will not work with you," is a negative approach. A more positive approach would be to determine a reward given upon smoking cessation. To ensure satisfactory results, contracts need to be evaluated frequently and perhaps renegotiated. This renegotiation can occur any time or during the formal evaluation process. What appeared to be fair and reasonable initially may not be so later. If a client discovers he or she cannot meet a specified commitment, you should discuss the difficulty and a new contract can be negotiated, drafted, and signed. This evaluation process will help ensure that the contract remains effective.

The following questions will help you troubleshoot while writing contracts:

1. Are the terms of the contract clear?
2. Is the contract fair?
3. Is the contract positive?
4. Is the target behavior clearly specified?
5. Does the contract provide for immediate reinforcement?
6. Is the reinforcement frequent and in small amounts?
7. Does the client understand the contract?
8. Is there a time specified for evaluation?

Feedback

Feedback is a powerful contributor to effective learning and client performance. It is any information about current or past behavior that can be used to improve performance and can be given verbally or nonverbally. It usually occurs after a client has asked a question or done something related to the exercise session. Feedback informs the client of the correctness of performance and recognizes effort. You will naturally respond and react to clients' behaviors, and they are greatly influenced by the way you behave toward them. They monitor their personal trainers' reactions and adjust their performance in accordance with what they interpret.

For feedback to be effective, a clearly defined standard of performance must be given. For example, a personal trainer defines the standard of performance for proper placement and movement of the arms in race walking during their explanation and demonstration of the skill. The client's performance is then measured and corrected according to the demonstrated criteria. The performance standard may need to be set at frequent intervals during instruction by continuing to explain and demonstrate. For the feedback to be effective and learning to occur, there must be a practice session that gives the client an opportunity to correct performance and reach the preset standard.

Research indicates that effective feedback has three characteristics: (1) it is specific; (2) it is contingent on performance; and (3) it provides corrective information for the learner. Specific feedback is clear about what was right and/or wrong. You may watch a client incorrectly perform a lat pulldown on the weight equipment and then exclaim, "That's not right, Susie!" Your response does not aid Susie's understanding of the performance, it only lets her know that it was wrong. By contrast, you might respond, "Not quite Susie. Let's reverse the position of your hands." Corrective feedback helps the client know what was wrong with the performance and what to do to get back on track. The number of different cues is infinite, and striving for unique ones will require your creativity and committed practice.

Feedback should not be given for every single move because too much of a good thing can have a negative effect; people tend to disregard excessive compliments. The feedback should match the achievement and specifically relate the response to the performance. For example, a personal trainer observing a client performing a biceps curl might respond with, "That's good," which is only a statement of general praise. However, an even more effective response would be, "That's it John, you're really isolating the biceps muscle now." This response gives the client specific information as to why the performance is correct. To maximize the effect, cues can be personalized by using a client's name, for instance, "That's the right idea, Jennie." Typical verbal cues are

Good	All right
Excellent	OK
Right	Very good
Correct	Fine

These words are less effective because they have been overused. Examples of other, more effective cues that you might use are

That's an effective thought.
You've got it.
You're on the money.
You are really with it today.
I'd give that move a 10.

Nonverbal feedback is far more effective than verbal feedback. Clients tune into facial expressions and gestures. When used properly, nonverbal cues are the epitome of personalization.

How else can a "thumbs up" signal and a generous smile be interpreted? Nonverbal positive feedback interactions include

Smiling	Touching
Making an "Okay" sign	Clapping
Nodding	Winking
Patting on the back	Thumbs up
Shaking hands	Applauding

Nonverbal negative feedback interactions include

Frowning	Looking away
Thumbs down	Rolling eyes
Shaking head	Grimacing
Drumming fingers	

A final and important point needs to be made regarding verbal and nonverbal feedback. As in all interpersonal communication, when both verbal and nonverbal cues are given, they must be congruent. For example, if you frown while telling a client that they are doing a great job, the two behaviors are incongruent and the conflicting messages are confusing. The client will receive a mixed message and will probably believe the frown rather than the words. On the other hand, when verbal and nonverbal cuing are congruently combined, you can have a powerful influence on the client.

STAGES OF LEARNING

Understanding the various stages of learning will help you teach more effectively. One of the most commonly cited learning models was developed by Fitts and Posner (1967), who theorized that there are three stages of learning for a motor skill: cognitive, associative, and autonomous. Within the **cognitive stage of learning,** learners make many errors and have highly variable performances. They know they are doing something wrong, but they do not know how to improve their performance. At this stage, participants seem terribly uncoordinated and consistently perform exercises incorrectly. Those in the **associative stage of learning** have learned the basic fundamentals or mechanics of the skill. Their errors tend to be less gross in nature and they can now concentrate on refining their skills. During this stage, exercise participants are able to detect some errors and the instructor needs to make only occasional corrections. During the **autonomous stage of learning** the skill becomes automatic or habitual. Learners can now perform without thinking and can detect their own errors. Driving a car, for example, is a very complex motor skill that over time is performed in the autonomous stage. The driver often is concentrating elsewhere and is able to recognize when mistakes are made. The type and amount of information that exercise participants can understand depends on their current stage within the learning process. An awareness of your client's stage of learning will enable you to employ the appropriate teaching strategy for each individual.

SUMMARY

Your relationships with clients are helping relationships throughout the stages of establishing and building rapport with them, gathering vital information, developing fitness goals, and implementing a plan to accomplish them. As a helper, you create conditions and use techniques that will help bring about the desired outcomes for the client. Merely possessing a fit body, technical skills, and a wide-based knowledge of health and fitness does not ensure your success. Probably the most crucial factor for determining a positive climate for the working relationship is the trainer's repertoire of communication skills. These skills include both verbal and nonverbal behaviors, such as attending, perceiving nonverbal messages, perceiving verbal messages, and verbal responding. These interpersonal communication skills can be learned, practiced, and mastered, and are important not only in the first stage of establishing rapport, but throughout the entire process.

Personal training is about behavioral change, which is the true measure of a successful trainer/client relationship. Every personal trainer is unique and brings into the relationship his or her own personal experience and opinions about what brings about lifestyle changes in people. Each client also is uniquely different. Therefore, you must be flexible in matching teaching techniques and changing strategies to meet the goals, needs, and personality of the client. A technique that is successful for one client does not ensure the same achievement or change for another. A skilled personal trainer will get to know the client and apply various techniques with wisdom, while another may resist to the point of discontinuing the relationship.

The flexibility required to do your job sometimes demands that you be deeply personal and at other times remain an objective observer. Being able to move freely along the full range of interpersonal skills and teaching techniques will permit you to respond appropriately at various stages of the relationship. On one hand, the process of sizing up and assisting a client toward a healthy lifestyle is naturally intuitive, but, on the other hand, it needs to be a deliberate, rational process.

REFERENCES

Bandura, A. (1977). *Social Learning Theory*. Englewood Cliffs, NJ: Prentice Hall.

Dick, W., Carey, L., & Carey, J.O. (2000). *The Systematic Design of Instruction* (5th ed.). New York:Addison-Wesley Publishing.

Fitts, P.M. & Posner, M.I. (1967). *Human Performance*. Belmont, CA: Brooks/Cole.

Good, F. & Brophy, J. (1999). *Looking in Classrooms* (8th ed.). Needham Heights, MA: Allyn & Bacon.

Hall, E.T. (1966). *The Hidden Dimension*. Garden City, CA: Doubleday.

Mehrabian, A. (1972). *Nonverbal Communication*. New York: Walter de Gruyter.

Rogers, C.R. et al. (1967). *The Therapeutic Relationship and Its Impact*. Madison: University of Wisconsin Press.

Truax, C.B. & Carkuff, R.F. (1967). *Toward Effective Counseling and Psychotherapy*. New York:Walter de Gruyter.

Wlodkowski, R. (1998). *Enhancing Adult Motivation to Learn*. San Francisco: Jossey-Bass.

SUGGESTED READING

Bolton, R. (1986). *People Skills*. Carmichael, CA: Touchstone Books.

Boothman, N. (2000). *How to Make People Like You in 90 Seconds or Less*. New York: Workman Publishing.

Carkhuff, R.R. & Anthony, W.A. (1999). *The Skills of Helping*. Amherst: Human Resource Development Press.

Covey, S.R. (1989). *The Seven Habits of Highly Effective People: Powerful Lessons in Personal Change*. New York: Simon & Schuster.

Covey, S.R. & Merrill, A.R., & Merrill, R.R. (1994). *First Things First*. New York: Simon & Schuster

Csikszentmihalyi, M. (1991). *Flow: The Psychology of Optimal Experience*. New York: HarperCollins.

Goleman, D. (1995). *Emotional Intelligence*. New York: Bantam Books.

Jacobson, D., Kauchak, D., & Eggen, P.D. (1992). *Methods for Teaching: A Skills Approach* (4th ed.). New York: Macmillan College Division.

Kauchak, D.P. & Eggen, P.E. (2002). *Learning and Teaching: Research-based Methods* (4th ed.). Needham Heights, MA: Allyn & Bacon.

Krumboltz, J. (1966). *Stating the Goals of Counseling* (Monograph No. 1). Fullerton: California

Personnel and Guidance Association.

Malouf, D. (1999). *Power Up Your People Skills: Communication in the New Millennium*. Australia. Australian Print Group.

Martens, R. (2004). *Successful Coaching* (3rd ed.). Champaign, IL: Human Kinetics.

Mosston, M. (1966). *Teaching Physical Education: From Command to Discovery*. Columbus: Merrill.

O'Connor, J. & McDermott, I. (2001). *Way of NLP*. London. Thorsons Publishing.

Okun, B.F. (2001). *Effective Helping: Interviewing and Counseling Techniques*. Belmont, CA: Wadsworth Publishing Company.

Rogers, C. (1995). *On Becoming a Person*. New York: Houghton Mifflin.

Vernacchia, R. et al. (1996). *Coaching Mental Excellence*. Portola Valley, CA: Warde Publishers.

CHAPTER 12

Musculoskeletal Injuries, Prevention, and First Aid

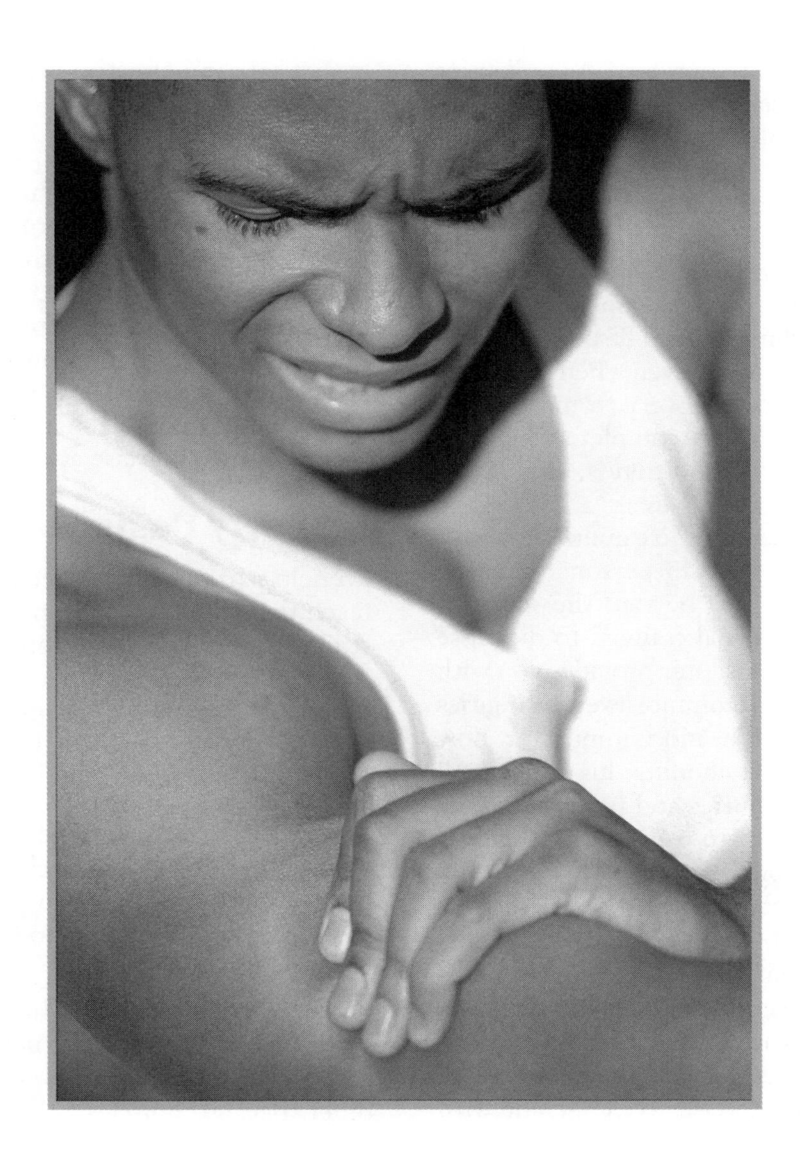

Although exercise can be enjoyable and provide numerous significant health benefits, any exercise program carries the potential for injury. Many health professionals, including physicians, athletic trainers, and physical therapists deal with injuries from exercise-related activities. With backgrounds in sport, medicine, and exercise science, these specialists are well prepared to give prompt diagnosis, treatment, and rehabilitation for exercise injuries. Considering the injury potential inherent in exercise, you need to know how injuries happen, how to prevent them, and how to provide first aid (depending on your YMCA's policy for handling emergencies) when they occur.

Musculoskeletal injuries are probably the most common injuries sustained by exercise participants. Unfortunately, they are also one of the leading causes for people to stop exercising. To help prevent musculoskeletal injuries, focus on developing programs that develop your participants' strength, endurance, and flexibility. However, injuries can still occur even when programs are properly designed. Recovery from an injury is often quicker and more complete when the participant is properly conditioned, facilitating rehabilitation of the injured area.

What can you do to minimize injuries for your members who participate in personal training programs? Although it is beyond the scope of practice for most personal trainers to diagnose and treat injuries, this chapter provides you with a basic understanding of common exercise injuries and health concerns and, more important, how to prevent them. Understanding this subject will help you recognize injuries and potential safety problems and allow you to react appropriately if you are confronted by them.

We begin this chapter by reviewing key factors related to injury prevention. The next section defines key anatomical and sports medicine terms. Then we briefly describe common musculoskeletal injuries, with a special section on muscle soreness and fatigue, and additional health problems related to exercise. We conclude with basic first aid for treating injuries.

PRINCIPLES OF INJURY PREVENTION

To achieve the many wonderful health benefits of exercise and physical activity, the body must be stressed beyond its normal fitness level. But those same potentially beneficial stresses can also harm the body if they are not properly monitored or prepared for. YMCA personal trainers can help minimize the risk of injuries in members with whom they work by following some principles of prevention—screening, using properly designed programs, hydration, appropriate clothing, the proper use of equipment, and understanding the impact of environmental factors. Although these recommendations might seem obvious, trainers and participants should review them regularly to ensure safe and effective programs.

Screening

Become familiar with the health screening procedures for members and program participants at your YMCA. Trainers and their participants need to be aware of conditions that could affect their exercise participation. Reproducible screening forms are located in appendix B. The more you and your participants know about their health and how it affects physical activity, the more likely they will be to exercise at an appropriate level.

Properly Designed Programs

To help participants reduce their risk of injury, teach them what an appropriate workload is for their fitness level. As mentioned in previous chapters, this information is part of a well-designed exercise program. Following are key factors in program design that will help prevent participant injury:

- **Biomechanics.** Teach controlled movements using proper biomechanics. Demonstrate proper technique in a complete, safe range of motion, and teach proper body alignment during all activity.
- **Muscular balance.** Muscles work in opposing pairs, making it vital to develop both pairs so that one does not overpower or overstretch the other. Because muscles help support the joints, balancing muscle groups often results in fewer injuries to the knees, hips, shoulders, and back. A properly designed program will work opposing pairs equally, as well as work both the left and right sides of the body equally.
- **Warm-up.** All exercise should be preceded by a 5- to 10-minute warm-up to prepare the

body for more vigorous activity. Beginners might require a longer, more gradual warm-up, while advanced participants might need a shorter warm-up period.

- **Pace.** Urge participants to work out at their own pace and within their physical capabilities. A beginner might sustain a strain or overuse injury by trying to participate at an intensity that is too high.
- **Cool-down.** A cool-down gradually returns the body to a low-intensity, preexercise level. This is usually accomplished by a gradual reduction in exercise intensity.
- **Flexibility.** Properly stretching the muscles used during exercise should always follow the cool-down. Stretching should be done in a pain-free range of motion that elongates muscles to the point where tension is felt, but not discomfort.

Hydration

Encourage participants to drink plenty of fluids (preferably water) at regular intervals during exercise. Water intake is necessary for replacing body fluid lost through perspiration and is therefore vital to preventing heat illnesses, as well as maximizing activity performance.

Mechanical Equipment

Trainers should teach members how to properly use exercise equipment and ensure that members use it properly each time. Before allowing members to use equipment, trainers should inspect it for signs of wear and breakage that could lead to injury.

Personal Equipment

Clothes and footwear are considered personal equipment. To perform at the optimum level safely, participants should do the following:

- **Wear comfortable clothes that allow adequate ventilation.** Clothing that is too tight or rough can irritate the skin, causing blisters, rashes, or even abrasions. Clothing should also be made of material that "breathes" to allow sweat to evaporate, which allows the body to cool. Do not allow participants to wear vinyl or rubber suits in an attempt to lose weight; these suits prevent sweat evaporation and cause the body's internal temperature to rise. This condition can result in heat exhaustion or, worse, heatstroke.
- **Wear comfortable, supportive footwear.** Properly constructed and fitted exercise footwear aids in shock absorption and stability, and minimizes potential foot and leg injuries. Shoes specifically developed for the activity the member is participating in are preferable, but a cross-training shoe is adequate for many fitness activities. Shoes should be supportive and cushioned appropriately for the activity, should have sufficient arch support, be flexible, and prevent excessive foot pronation or supination. Most shoes maintain their support and cushion qualities for about six months if a person exercises several times a week and does not use the shoes for other activities. Encourage participants to invest in high-quality exercise footwear.

Environmental Considerations

Personal trainers should monitor the environment to ensure that it is safe for exercise. In particular, advise members to be cautious when exercising in the heat and cold. Exercising in hot and humid conditions can cause adverse reactions such as heat cramps, heat exhaustion, and heatstroke, so moderation and proper hydration are vital. Members should be aware of the possibility of hypothermia (low core body temperature) and frostbite when exercising in cold environments. Layering clothes and wearing hats, mittens, and ear and nose protection will prevent the majority of cold-related injuries.

ANATOMICAL AND SPORTS MEDICINE TERMS

To fully understand the intricacies of injuries, you must become familiar with a few anatomical and medical terms. Let's start by taking a look at the structure of a joint (figure 12.1). Knees, elbows, and other joints consist of bones, cartilage, muscles, tendons, and ligaments.

Tendons and ligaments are the structures that hold joints together. Ligaments act as guy wires, connecting bone to bone. They function as the joint's primary stabilizers, and muscles serve as backup supporters. Without ligaments and muscles, bones in a joint would easily dislocate or separate. Tendons connect muscles to bones

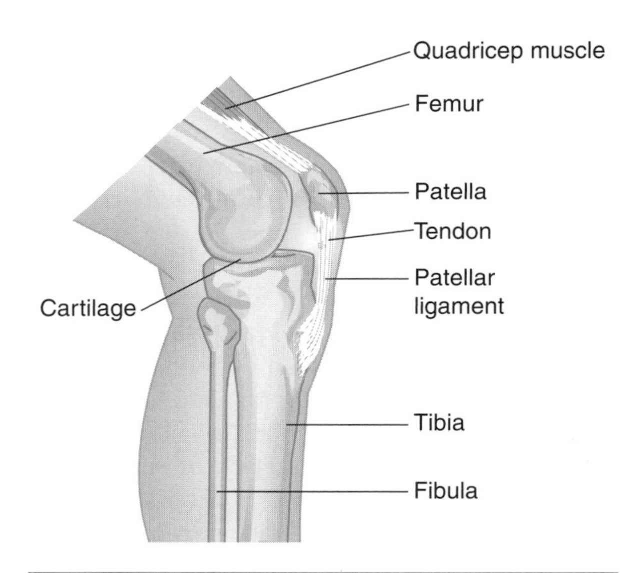

Figure 12.1 Structures of the knee joint.

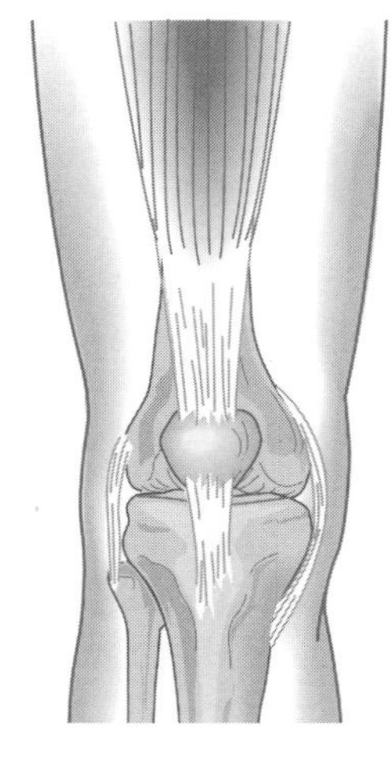

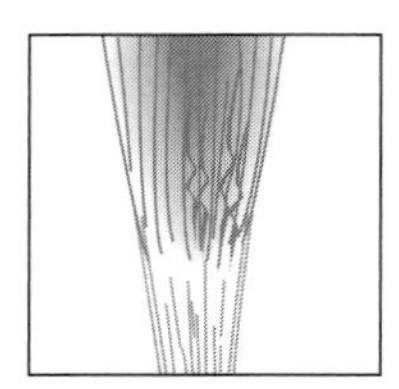

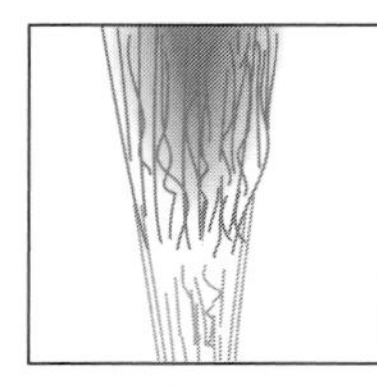

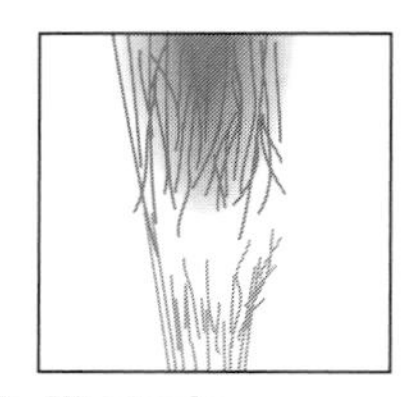

Figure 12.2 Three types of muscle strains.

and help make a joint move. And to protect a joint's integrity, cartilage acts as a shock absorber and prevents the bones from abrading (wearing down).

With this basic anatomy in mind, let's discuss terms that you will undoubtedly come across when reading sports medicine information.

- **Strains.** Stretching and tearing injuries that affect muscles and tendons. A strain often results when a sudden or persistent stretch forces a muscle or tendon beyond its normal stretching limit. Among the structures strained most often are the calf muscles, the Achilles tendon, the quadriceps muscles, the hamstring muscles, the shoulder muscles, and the low back.

  Depending on their severity, strains are classified in one of three categories (see figure 12.2). A grade I strain stretches muscle or tendon fibers with minimal tearing. Symptoms include little or no swelling, point tenderness at the site of the injury, and mild pain when the muscle or tendon is stretched or contracted. In a grade II strain, stretched muscle or tendon fibers are also partially torn. Grade II symptoms include pain, swelling, and possibly a slight indentation at the site of the strain. Grade III strains involve extensive tearing of muscle or tendon fibers and cause pain, swelling, and an obvious indentation at the injury site.

- **Sprains**. Stretching and tearing injuries of the ligaments. A common cause of sprains is a sudden twisting movement that stretches or tears the ligament fibers. Sprains, like strains, can be classified according to severity, with various levels of pain, swelling, and disability (see figure 12.3).

- **Tendinitis.** An inflammation or irritation of a tendon resulting from overuse or a forceful stretch. Tendons most affected by tendinitis are the Achilles tendon and the elbow and shoulder tendons.

- **Chondromalacia.** A softening or abrading of joint cartilage as a natural part of aging (wear and tear) or as a result of direct injury.

- **Periostitis.** An inflammation or irritation of the membrane that covers the bones.

- **Foot pronation.** A structural condition in which the foot rolls inward, under the ankle (see figure 12.4).

With an understanding of these general terms, we can discuss specific injuries sustained by exercise participants.

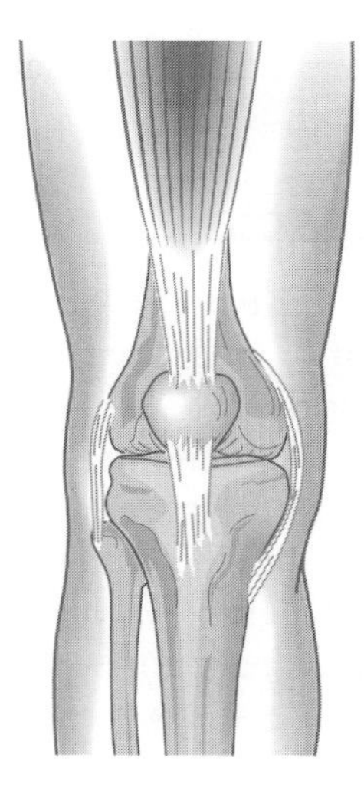

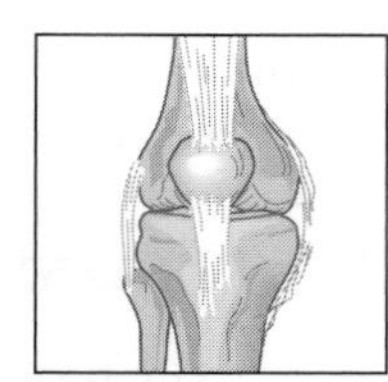

Grade I sprain
Ligament(s) stretched slightly with a few fibers possibly torn

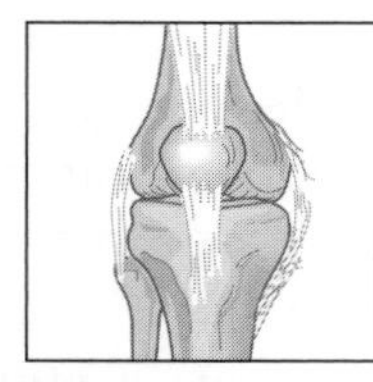

Grade II sprain
Ligament(s) stretched and partially torn

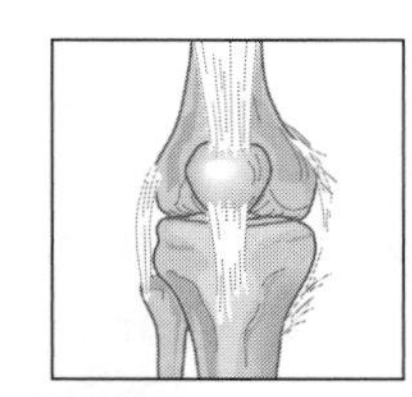

Grade III sprain
Ligament(s) torn completely

Figure 12.3 Three types of ligament sprains.

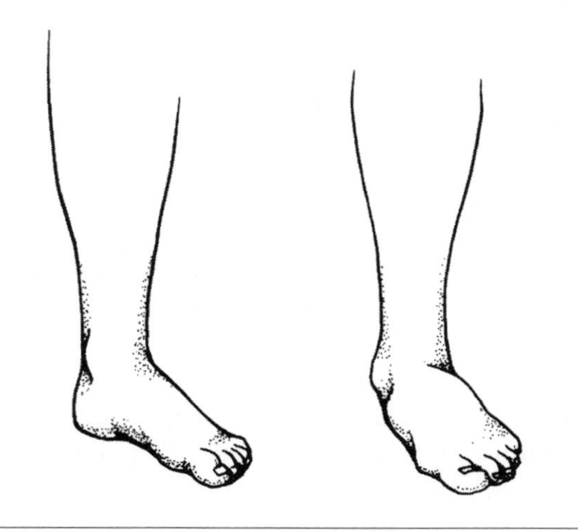

Figure 12.4 Comparison of a normal and a pronated foot.

EXERCISE-RELATED INJURIES

Most musculoskeletal injuries related to exercise fall into the category of overuse syndrome. Overuse injuries occur when the body is subjected to abnormal, constant, or repetitive stress or is inadequately prepared for a particular activity. It's easy to understand why overuse injuries can occur with repetitive activities (lifting, jumping, running) and stressful movements (twisting, lunging). People who are out of shape or are participating at a level too advanced for their physical capabilities are also prone to overuse syndrome. Be aware of the following signs and symptoms that indicate injury:

- Persistent pain, even when the body part is resting
- Swelling and discoloration
- Increased pain when body weight is placed on the injury
- Joint pain
- Pain or tenderness when the injured area is touched lightly
- Deviations in normal movement patterns

Common exercise-related overuse injuries are shin splints, calf muscle strain, Achilles tendinitis, bone bruises, stress fractures, arch strain, patellar (kneecap) chondromalacia, impingement syndrome, and carpal tunnel syndrome. Let's take a look at each to find out why and how it happens.

Shin Splints

Shin splints is a catchall phrase used to describe aching pain in the front of the lower leg. It can be caused by a strain to lower-leg muscles or tendons, by shin bone periostitis, or by a stress fracture. Some causes of shin splints include the following:

- **Abnormal foot positioning.** The foot might be tilted in (pronated), which puts stress on the calf muscles and tendons.
- **Muscle imbalance.** The muscles on the front of the leg might not be equal in strength to the muscles on the back of the leg, causing the weaker of the two to suffer from strain.
- **Excessive shock transmitted through the lower leg.** Unyielding floor surfaces or poorly padded shoes force the leg to bear the brunt of the impact shock.

Calf Muscle Strain and Achilles Tendinitis

In the back of the lower leg, potential problem areas include the calf muscle and the Achilles tendon at its base. Injuries to both areas are felt as aching or sharp pain. Calf strains are felt in the muscle belly, and Achilles tendinitis is felt in the upper-heel area. Standing or jumping on the toes, rocking back, or walking on the heels can be painful in both conditions. Causes of calf muscle strain and Achilles tendonitis include the following:

- Shortened calf muscle or Achilles tendon. Some people naturally have short calf muscles or tendons. Others have worn high-heeled shoes that let the calf muscles and tendons shorten. In either case, stretching the muscle or tendon beyond its normal limits can result in a strain.
- Inadequate stretching in warm-up or cool-down.
- Repeated stress.
- Landing on the balls of the feet without letting the heels touch the floor.

Bone Bruises, Stress Fractures, and Arch Strain

Because of the pounding the foot often experiences during exercise, it is another site of frequent injury. Hard floors and improperly fitting shoes or shoes with insufficient padding can contribute to all overuse injuries, including injuries of the feet. Foot stress most often appears as a bone bruise, a stress fracture, or an arch strain.

Bone bruises and stress fractures can occur at the heel or ball of the foot. Bone bruises are commonly felt on the sole of the foot, whereas stress fractures at the ball of the foot are usually felt on the top of the foot. Stress fractures become more painful with exercise. Common causes of bone bruises and stress fractures include poorly padded shoes and nonyielding floor surfaces that force the foot to absorb excessive shock. Another cause is deviations in proper running gait.

Arch strain is pain felt on the sole of the foot between the heel and the ball. It is most often the result of a strain to the plantar fascia that spans the area. Some causes of arch strain include flat feet and inadequate arch support.

Patellar Chondromalacia

The knee, like the foot and the ankle, is subjected to the shock of the body pounding against the floor or the repeated bending during strength training. A common knee problem in exercise programs is patellar (kneecap) chondromalacia, in which the cartilage surface on the back of the kneecap becomes irritated and begins to crack and flake. It is most noticeable as a pain under the kneecap that is felt when climbing stairs, sitting in one position for a prolonged period, squatting, kneeling, or bending at the knee.

Causes of patellar chondromalacia include the following:

- Kneecap that doesn't ride properly in its groove on the thigh bone (especially in people with knock-knees or bowlegs)
- Natural wear and tear on the joint from aging
- Direct blow to the top of the kneecap
- Excessive kneeling or squatting

Impingement Syndrome

In shoulder impingement syndrome, swollen rotator cuff muscles and the bursa are "pinched" by the scapula when the arm is abducted (moved away from the center of the body). This syndrome makes it difficult to perform exercises when the arms are raised over the head or abducted. Exercises such as overhead presses, military presses, and lat pull-downs may aggravate this condition.

Causes of impingement syndrome include prior shoulder dislocation injury, which causes discomfort when the shoulder is placed in an abducted and externally rotated position such as the starting position of a bench press. Overstretched front or anterior ligaments of the shoulder can also cause impingement syndrome.

Carpal Tunnel Syndrome

Most commonly seen as an occupational illness, carpal tunnel syndrome occurs in people who perform repetitive tasks such as working at a computer keyboard. It also can result from weight training and other athletic activities. People with carpal tunnel syndrome might complain of numbness in the middle fingers of the hand, usually after repetitive work using the wrist and finger-flexor muscles. Stretching to keep these muscles flexible can help prevent this type of injury.

Causes of carpal tunnel syndrome include:

- Repetitive tasks such as typing or working at a cash register
- Weight training
- Engaging in athletic activities that involve extensive use of the wrist and finger-flexor muscles

A summary of the overuse injuries common to exercisers and their causes and symptoms is presented in table 12.1. Other musculoskeletal problems common to exercisers are muscle soreness and muscle cramps.

MUSCLE SORENESS AND FATIGUE

Muscle soreness and fatigue is inevitable for anyone who exercises, particularly newcomers. Most often it occurs in people who begin to participate after a period of inactivity or those attempting a higher level of difficulty. The muscles and tendons are forced to work harder than they are accustomed to, and the result is a general aching pain that can last from one to three days.

Muscle Soreness

Two general types of exercise-related muscle soreness exist. The first type, immediate soreness, is felt during exercise or immediately afterward. This type of soreness appears to be most directly related to lactic acid that has built up in the muscle and leaked out of the muscle cells. Usually the body removes this excess lactic acid 30 to 60 minutes after a training session. Immediate soreness might also be due to increased muscle acidity or chemical energy depletion.

The second type of soreness persists for one to three days following a training session. Immediately following a hard strength training session the muscles might feel tight or fatigued, but not necessarily sore. However, the following day the exerciser might experience considerable muscle soreness, which could persist for another day or two. This is known as delayed onset muscle soreness (DOMS). DOMS is most likely caused by microtrauma (microscopic tears) in the muscle or connective tissue. The body usually requires several days to complete the repairing and building processes. DOMS is typically associated with eccentric muscle contractions.

Muscle Fatigue

The reasons for fatigue are varied, but they relate primarily to the intensity and duration of exercise. Skeletal muscle eventually fatigues after a period of work or exercise. During heavy strength training, the primary causes of muscle fatigue are the depletion of anaerobic energy supplies and the accumulation of anaerobic byproducts such as lactic acid. However, even when a muscle is fatigued to the point that it can no longer contract concentrically, a two-minute recovery period is usually sufficient to replace the anaerobic energy stores and remove the anaerobic byproducts.

Causes of muscle soreness and fatigue include the following:

- Injury or strain to the muscle or tendon
- Insufficient supply of oxygen to working muscles
- Insufficient levels of potassium, sodium, or other minerals in the body that are used in muscle contraction; insufficient supplies disrupt normal function

ADDITIONAL EXERCISE-RELATED HEALTH PROBLEMS

In addition to suffering musculoskeletal injuries, exercise participants might encounter other health problems. Participants might suffer from blisters, abrasions, fainting, and heat illnesses. Knowing the causes of these conditions can help you and your participants prevent them.

- **Blisters.** Blisters are caused by friction between the skin and the shoe or sock. The friction causes the outer and middle skin layers to

Table 12.1 Common Overuse Injuries

Injury	Common causes	Symptoms
Shin splints	Abnormal foot positioning Muscle imbalance Excessive impact shock	Dull ache in the lower leg after workout Pain on moving the foot up and down
Strains	Inadequate stretching Stretching muscles beyond their normal limits Landing on balls of feet without heels touching floor	Grade I – some tenderness, no swelling Grade II – tenderness at site, painful movement, swelling if not treated Grade III – immediate loss of function, swelling
Sprains	Sudden twisting movements	Grade I – some tenderness, no swelling Grade II – tenderness at site, painful movement, swelling if not treated Grade III – immediate loss of function, swelling
Tendinitis	Inadequate stretching Repeated stress	Tenderness
Bone bruises	Hard surfaces Poorly padded shoes	Pain at the heel or ball of the foot
Stress fractures	Hard surfaces Deviated running gait Poorly padded shoes	Pain at the fracture site Increased pain with exercise
Arch strain	Flat feet Inadequate arch support	Pain on the sole of the foot, between the heel and ball
Patellar chondromalacia	Excessive kneeling/squatting Direct blow to the kneecap Knock-knees/bowlegs Natural wear and tear	Pain underneath the kneecap
Impingement syndrome	Prior shoulder dislocation Overstretched front or anterior shoulder ligaments	
Carpal tunnel syndrome	Repetitive tasks Weight training or other athletic activities	Numbness of middle fingers
Muscle soreness—immediate	Buildup of lactic acid	Immediate discomfort
Muscle soreness—delayed	Microtrauma of muscle tissue	Discomfort 1 to 3 days after training

rub together and consequently to separate and fill with fluid. Blisters are caused by improperly fitting shoes (too tight or too loose), shoes constructed of an unyielding material (especially new shoes), and shoes with poor ventilation.

- **Abrasions.** Abrasions, like blisters, are often caused by friction between the skin and another surface, such as a mat, floor, or carpet. Abrasions are caused by subjecting unprotected skin to an abrasive surface, either continuously or forcefully.

- **Fainting.** Fainting is a condition in which a person partially or totally loses consciousness for a short time. Symptoms leading to fainting might include dizziness, nausea, sweating, cold skin, or paleness. Lack of blood supply to the brain, resulting from fatigue, illness, injury, or shock causes fainting.

- **Heat exhaustion.** Heat exhaustion occurs when the body is subjected to a progressive loss of body fluid through sweating. Symptoms might include profuse sweating, pale or clammy skin, headache, dizziness, nausea, fatigue, or fainting. The loss of body fluids through sweating during vigorous activity in a hot environment and the failure to replace them causes shock and circulation problems, enacting heat exhaustion.

- **Heatstroke.** Heatstroke is a condition in which the body's temperature suddenly rises uncontrollably. It is characterized by hot, red skin (moist or dry), extremely high body temperature, and a disruption in the sweating mechanism.

Causes of heatstroke include the following:

- Failure to replace the body fluids lost through sweating during vigorous activity
- Exercising in a hot, humid environment, which reduces the amount of perspiration that can evaporate from the body
- Exercising when you have a fever

Now that you know the potential injuries and health problems related to exercise, let's take a look at what you can do to prevent and minimize them.

FIRST AID

If one of your participants sustains an injury, you must be prepared to handle it. Beware of treating injuries, however; you could leave yourself vulnerable to lawsuits. Improper treatment can lead to further injury or infection. Therefore, for your participants' and your own protection, limit treatment to first aid basics.

You should obtain certification in first aid and cardiopulmonary resuscitation (CPR). Through certification you will learn how to properly care for minor injuries (scrapes, cuts, blisters), serious injuries (fractures, bleeding), and life-threatening problems (heart failure, choking). First aid classes generally require 4 to 8 hours of training, and CPR certification requires 4 to 12 hours of instruction.

Any time you suspect a serious injury or illness, follow the emergency procedures set by your YMCA and urge the affected participant to seek medical attention. If an injury or illness occurs, what can you do initially to help relieve pain and minimize further complications? If a musculoskeletal injury occurs, you should use R-I-C-E (rest, ice, compression, and elevation) to minimize pain and swelling.

1. **Rest.** For mild injuries, the participant should stop moving until the pain subsides. Activity usually can be resumed once the participant can move the injured area without pain or discomfort. For more severe injuries, rest should be prescribed until a physician gives medical clearance for resuming participation.

2. **Ice.** Ice minimizes pain and swelling. Always keep a cooler of ice and plastic bags handy. Ice should be applied directly to the injured area for 15 to 20 minutes. Crushed ice in a plastic bag works best because it can conform to the body. Avoid using commercial chemical ice. It does not cool as well, and it can cause chemical burns if its container is punctured.

3. **Compression.** Wrap an elastic bandage over the ice, starting at the point farthest away from the body and wrapping toward the body with even pressure (for example, for the ankle, start at the toes and wrap up to the lower leg). Be sure the wrap applies pressure, but is not so tight that it cuts off the circulation. Properly applied compression minimizes swelling.

4. **Elevation.** Raise the injured part above the level of the heart. When used in conjunction with ice and compression, elevation can help minimize swelling.

For blisters, apply ice to reduce the heat created by the friction between the skin layers. To minimize further pressure and irritation to the area, tape a donut-shaped piece of felt or foam rubber over the blister (see figure 12.5). Do not, however, attempt to open and drain blisters. This could lead to infection if not performed properly.

For muscle soreness and cramps, gradual, sustained stretching can help relax the affected muscles. The muscles should be stretched for 15 to 30 seconds, just to the point of slight discomfort. Holding this stretch several times might help relieve the pain associated with soreness or cramps.

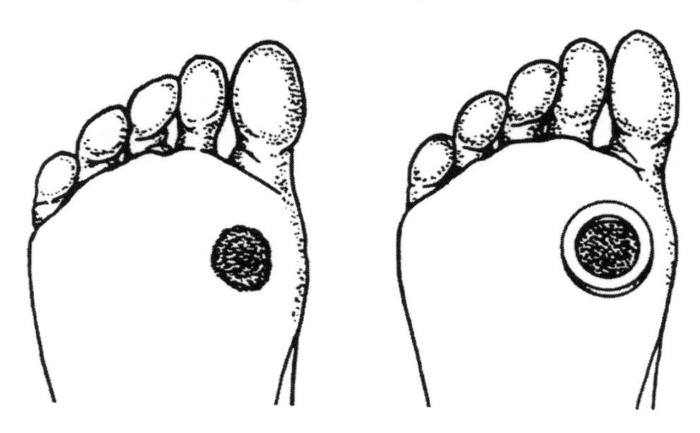

Figure 12.5 Application of a donut-shaped piece of foam rubber to a blister.

Participants experiencing heat illnesses, fainting, or shock should lie down. Those suffering from heat illness should be given water to drink (if conscious) and moist towels to cool the body. You should monitor breathing and heart rate as needed and notify the appropriate YMCA staff.

By applying the information and the principles in this chapter, you should be able to create a safe environment in which you and your participants can enjoy exercise. Remember, the key to preventing injuries is to exercise caution in designing workout sessions, in teaching proper technique, and in limiting participation. If an injury does occur, use R-I-C-E and consult a sports medicine specialist as necessary. With proper planning, you can reduce your members' risk of injury and responsibly care for any injuries that do happen.

CHAPTER 13

Administrative Notes

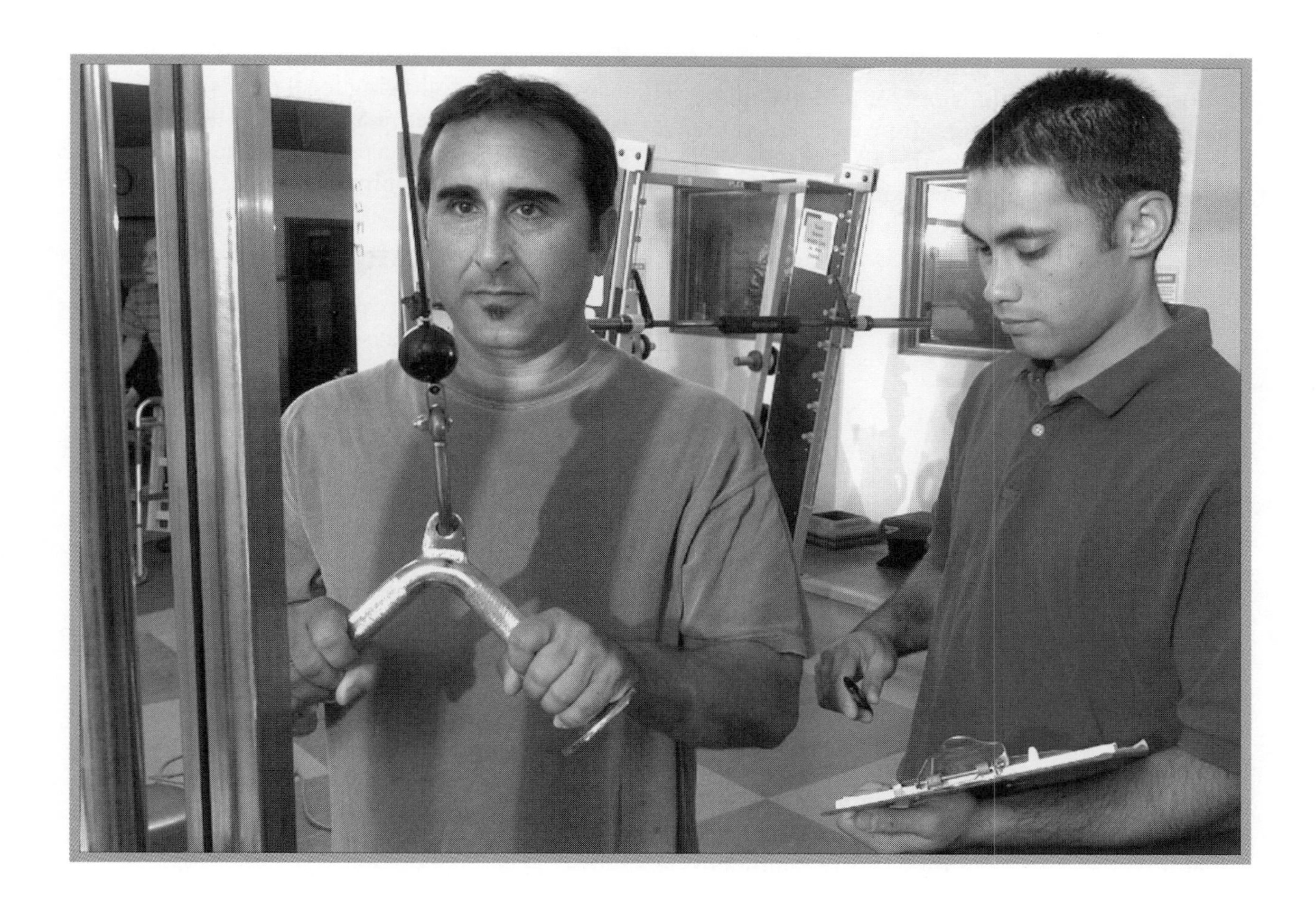

The preceding chapters present personal training guidelines and principles from the exercise and behavioral sciences. Applying these guidelines will make your program safer, well rounded, and more enjoyable for participants. However, in addition to developing knowledge of the exercise sciences, you should also consider administrative duties as you plan your programs. Most YMCAs have established guidelines for these administrative procedures, so in most cases your role is one of understanding what is expected, carrying out procedures in the exercise facility, and giving the YMCA administration input based on your training experience. Just as your participants benefit from the guidelines you apply from the exercise sciences, your overall program benefits from your attending to these administrative tasks. The tasks discussed here include

- legal liability,
- negligence,
- promotion,
- participant education,
- program evaluation,
- training guidelines for members, and
- instructor supervision.

LEGAL LIABILITY

In every exercise venture there exists the possibility that a participant might be injured, perhaps for reasons beyond your control. To avoid the risk of liability, the YMCA of the USA recommends that you do the following:

- Distribute health screening (PAR-Q) forms to all participants.
- Require participants to obtain physician clearance if they have a medical condition or high-risk profile, undergo fitness testing, and encourage them to follow an exercise program appropriate for their level of fitness.
- Teach safe exercises and proper technique.
- Maintain facilities and equipment in good working order.
- Make sure you have adequate insurance protection.

Use the reproducible health screening forms that appear in appendix B.

By law, you are required to fulfill certain responsibilities for the welfare of your participants. You owe it to your participants to perform certain duties, and your compliance is important if a participant is injured in your class and files a lawsuit. The following legal duties are adapted from *ACEP's Guide to Sport Law* (1985) by Gary Nygaard and Thomas Boone. The duties have been modified to apply to personal training.

Proper Technique

As you know, there are proper and improper ways to structure an exercise session. These include format (warming up, cardiorespiratory work, muscle conditioning, and cooling down); proper exercise movement selection; and appropriate frequency, intensity, and duration of exercise. Failure to teach a safe, progressive program infringes on members' right to trust you as a knowledgeable instructor.

Hand in hand with teaching proper exercise techniques should be warning participants about what could happen if they do not follow your instructions. For example, let's say that you have properly explained the physiological rationale for progressively increasing the intensity, frequency, and duration of workouts. You should also warn participants that if they exceed their predetermined intensity, symptoms of distress could stop the workout altogether. All explanations of the proper ways to exercise should be accompanied by appropriate warnings of the possible consequences if participants don't heed your instructions.

Adequate Supervision

You have learned about the importance of observing your program participants. You owe it to your participants to be continually on the lookout for improper exercise techniques and signals of overexertion. Do not leave participants during an exercise session in which direct supervision is needed—you are in charge, and it is your responsibility to be present and prepared at all times.

Sound Planning

The primary goal of personal training is, of course, for participants to achieve training benefits. Progress toward this goal must be made slowly and in increments established to meet each person's fitness level. Sound planning requires that you cover every detail in advance, from providing a safe exercise environment to teaching safe exercises to thinking through emergency procedures.

Inherent Risks

Participants must know the risks inherent in physical activity, both those that accompany any type of exercise and those specific to their programs. For example, vigorous cardiorespiratory exercise carries the risk of muscular and cardiac problems. An inherent risk is generally defined as one incurred while working out in a safe facility with a qualified instructor. The qualified instructor is aware of and understands the inherent risks of exercise and does everything in his or her power to minimize them. Take the time to discuss inherent risks with participants at your first session, and repeat the warnings periodically. Ensure that participants sign informed consent forms to engage in such activities.

Safe Workout Environment

The more sensitive you are to creating a safe workout environment, the more protected your participants will be. Before each training session begins you should check the facility for unsafe conditions, including water, dirt, or loose weights on the floor, uneven surfaces, poor ventilation, and so on.

Additional hazards could include items such as structural columns, projections hanging from the ceiling, or equipment from other programs left sitting out. Point out the potentially dangerous features of the facility. In any setting, don't forget to consider the temperature of the facility before starting the workout.

Proper Training and Certification

The better trained you are and the more carefully you carry out proper training techniques, both in carrying out your instructor duties and in the face of an injury or crisis, the better your legal protection will be if an injury occurs. Certification from a nationally recognized organization like the YMCA of the USA provides evidence of your competency. The YMCA of the USA recommends that all personal trainers working in YMCAs be certified as YMCA Personal Training Instructors.

First Aid and Emergency Response Plans

How well your emergency response system works depends on the procedures your YMCA has set up and your ability to carry them out. You should prepare in advance to effectively handle injuries or accidents. In a situation demanding first aid, remember that you could be judged negligent if you do nothing, but you are likely to be found just as negligent if you select the correct action but perform it incorrectly.

You must be certified to administer cardiopulmonary resuscitation (CPR) and to use an automated external defibrillator (AED). First aid training is recommended as well. Review your skills periodically and renew your certifications as required. Keep a well-supplied first aid kit on hand. If possible, have access to another room where first aid can be given. Plan what will happen if a participant is injured.

Your YMCA should have a plan of action for contacting medical personnel if a person needs further medical treatment. This plan will depend on available resources such your community's emergency medical services (EMS), a local medical center, or a private physician. Emergency telephone numbers should be accessible at all times, and you should be prepared to give a complete description of the situation over the phone. The more details you can provide, the better.

Record Keeping

If an incident occurs, you should notify the risk manager at your YMCA who will contact your Y's insurance provider. You may be asked to file a written report of what happened and exactly what actions were taken or care provided. If your YMCA doesn't have a standard accident report, model forms can be obtained from the National Safety Council. When you fill in a report, keep your description simple, yet thorough. Record the information completely, precisely, accurately, and objectively. A written report will help you recall the details of the situation if a participant decides to press charges against you or your YMCA.

Evaluate the accident or injury to determine the cause or contributing factors. Once these have been identified, do all you can to correct them or eliminate them from your program.

NEGLIGENCE

If a participant sues you and/or your YMCA and your case is brought to trial, your behavior will be judged in light of whether you fulfilled your duties with reasonable care. The most common lawsuit brought against fitness instructors is one of negligence. You were negligent if you failed to act as a reasonable and prudent instructor would have acted in a similar situation. In trying to confirm whether you were negligent, the plaintiff must prove four factors:

Presence of the duty—Did you owe the participant the duty in question? Were you obligated to perform the action?

Breach of duty—Was that duty breached (unfulfilled)? Did you do the proper thing, but do it incorrectly, or did you omit to do something?

Cause of the injury—Was your breach of duty a contributing cause?

Extent of the injury—What was the actual extent of the injury?

All four factors must be proven before you can be found negligent. If any one of the factors is missing, liability cannot be charged. Check whether your YMCA provides liability insurance. If not, it is advisable to add a clause to your personal insurance policy that will protect you if necessary.

In summary, participation in physical activity has risks, and it is your responsibility to help protect against them. Meet the challenge of your responsibilities by thinking through your entire program, giving maximum attention to the welfare of your participants. Know your legal duties before leading your first training session.

PROMOTION

Advertising and promoting personal training programs are probably taken care of by others on your YMCA staff, but you should always be on the lookout for new marketing strategies, and you might want to share some of the ideas presented here with your marketing staff.

The two main considerations in advertising are cost and time. Ideally, the money and the time invested in advertising will be proportional to the number of people attracted to the program. Two methods for advertising your personal training program are printed materials and word of mouth.

Printed Materials

Printed promotion can include flyers, news releases, brochures, and so on. When writing the promotional copy, include all of the pertinent information about the personal training program: your credentials, where and when sessions are held, and what benefits participants can expect to gain. If you create flyers, make them attractive. If possible, have them professionally printed. Obtain permission from your superior to post them in strategic locations for the audience you are trying to reach. If you are trying to reach the employees of a certain company, seek permission from the company to distribute your notices. Most businesses have a centrally located lounge or eating area with a bulletin board for notices. Posting a flyer there will help publicize your message.

News releases should be brief and descriptive and approved by YMCA management for distribution. Hand deliver them, if possible, to the local newspaper. Don't forget weekly papers, which often look for local news and are more likely to print public service announcements.

Word of Mouth

Perhaps the most effective kind of advertising is word of mouth, which also is the least expensive. Ask people in charge of groups you are interested in reaching to make announcements about your program. You'll need to prepare these brief, concise announcements and see that they are delivered to the appropriate people.

Those who have worked with you before are good sources of free advertising. Personal testimonials about the fitness and fun derived from your sessions will be just as effective (if not more so) than all of the written ad copy you can generate. Consider having a participant go with you to promote your program.

PARTICIPANT EDUCATION

Instructors should enhance their programs with health and fitness information from reliable sources. Handouts, posters, charts, and pictures add to the fitness experience for participants, and can help create a pleasant workout environment. You don't need to be an expert on every topic of exercise and fitness, but you should be prepared to refer participants to reliable sources of information. These sources should be written in nontechnical, understandable language. If you are not sure you can compile an appropriate reference list, seek local experts from universities, schools, hospitals, volunteer agencies, and so on.

The YMCA of the USA has developed a series of 22 health and fitness tips to supplement exercise workouts for personal training participants. These tips are presented in outline format in appendix A for instructors to use when discussing these topics as part of a member's training session. The topics are as follows:

1. Orientation to exercise
2. What change you can expect and how soon you can expect it!
3. Changing exercises to fit your needs
4. Exercise exertion
5. Warm-up and cool-down
6. What is physical fitness?
7. Aerobic exercise for older adults
8. Good form and posture
9. Walking as cardiorespiratory exercise
10. Choosing exercise footwear
11. Choosing exercise apparel
12. Building muscular strength for daily activities
13. Exercises to avoid and exercises to modify
14. Exercise for relaxation
15. Setting reasonable weight control goals
16. Exercise in hot weather
17. Exercise in cold weather
18. Other programs of interest at your YMCA
19. Motivating yourself to exercise
20. The basics of nutrition
21. Hydration
22. Self-esteem and relating to others

Not all instructors feel comfortable discussing all of these topics, but this should not prevent them from providing educational information to their participants. There are many alternatives. Handouts can be used to present information. Other YMCA staff could be scheduled to discuss fitness tips or YMCA news.

DVDs, videotapes, and Internet Web sites provide other teaching tools for you to consider. The subject matter can be used in its entirety or broken down into small segments for several sessions. You could schedule a special event every few months and show an entire video. Running a video update of fitness hints in the YMCA lobby can pass along information as well.

PROGRAM EVALUATION

To measure your program's success, both a trained observer and your participants must conduct periodic evaluations. Use all available data to determine how you are doing in each area of your program. Honestly evaluate questions such as, Do participants attend regularly? Do they enjoy themselves? If the answer is no, you need to develop a plan for making improvements.

To evaluate your program, develop two checklists, one for an observer, most likely your supervisor, and one for participants. Ask them to identify both strong areas and areas that need improvement. The more input you get, the better your program can become.

TRAINING GUIDELINES FOR MEMBERS

Quality is sometimes defined as conformance to stated objectives. If this is so, then the first step to a quality personal training program is to make the training objectives clear to the participants, providing specific guidelines for exercising in the fitness facility. These guidelines can be presented verbally, in a participant policy handout, and in a member orientation program. They also should be posted (in large print) in a prominent location.

Training guidelines might be different for cardiorespiratory equipment, weight machines, and free weights, and they could include rules for appropriate exercise attire, spotters for high-risk exercises, age requirements, returning dumbbells to racks, placing barbell plates on weight trees, stripping barbells when finished, carrying gym bags, wearing headsets, and so on. The following list shows sample guidelines.

Training Facility Guidelines

- Wear appropriate exercise attire, including shirts and shoes, at all times.
- Put equipment back when you are finished.
- Do not bring food or beverage into the exercise facility.
- Do not bring children into the exercise facility.
- Youth ages 7 to 16 may use the facility after orientation and with adult supervision.
- Use collars on all free-weight bars.
- Do not allow socializing to interfere with others.
- Respect staff and members in the exercise facility.

Personal Behavior Guidelines

- Please train quietly.
- Please respect the YMCA staff and other members using the facility.
- Please use proper technique on all exercise machines.
- Please wipe down machines after each use.
- Please complete and file your workout card each training session.

Strength Training Guidelines

- Perform each exercise in a slow and controlled manner.
- Perform each exercise through a full range of joint movement.
- Perform each exercise for one to three sets of 8 to 12 repetitions.
- When you are able to complete 12 repetitions, increase the resistance by 5 percent or less.
- Exhale during lifting movements and inhale during lowering movements.

In addition to posting training guidelines, we recommend that you display signs that promote proper exercise technique.

INSTRUCTOR SUPERVISION

If you supervise instructors who conduct personal training programs, make sure that all instructors are aware of what is expected of them in their roles as personal trainers. Upon hiring personal trainers, clearly inform them of the rules and procedures for carrying out their duties. The following list shows sample guidelines for personal training instructors.

- **Attire.** All personal training staff are expected to wear staff shirts and identification name tags when on duty. They should complete their instructional outfits with athletic shoes and exercise shorts or sweat pants.
- **Absence.** Any staff member who cannot report to work at the assigned time is responsible for contacting their participants, and possibly arranging a replacement from the staff list. He or she should not wait until the last minute to notify a substitute. Staff members must report all schedule changes to the health and fitness director.
- **Attitude.** The most important characteristic of a successful personal training staff member is a good attitude toward the job responsibilities and toward the participants. All staff should exhibit a

positive attitude, a high level of enthusiasm, and a genuine interest in each participant's progress.

- **Certification.** All personal training staff must have current CPR and YMCA of the USA Personal Training Instructor certification.
- **Cleanliness.** The personal training staff is responsible for keeping the training center neat, clean, and cheerful. Whenever necessary, staff should wipe down machines (metal, plastic, and vinyl), pick up papers, organize the files, and keep cleanser bottles and towels at every workstation.
- **Emergencies.** All personal training staff must read, understand, and follow the YMCA emergency procedures.
- **First aid.** All personal training staff must be aware that a first aid kit and ice packs are located inside the fitness center desk. The emergency telephone numbers are located above the telephone.
- **Hours.** Part-time personal training staff usually work no more than 20 hours per week. Work schedules begin and end on the hour or the half-hour. Staff must report to work on time and leave work as scheduled.
- **Instruction.** The YMCA exercise facility is an instructional facility where the goal is to teach concepts as well as skills. Staff should share the "why" as well as the "how" with participants. Staff must communicate clearly and concisely with members so that members will train with good form and will understand what they are doing.
- **Knowledge.** All personal training staff are expected to learn the basic and advanced principles and procedures for safe and effective fitness training. In addition to participating in required training events and certifications, staff should read and refer to the this text for information on training benefits, research, recommendations, exercise execution, program design, and related topics.
- **On-the-job behavior.** Whenever staff work with members in the fitness center, it is their responsibility to be attentive and helpful. This includes teaching, modeling, providing feedback, sharing new concepts, recording, observing, and assisting members.
- **Personal workouts.** All personal training staff are encouraged to serve as role models by training regularly and correctly. However, staff should not perform their personal workout during scheduled work hours.
- **Problems.** Staff should neither ignore nor inflate problems. They should deal with problems immediately if it is within their scope of responsibility. If not, they should bring the problems to the attention of their supervisor to be resolved together. Staff should document all member issues or complaints on an incident form.
- **Reference.** The main reference text for staff is the *YMCA Personal Training Manual, Second Edition.*
- **Time cards.** Each staff member should complete a time card every time she or he begins and ends a work shift. The staff member should fill in the date and the hours worked.
- **YMCA information.** We encourage staff to become knowledgeable about general YMCA policies and procedures, as well as about other YMCA programs and activities to promote to participants.

Appendix A

HEALTH AND FITNESS TIPS FOR MEMBERS

This appendix contains 22 outlines of a range of health and fitness topics that you can use with all members, including your personal training participants. Use these outlines to help you organize what you say about these topics.

Topic 1: Orientation to Exercise

I. Why people exercise

A. To feel good

B. To meet people

C. To have fun

D. For medical reasons

E. To look good

F. To lose weight

II. Physical benefits

A. Improves cardiorespiratory efficiency

B. Improves metabolism

C. Improves body composition and benefits internal organs

D. Improves joint and muscle flexibility

E. Increases bone strength

F. Increases muscle strength

G. Improves balance and coordination

H. Promotes relaxation

III. Mental benefits

A. Increases knowledge of healthy habits

B. Increases knowledge of fitness goals

C. Increases knowledge of safe and efficient movement

D. Increases knowledge of one's own abilities

IV. Social and emotional benefits

A. Increases opportunities to meet people

B. Encourages participation in a supportive atmosphere

C. Increases self-esteem

D. Improves body image

V. Spiritual benefits

A. Increases respect for and appreciation of self and others

B. Provides opportunity to let go of daily concerns, to get in touch with yourself, and to enjoy other people

C. Encourages you to be uniquely you

Topic 2: What Change You Can Expect and How Soon You Can Expect It!

I. Progress

A. You will progress at your own rate (influenced by your health, heredity, and motivation).

B. Change will occur, particularly if you

- participate regularly,
- work at your own pace,
- set realistic goals and make adjustments for day-to-day changes in your health status,
- are free from pressure to compete, and
- measure and celebrate your progress.

II. Regression

A. Beginners often overestimate the amount of change to expect.

B. Change in the first weeks might be very noticeable.

C. A plateau period of several weeks might follow, which is normal.

D. The plateau period is followed by slow, gradual change.

III. Common changes after four to six weeks of regular participation

A. You feel better physically.

B. It is easier to reach high shelves or your feet and to fasten and unfasten seat belts.

C. House and yard work is easier and less exhausting.

D. It is easier to go up and down stairs.

E. Chronic back pain decreases.

F. Sport performance improves.

G. You feel better about life.

Topic 3: Changing Exercises to Fit Your Needs

I. Taking into account differences in shape, health status, and fitness level

A. Change exercise to "fit" your individual length and circumference of limbs and trunk.

B. Follow your doctor's recommendations for exercise based on your health status.

C. Take advantage of opportunities for fitness assessment.

II. Changing exercises for differences in shape

A. People with short arms and legs should reach toward instead of to the designated spot; static stretching might be difficult.

B. People with long arms and legs need a slower movement tempo and more space.

C. People with excess weight should exercise at a lower intensity.

III. Changing exercises for differences in fitness level

A. Exercise position and intensity should match your fitness level.

B. Exercise intensity should increase gradually as your fitness level improves.

Topic 4: Exercise Exertion

I. How to measure exertion

A. Target heart rate using pulse count

B. Rating of perceived exertion scale

C. Talk test

II. Factors affecting exercise heart rate (HR)

A. Age

B. Weather (HR rises faster in warm weather)

C. Health status (HR rises faster when you are sick)

D. Medications

III. Reasonable levels of exertion

A. 55 to 65 percent for beginners

B. 70 to 80 percent for the regularly active

C. 80 to 90 percent for well-conditioned adults

IV. Blood pressure

A. Blood pressure increases during exercise.

B. Resting blood pressure gradually decreases with regular exercise participation.

C. Heart rate and blood pressure are not directly related.

Topic 5: Warm-Up and Cool-Down

I. Reasons for warm-up

A. Increase heart rate and muscle temperature

B. Loosen joints

C. Prevent injury
D. Get mentally ready for activity

II. Components of warm-up

A. Part 1: Active movements to get blood moving and warm muscles; 3 to 6 minutes
B. Part 2: Move each joint through full range of motion, gently stretch major muscle groups, and keep heart rate elevated; 5 to 10 minutes

III. Reasons for cool-down

A. Allow heart rate to gradually drop to preexercise level
B. Allow blood flow to move from large leg muscles to other organs and muscles
C. Stretch major muscle groups
D. Enjoy a period of relaxation

IV. Components of cool-down

A. Easy exercise at a moderate pace, such as walking
B. Sustained stretches of major muscle groups to prevent soreness or tightness
C. Relaxation period

Topic 6: What Is Physical Fitness?

I. Different things to different people

A. Feeling good
B. Being active without feeling fatigued
C. Coping with daily stresses and problems with a more relaxed attitude
D. Participating in daily activities with ease and enjoyment
E. Improving components of physical fitness: muscular strength and endurance, aerobic conditioning, flexibility, body composition, and relaxation

II. Muscular strength and endurance

A. Definition
B. Examples

III. Cardiorespiratory fitness: Aerobic conditioning

A. Definition
B. Examples, including continuous and discontinuous activities

IV. Flexibility of muscles and joints

A. Definition of joint range-of-motion exercise
B. Definition of muscle flexibility exercise
C. Examples of different kinds of flexibility exercises

(Relaxation is covered in Topic 14; body composition is covered in Topic 15.)

Topic 7: Aerobic Exercise for Older Adults

I. What is aerobic exercise?

A. Energizing movement for all ages
B. Large-muscle activity that lasts more than three minutes
C. Activity that increases heart and breathing rates
D. Can be done in a chair, a pool, and an open indoor or outdoor space
E. Some examples of aerobic exercise are swimming, walking, dancing, biking, running, and aerobics

II. Frequency (how often)

A. A minimum of three times a week
B. A maximum of five times a week

III. Intensity (how hard)

A. Harder is not better; moderate pace is fine
B. Heart rate in target range (55 to 90 percent maximum HR) or perceived exertion is fairly light to very hard
C. Able to talk comfortably
D. Should not leave you exhausted

IV. Duration (how long)

A. Beginners or during recovery from illness: up to 15 minutes

B. Two options for healthy, conditioned adults
    1. 30 to 45 minutes, three times a week
    2. 15 to 30 minutes, four or five times a week

Topic 8: Good Form and Posture

I. Reasons for moving with good form

A. Save energy

B. Prevent injury

C. Feel better and express positive self-image

II. Proper body alignment

A. Standing posture
    1. Weight carried by bones
    2. Alignment of ear, shoulder, hip joint, knee, and ankle form a straight line when body is viewed from the side

B. Sitting posture
    1. Alignment of ear, shoulder, and hip form a straight line
    2. Knees and feet are apart with feet flat on floor

III. Movement mechanics

A. Walking
    1. Good alignment
    2. Smooth weight transfer
    3. Opposition arm swing
    4. Eyes focused forward instead of down

B. Lifting
    1. Feet apart
    2. Bent knees (instead of hips)
    3. Lifted weight held close to body

C. Carrying
    1. Weight held close to body
    2. Weight centered

D. Pushing and pulling
    1. Feet in stride position
    2. Bent knees (instead of hips), knees in line with feet
    3. Hands and arms kept over space between feet
    4. Body weight shifted forward (push) or backward (pull)

E. Rising from floor or chair
    1. Weight kept over feet
    2. Arms used to push on knees or against chair, if necessary
    3. Weight kept over feet by bending and straightening knees and hips
    4. Body lifted slowly to avoid dizziness

Topic 9: Walking As Cardiorespiratory Exercise

I. Variety of walking programs

A. YMCA Walk Reebok programs

B. YMCA self-guided walking programs

C. YMCA walking clubs

II. Benefits of walking

A. Familiar movement that can be done many places at a time convenient to the individual

B. Strengthens bones

C. Improves cardiorespiratory fitness

D. Easy to adjust to individual fitness level

E. Burns calories

III. Sample walk program (see *YMCA Walk Reebok Instructor Manual*)

Topic 10: Choosing Exercise Footwear

I. Reasons for selecting footwear carefully

A. Appropriate shoes that fit well prevent injury.

B. Better fit increases foot comfort.

II. Being a wise shopper

A. Stores that specialize in athletic shoes are more likely to have a range of sizes and salespeople who are better trained to help you.

B. Always try on both shoes for fit and comfort; walk in them in the store before you pay for them.

III. Types of shoes

A. Aerobic and cross-training shoes are lighter in weight, have soles that accommodate side-to-side stepping, and provide additional cushioning under the ball of the foot.

B. Walking shoes have smoother and stiffer soles, lower heels, and more solid support in the uppers.

C. Running shoes have flexible soles, higher heels, and less support at the toe of the shoe.

IV. Choosing shoes

A. Well-cushioned heel

B. Firm heel counter

C. Adequate internal cushioning (insole)

D. Resilient and pliable outer sole

E. Leather or mesh upper construction

F. Roomy toe box

G. Adequate arch support

H. Comfortable fit

Topic 11: Choosing Exercise Apparel

I. General considerations

A. Material should absorb perspiration.

B. Cut should prevent chafing.

C. Fit should allow comfortable, full range of motion.

II. Underwear

A. An absorbent fabric like cotton is preferred.

B. Garments should provide support without being too tight or binding.

III. Socks

A. Look for a snug fit without rough toe seams.

B. Cotton and wool socks absorb moisture, but might cause blisters in presence of profuse sweating.

C. To wick moisture away from the foot, wear silk, nylon, or polypropylene next to the skin.

D. Add extra cushioning, if needed, by wearing a second pair of socks made of wool or lightly padded terry cloth.

IV. Exercise clothing

A. Wear shorts, tights, or pants designed for the particular type of exercise.

B. Clothing made with microfiber material is light, allowing for easy movement, and wicks perspiration away from the body for a cooling effect.

Topic 12: Building Muscular Strength for Daily Activities

I. **Daily living** depends on muscular strength: Use it, don't lose it!

II. **Knee extension** in seated or standing position builds the quadriceps strength needed to climb stairs or get out of cars or deep chairs.

III. **Biceps curls and triceps exercises** build the arm strength needed for lifting and lowering, pushing, pulling, and carrying objects.

IV. **Arm and leg exercise** improves posture and builds the strength needed for sports and daily yard- and housework.

V. **Abdominal curls** (plus variations) improve posture and stabilize trunk movements.

VI. **Forced expiration exercises** build diaphragm strength to improve depth of breathing and elimination function (bowel movement). Avoid hyperventilation.

Topic 13: Exercises to Avoid and Exercises to Modify

Almost any exercise can be harmful if it is improperly executed or if it is repeated too often (repetitive motion syndrome). However, several exercises should be avoided, including some we have learned in past exercise experiences. As our knowledge of the body and how it works advances, we sometimes learn that we have been doing certain things incorrectly.

I. Exercises to avoid

A. Standing, straight-leg toe touches can cause back and knee injury. Do single-leg raises lying on your back instead.

B. Deep knee bends can cause knee injury. Do knee dips instead, keeping heels on the floor.

C. Standing windmills can cause back injury.

D. Double-leg lifts can cause low back injury and hernias. Keep the knee of one leg bent and the foot on the floor while lifting the other leg.

E. Straight-leg sit-ups can cause back injury. Do abdominal curls with knees bent.

F. Sit-ups with feet stabilized (i.e., held down by a partner) can cause back injury. Do abdominal curls lifting only the shoulders (or upper trunk) from the floor.

G. Head or neck circles can cause damage to nerves in the neck and dizziness. Do isolated neck exercises: Turn right and left, center and down, center and diagonally down to the right or left; draw chin and head in and forward, tilt head side to side.

II. Important modifications to all exercise

A. Protect the back by keeping it upright; bend at the knees instead of bending at the waist.

B. Protect the knees by keeping them lined up with the toes.

C. Protect the arch of the foot by taking weight on the heel, then shifting weight toward the toes.

D. Protect the back and arm joints by bending (flexing or extending) or turning (rotation), but not both.

E. There are other modifications related to common performance errors.

Topic 14: Exercise for Relaxation

I. Importance of relaxation exercise

A. Physiological changes

1. Reduced blood pressure
2. Increased release of endorphins, which act as natural sedatives
3. Reduced muscle tension

B. Psychological changes

1. Release of worries and anxiety (letting go)
2. Reduced depression
3. Increased feelings of well-being

II. Dynamic relaxation

A. Relaxation effect of active exercise is caused by endorphin release.

B. Effect occurs with:

1. Noncompetitive, energetic activity
2. Natural spontaneous laughter and enjoyment experienced with activity
3. Balance of a challenging activity requiring coordination, such as lifting the knee and tapping it with the opposite hand, with an easy, no-fail activity like marching in place and clapping

III. Static relaxation

A. Quiet breathing, guided muscle contraction–relaxation exercise, or exercise like tai chi and yoga.

B. Guided imagery or meditation

Topic 15: Setting Reasonable Weight Control Goals

I. Diet

A. Weight loss occurs with increased caloric expenditure or decreased caloric intake or both.

B. Adults should drink six to eight 8-ounce glasses of water a day.

C. A safe rate of weight loss is one to two pounds a week.

D. Spot reducing is a fallacy.

E. Weight will be lost according to genetic design and order of gain.

F. Change diet by eating more nutritious foods, consuming less, and reducing fat intake.

II. Exercise

A. 3,500 calories equals one pound of fat.

B. Calories are "burned" during all types of physical activity; aerobic activity typically "burns" more calories than other forms of exercise.

C. Combine exercise with diet modifications to lose weight and build muscle mass.

D. Real weight may not change, but body composition—that is the amount of fat versus lean weight—will change.

Topic 16: Exercise in Hot Weather

I. Heat stress—Heat reactions can occur in any season under the right conditions. Heat stress is caused by a combination of factors:

A. Increased humidity

B. Increased temperature

C. Lack of wind

D. Solar radiation

E. Age (older adults are more prone to heat stress)

II. Precautions

A. Wear a hat with good ventilation (e.g., a hat made of loosely woven straw or natural fiber).

B. Wear loose, absorbent (preferably cotton), light-colored clothes. Avoid wearing clothes that hold heat next to the skin, such as clothing made of nylon.

C. Exercise during a cooler part of the day.

D. Drink plenty of cool water.

E. Reduce exercise intensity.

III. Symptoms to watch for

A. Dizziness

B. Confusion or loss of consciousness

C. Hot, dry skin

D. Nausea

E. Muscle cramps

IV. Remedies

A. Get out of the sun and heat!

B. Drink plenty of fluids.

C. Cool the body gradually with water or a breeze (fan).

D. Seek immediate medical aid if heatstroke symptoms occur (hot, dry skin; loss of consciousness; high body temperature).

Topic 17: Exercise in Cold Weather

I. Hypothermia can occur in any season under the right conditions. Hypothermia is caused by a combination of factors

A. Decreased temperature

B. Increased humidity or moisture

C. Increased wind

D. Age (older adults are more prone to hypothermia)

II. Precautions

A. Wear clothes that allow freedom of movement.

B. Wear clothes in layers.
C. Wear clothes made from materials with a high insulating value, such as wool or down.
D. Wear hats that cover ears and wear mittens instead of gloves.
E. Wear a breathing mask on colder days.
F. Keep your neck and chest covered.
G. Exercise during warmer parts of the day, and avoid becoming chilled.

Guard against outdoor exercise on days when the windchill reading drops below 10 degrees Fahrenheit.

III. Symptoms of hypothermia

A. Marked shivering
B. Numbness, loss of feeling
C. Marked muscular weakness
D. Drowsiness or loss of consciousness
E. Low body temperature
F. Personality change, impaired judgment, or mental confusion

IV. Remedies

A. Remove wet or frozen clothing.
B. Provide extra clothing, blankets, or the warmth of another body.
C. Move to a warm place indoors.
D. Provide warm, nonalcoholic drinks.
E. Warm the skin gradually in warm—not hot—water, and then dry thoroughly.

Topic 18: Other Programs of Interest at Your YMCA

Outline the programs currently offered at your YMCA.

Topic 19: Motivating Yourself to Exercise

I. Review personal goals and personal benefits of exercise based on your experience and your participants' experiences.

II. Give reasons people drop out of exercise programs.

A. No benefit experienced with exercise
B. Injury from muscle overuse or strains
C. Other activities in life take priority
D. Exercise program not enjoyable
E. Exercise program not challenging or interesting
F. Others

III. Identify the motivational techniques that work best for each participant.

A. Mention some of the common ways to motivate yourself to exercise:
   1. Get support from family and friends.
   2. Find a buddy to exercise with.
   3. Choose a regular time to exercise that fits well in your schedule.
   4. Set short- and long-term goals.
   5. Keep records on how long and often you exercise and your progress.
   6. Vary the type of exercise you do and where you do it.

B. Ask each participant to identify specific techniques that work well for him or her.

Topic 20: Basics of Nutrition

I. Age and nutrition

A. Calorie needs typically decrease with age.
B. Rate of metabolism declines with age.

II. Roles nutrients play in physical activity

A. Carbohydrate is the primary source of energy.
B. Fat and protein are energy producers after the body's glycogen stores are depleted.

C. Protein, minerals, vitamins, and water are essential to metabolic processes that produce energy.

III. Proper eating habits

A. Eat a balanced diet that contains grains, fruits and vegetables, dairy products, and meats.

B. Eat fewer "empty" calories, i.e., foods such as candy or alcohol that have lots of calories but little nutritional value.

IV. Fat

A. Less healthy fat sources are saturated and trans fat and are found in foods such as animal fat, organ meat, tropical oils (coconut), eggs, whole milk, butter, and cream.

B. Better fat sources are polyunsaturated fat and are found in foods such as safflower, olive, canola, and sunflower oils.

C. Check the labels of processed foods (including "low-fat" foods) and baked goods for the types of fat used.

Topic 21: Hydration

I. The body's water needs

A. Water is used for metabolic processes: to produce energy, build muscle, repair tissue, and maintain body temperature.

B. Fluid retention is related to heart problems or inactivity, not excessive water intake.

C. Extra water is needed during warm weather, illness, and before and after vigorous exercise.

II. How much?

A. Adults should drink six to eight 8-ounce glasses of water a day.

B. Thirst is not a good gauge of water need; although thirst might be quenched, our bodies usually need more water, especially when we are active.

III. When?

A. Drink water throughout the day.

B. Drink water before, during, and after exercise.

C. Even if you fear incontinence, don't stop drinking water; instead, plan ahead and locate restrooms before you need them.

D. Do Kegel exercises to help control incontinence.

Topic 22: Self-Esteem and Relating to Others

I. Self-concept

A. We all develop concepts of how well we do in many different areas in life; we are good in some, not so good in others.

B. The one area that affects our ability to succeed in all the others is our ability to relate to other people.

II. Self-esteem and helping others

A. We must first feel good about ourselves.

B. When we feel good about ourselves, we can help others.

III. How to increase self-esteem

A. We need to take steps to build our self-esteem and avoid self-destructive messages.

B. We can choose to build on the positive aspects of those around us.

Appendix B

HEALTH SCREENING, MEDICAL CLEARANCE, AND INFORMED CONSENT FORMS

The following four forms are taken from *YMCA Healthy Lifestyle Principles Manual, Fourth Edition*, and *YMCA Fitness Testing and Assessment Manual.* They can be reproduced and used as needed for your YMCA classes. The screening forms should be administered when participants enter a program and yearly thereafter. Copies of all completed participant forms should be retained in a records file for at least three years.

1. **Form I**—Health Screen (PAR-Q & YOU)

Form I is the Physical Activity Readiness Questionnaire developed by the Canadian Society for Exercise Physiology. It asks for general information about the participant's physical condition. Instruct members to follow the recommendations based on their answers before participating in YMCA fitness testing or exercise programs.

2. **Forms II and IIa**—Medical Clearance and Testing/Program Description

The Medical Clearance form is used by the participant's physician to report restrictions that should be placed on the participant during fitness testing or exercise programs. In addition to form II, the physician should see form IIa, which describes generally the YMCA fitness testing and exercise programs and the risks associated with each.

3. **Form III**—Informed Consent for Fitness Testing

The Informed Consent for Fitness Testing form ensures that the participant is aware of the risks involved in the fitness testing procedures. It documents that a description of the testing procedures has been read and that all questions concerning those procedures have been answered satisfactorily.

4. **Form IV**—Informed Consent for Exercise Participation

The Informed Consent for Exercise Participation form ensures that the participant is aware of the risks involved in exercise. It documents that the description of the exercise program has been read and all questions concerning the exercise program have been answered to the participant's satisfaction.

WHEN AND HOW TO USE THE FORMS

The Health Screen form (form I) should be completed before a participant starts a program, even if it is an education class. The information obtained on this form is valuable for educating participants about potential health and cardiovascular risks. Form I is not intended to be a medical exam, but simply a self-clearance tool to review key health information.

If a potential participant requires medical clearance, use form II. It allows a physician to indicate that he or she thinks the person is capable of participating in the YMCA's exercise programs. Form IIa provides a description of the YMCA exercise programs.

The informed consent forms (forms III and IV) are designed to notify participants of the inherent risks of fitness testing and exercise programs. Form III, Informed Consent for Fitness Testing, should be given to anyone registering for a fitness test. It should be read and signed before testing starts. Form IV, Informed Consent for Exercise Participation, should be given to any participant in a supervised exercise program. It should be read and signed before exercise starts.

Form I

Physical Activity Readiness
Questionnaire - PAR-Q
(revised 2002)

PAR-Q & YOU

(A Questionnaire for People Aged 15 to 69)

Regular physical activity is fun and healthy, and increasingly more people are starting to become more active every day. Being more active is very safe for most people. However, some people should check with their doctor before they start becoming much more physically active.

If you are planning to become much more physically active than you are now, start by answering the seven questions in the box below. If you are between the ages of 15 and 69, the PAR-Q will tell you if you should check with your doctor before you start. If you are over 69 years of age, and you are not used to being very active, check with your doctor.

Common sense is your best guide when you answer these questions. Please read the questions carefully and answer each one honestly: check YES or NO.

YES	NO		
☐	☐	1.	**Has your doctor ever said that you have a heart condition and that you should only do physical activity recommended by a doctor?**
☐	☐	2.	**Do you feel pain in your chest when you do physical activity?**
☐	☐	3.	**In the past month, have you had chest pain when you were not doing physical activity?**
☐	☐	4.	**Do you lose your balance because of dizziness or do you ever lose consciousness?**
☐	☐	5.	**Do you have a bone or joint problem (for example, back, knee or hip) that could be made worse by a change in your physical activity?**
☐	☐	6.	**Is your doctor currently prescribing drugs (for example, water pills) for your blood pressure or heart condition?**
☐	☐	7.	**Do you know of any other reason why you should not do physical activity?**

If you answered

YES to one or more questions

Talk with your doctor by phone or in person BEFORE you start becoming much more physically active or BEFORE you have a fitness appraisal. Tell your doctor about the PAR-Q and which questions you answered YES.

- You may be able to do any activity you want — as long as you start slowly and build up gradually. Or, you may need to restrict your activities to those which are safe for you. Talk with your doctor about the kinds of activities you wish to participate in and follow his/her advice.
- Find out which community programs are safe and helpful for you.

NO to all questions

If you answered NO honestly to all PAR-Q questions, you can be reasonably sure that you can:

- start becoming much more physically active – begin slowly and build up gradually. This is the safest and easiest way to go.
- take part in a fitness appraisal – this is an excellent way to determine your basic fitness so that you can plan the best way for you to live actively. It is also highly recommended that you have your blood pressure evaluated. If your reading is over 144/94, talk with your doctor before you start becoming much more physically active.

DELAY BECOMING MUCH MORE ACTIVE:

- if you are not feeling well because of a temporary illness such as a cold or a fever – wait until you feel better; or
- if you are or may be pregnant – talk to your doctor before you start becoming more active.

PLEASE NOTE: If your health changes so that you then answer YES to any of the above questions, tell your fitness or health professional. Ask whether you should change your physical activity plan.

Informed Use of the PAR-Q: The Canadian Society for Exercise Physiology, Health Canada, and their agents assume no liability for persons who undertake physical activity, and if in doubt after completing this questionnaire, consult your doctor prior to physical activity.

No changes permitted. You are encouraged to photocopy the PAR-Q but only if you use the entire form.

NOTE: If the PAR-Q is being given to a person before he or she participates in a physical activity program or a fitness appraisal, this section may be used for legal or administrative purposes.

"I have read, understood and completed this questionnaire. Any questions I had were answered to my full satisfaction."

NAME ________________________________

SIGNATURE ________________________________ DATE ________________

SIGNATURE OF PARENT ________________________________ WITNESS ________________
or GUARDIAN (for participants under the age of majority)

Note: This physical activity clearance is valid for a maximum of 12 months from the date it is completed and becomes invalid if your condition changes so that you would answer YES to any of the seven questions.

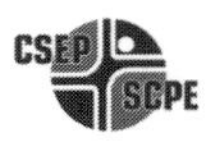

Supported by: 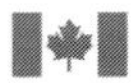 Health Canada Santé Canada

continued on other side...

...continued from other side

PAR-Q & YOU

Physical Activity Readiness
Questionnaire - PAR-Q
(revised 2002)

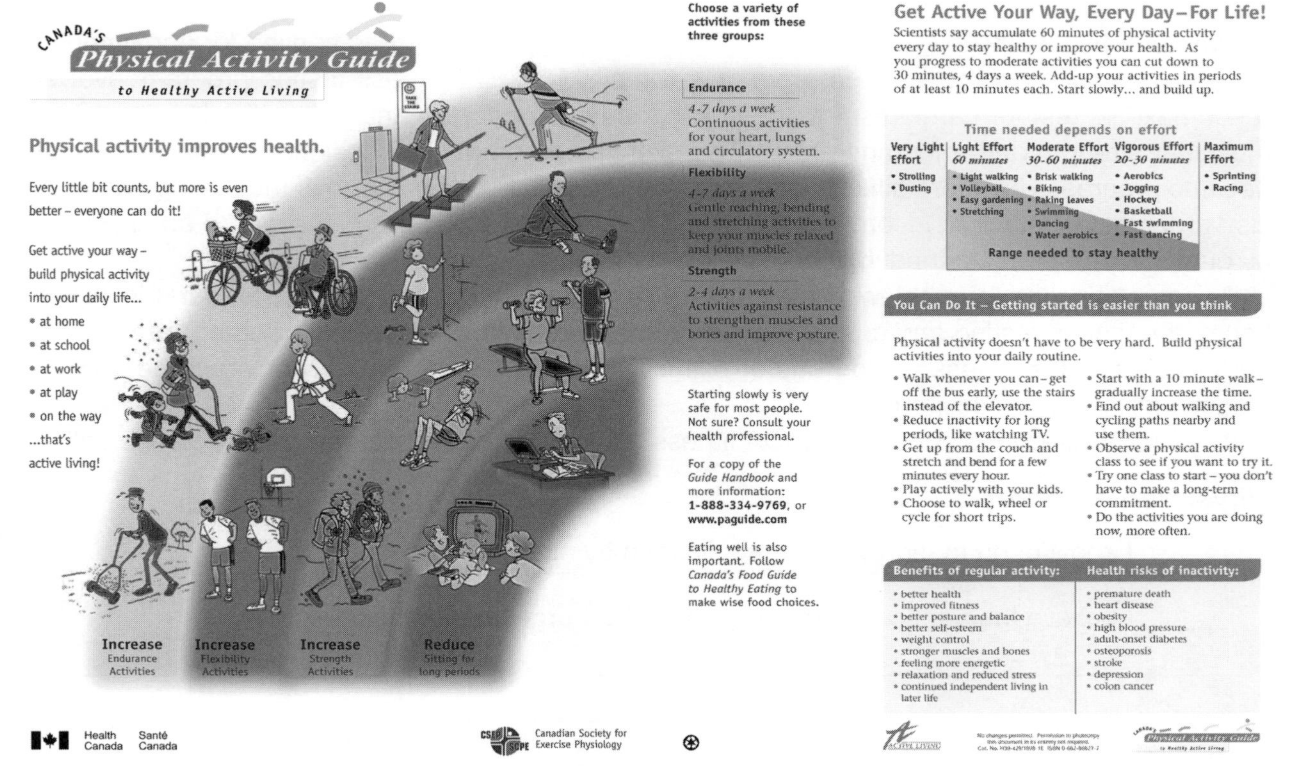

CANADA'S **Physical Activity Guide** to Healthy Active Living

Physical activity improves health.

Every little bit counts, but more is even better – everyone can do it!

Get active your way – build physical activity into your daily life...

- at home
- at school
- at work
- at play
- on the way

...that's active living!

Choose a variety of activities from these three groups:

Endurance
4-7 days a week
Continuous activities for your heart, lungs and circulatory system.

Flexibility
4-7 days a week
Gentle reaching, bending and stretching activities to keep your muscles relaxed and joints mobile.

Strength
2-4 days a week
Activities against resistance to strengthen muscles and bones and improve posture.

Increase Endurance Activities | **Increase** Flexibility Activities | **Increase** Strength Activities | **Reduce** Sitting for long periods

Starting slowly is very safe for most people. Not sure? Consult your health professional.

For a copy of the *Guide Handbook* and more information: **1-888-334-9769**, or **www.paguide.com**

Eating well is also important. Follow *Canada's Food Guide to Healthy Eating* to make wise food choices.

Get Active Your Way, Every Day–For Life!

Scientists say accumulate 60 minutes of physical activity every day to stay healthy or improve your health. As you progress to moderate activities you can cut down to 30 minutes, 4 days a week. Add-up your activities in periods of at least 10 minutes each. Start slowly... and build up.

Time needed depends on effort

Very Light Effort	Light Effort *60 minutes*	Moderate Effort *30-60 minutes*	Vigorous Effort *20-30 minutes*	Maximum Effort
• Strolling	• Light walking	• Brisk walking	• Aerobics	• Sprinting
• Dusting	• Volleyball	• Biking	• Jogging	• Racing
	• Easy gardening	• Raking leaves	• Hockey	
	• Stretching	• Swimming	• Basketball	
		• Dancing	• Fast swimming	
		• Water aerobics	• Fast dancing	

Range needed to stay healthy

You Can Do It – Getting started is easier than you think

Physical activity doesn't have to be very hard. Build physical activities into your daily routine.

- Walk whenever you can – get off the bus early, use the stairs instead of the elevator.
- Reduce inactivity for long periods, like watching TV.
- Get up from the couch and stretch and bend for a few minutes every hour.
- Play actively with your kids.
- Choose to walk, wheel or cycle for short trips.
- Start with a 10 minute walk – gradually increase the time.
- Find out about walking and cycling paths nearby and use them.
- Observe a physical activity class to see if you want to try it.
- Try one class to start – you don't have to make a long-term commitment.
- Do the activities you are doing now, more often.

Benefits of regular activity:	Health risks of inactivity:
• better health	• premature death
• improved fitness	• heart disease
• better posture and balance	• obesity
• better self-esteem	• high blood pressure
• weight control	• adult-onset diabetes
• stronger muscles and bones	• osteoporosis
• feeling more energetic	• stroke
• relaxation and reduced stress	• depression
• continued independent living in later life	• colon cancer

Health Canada Santé Canada

Canadian Society for Exercise Physiology

Active Living

Source: *Canada's Physical Activity Guide to Healthy Active Living*, Health Canada, 1998 http://www.hc-sc.gc.ca/hppb/paguide/pdf/guideEng.pdf

FITNESS AND HEALTH PROFESSIONALS MAY BE INTERESTED IN THE INFORMATION BELOW:

The following companion forms are available for doctors' use by contacting the Canadian Society for Exercise Physiology (address below):

The **Physical Activity Readiness Medical Examination (PARmed-X)** – to be used by doctors with people who answer YES to one or more questions on the PAR-Q.

The **Physical Activity Readiness Medical Examination for Pregnancy (PARmed-X for Pregnancy)** – to be used by doctors with pregnant patients who wish to become more active.

References:
Arraix, G.A., Wigle, D.T., Mao, Y. (1992). Risk Assessment of Physical Activity and Physical Fitness in the Canada Health Survey Follow-Up Study. **J. Clin. Epidemiol.** 45:4 419-428.
Mottola, M., Wolfe, L.A. (1994). Active Living and Pregnancy, In: A. Quinney, L. Gauvin, T. Wall (eds.), **Toward Active Living: Proceedings of the International Conference on Physical Activity, Fitness and Health.** Champaign, IL: Human Kinetics.
PAR-Q Validation Report, British Columbia Ministry of Health, 1978.
Thomas, S., Reading, J., Shephard, R.J. (1992). Revision of the Physical Activity Readiness Questionnaire (PAR-Q). **Can. J. Spt. Sci.** 17:4 338-345.

To order multiple printed copies of the PAR-Q, please contact the:

Canadian Society for Exercise Physiology
202-185 Somerset Street West
Ottawa, ON K2P 0J2
Tel. 1-877-651-3755 • FAX (613) 234-3565
Online: www.csep.ca

The original PAR-Q was developed by the British Columbia Ministry of Health. It has been revised by an Expert Advisory Committee of the Canadian Society for Exercise Physiology chaired by Dr. N. Gledhill (2002).

Disponible en français sous le titre «Questionnaire sur l'aptitude à l'activité physique - Q-AAP (revisé 2002)».

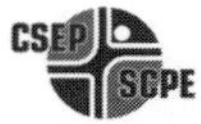

Supported by: 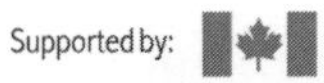 Health Canada Santé Canada

Source: Physical Activity Readiness Questionnaire (PAR-Q) © 2002. Reproduced with permission from the Canadian Society for Exercise Physiology. http://www.csep.ca/forms.asp.

Form II

Medical Clearance Form

Dear Doctor:

(Name of applicant) ______________________ has applied for enrollment in the fitness testing and/or exercise programs at the YMCA. The fitness testing program involves a submaximal test for cardiorespiratory fitness, body composition analysis, a flexibility test, and muscular strength and endurance tests. The exercise programs are designed to start easy and become progressively more difficult over time. A more detailed description of the testing and exercise programs is attached in form IIa. All fitness tests and exercise programs will be administered by qualified personnel trained in conducting exercise tests and exercise programs.

By completing the form below, however, you are not assuming responsibility for our administration of the fitness testing and/or exercise programs. If you know of medical or other reasons why participation in the fitness testing and/or exercise programs by the applicant would be unwise, please indicate so on this form.

If you have questions about the YMCA fitness testing and/or exercise programs, please call.

Physician's Report

______ I know of no reason why the applicant may not participate.

______ I believe the applicant can participate, but I urge caution because

____

____

______ The applicant should not engage in the follow activities:

____

____

______ I recommend that the applicant NOT participate.

Physician signature ______________________ Date __________

Address ______________________ Telephone __________

City and state ______________________ ZIP __________

Form IIa

Description of Fitness Testing and Exercise Programs

Dear Doctor:

The YMCA fitness testing and/or exercise programs for which the participant has applied are described as follows:

- **Fitness testing.** The purpose of the fitness testing program is to evaluate cardiorespiratory fitness, body composition, flexibility, and muscular strength and endurance. The cardiorespiratory fitness test involves a submaximal test that may include a bench step test, a cycle ergometer test, or a one-mile walk for best time test. Body composition is analyzed by taking several skinfold measurements to calculate percentage of body fat. Flexibility is determined by the sit-and-reach test. Muscular strength and upper-body endurance may be evaluated by the one-minute, bent-knee sit-up test or the bench press test.
- **Exercise programs.** The purpose of the exercise programs is to develop and maintain cardiorespiratory fitness, body composition, flexibility, and muscular strength and endurance. A specific exercise plan will be given to the participant based on needs and interests and your recommendations. All exercise programs include warm-up, exercise at target heart rate, and cool-down (except for muscular strength and endurance training, in which target heart rate is not a factor). The programs might involve walking, jogging, swimming, or cycling (outdoor and stationary); participation in exercise fitness, rhythmic aerobic exercise, or choreographed fitness classes; or calisthenics or strength training. All programs are designed to place a gradually increasing workload on the body in order to improve overall fitness and muscular strength. The rate of progression is regulated by exercise target heart rate or perceived effort of exercise or both.

In both the fitness testing and exercise programs, the reaction of the cardiorespiratory system cannot be predicted with complete accuracy. There is a risk of certain changes occurring during or after exercise. These changes might include abnormalities of blood pressure or heart rate or both. YMCA exercise instructors are certified in CPR, and emergency procedures are posted in the exercise facility.

In addition to your medical approval and recommendations, the participant will be asked to sign informed consent forms that explain the risks of fitness testing and exercise participation before the programs are initiated.

Form III

Informed Consent for Fitness Testing

Name ____
(Please print)

The purpose of the fitness testing program is to evaluate cardiorespiratory fitness, body composition, flexibility, and muscular strength and endurance. The cardiorespiratory fitness test involves a submaximal test that may include a bench step test, a cycle ergometer test, or a one-mile walk test. Body composition is analyzed by taking several skinfold measurements to calculate percentage of body fat. Flexibility is determined by the sit-and-reach test. Muscular strength and upper-body endurance could be evaluated by the one-minute, bent-knee sit-up test or the bench press test.

I understand that I am responsible for monitoring my own condition throughout the tests, and should unusual symptoms occur, I will cease my participation and inform the instructor of the symptoms.

In signing this consent form, I affirm that I have read it in its entirety and that I understand the description of the tests and their components. I also affirm that my questions regarding the fitness testing program have been answered to my satisfaction.

In the event that a medical clearance must be obtained before I participate in the fitness testing program, I agree to consult with and obtain written permission from my physician before beginning any fitness tests.

Also, in consideration for being allowed to participate in the fitness testing program, I agree to assume the risk of such testing, and further agree to hold harmless the YMCA and its staff members conducting such testing from any and all claims, suits, losses, or related causes of action for damages, including, but not limited to, such claims that may result from my injury or death, accidental or otherwise, during, or arising in any way from, the testing program.

Date ____________________ ____
(Signature of participant)

Date ____________________ ____
(Person administering tests)

Form IV

Informed Consent for Exercise Participation

I desire to engage voluntarily in the YMCA exercise program in order to attempt to improve my physical fitness. I understand that the activities are designed to place a gradually increasing workload on the cardiorespiratory system and to thereby attempt to improve its function. The reaction of the cardiorespiratory system to such activities can't be predicted with complete accuracy. There is a risk of certain changes that might occur during or after the exercise. These changes might include abnormalities of blood pressure or heart rate.

I understand that the purpose of the exercise program is to develop and maintain cardiorespiratory fitness, body composition, flexibility, and muscular strength and endurance. A specific exercise plan will be given to me, based on my needs and interests and my doctor's recommendations. All exercise programs include warm-up, exercise at target heart rate, and cool-down. The programs might involve walking, jogging, swimming, or cycling (outdoor and stationary); participation in exercise fitness, rhythmic aerobic exercise, or choreographed fitness classes; or calisthenics or strength training. All programs are designed to place a gradually increasing workload on the body in order to improve overall fitness. The rate of progression is regulated by exercise target heart rate and perceived effort of exercise.

I understand that I am responsible for monitoring my own condition throughout the exercise program and should unusual symptoms occur, I will cease my participation and inform the instructor of the symptoms.

In signing this consent form, I affirm that I have read it in its entirety and that I understand the nature of the exercise program. I also affirm that my questions regarding the exercise program have been answered to my satisfaction.

In the event that a medical clearance must be obtained before I participate in the exercise program, I agree to consult with and obtain written permission from my physician before I begin an exercise program.

Also, in consideration for being allowed to participate in the YMCA exercise program, I agree to assume the risk of such exercise, and further agree to hold harmless the YMCA and its staff members conducting the exercise program from any and all claims, suits, losses, or related causes of action for damages, including, but not limited to, such claims that may result from my injury or death, accidental or otherwise, during, or arising in any way from, the exercise program.

Date ____________________ ____

(Signature of participant)

Please print:

Name ____ Date of birth ____________________

Address ____

Telephone ______________________________

Name of personal physician ____

Physician's address ____

Physician's phone ______________________________

Limitations and medications ____

Glossary

The following is an alphabetical listing of common personal training terms, with a brief definition of each. It is meant to help you better understand materials from the field of health and fitness.

abduction—Sideways movement away from the body.

adduction—Sideways movement toward the body.

antagonist muscle—Muscle that lengthens as the prime mover muscle shortens. The triceps is the antagonist muscle to the biceps.

assisted training—An advanced strength training technique in which a partner helps the exerciser perform a few additional repetitions at the completion of the exercise set.

ATP (adenosine triphosphate)—The chemical compound that releases the energy for muscle contraction.

atrophy—Decrease in muscle cross-sectional size.

bodybuilder—Person who follows a strength training program designed to develop greater muscle size.

body composition—The ratio of lean weight (muscle, bone, and so on) to fat weight. Ideally, males should be less than 15 percent fat, and females should be less than 20 percent fat.

body weight exercises—Exercises such as push-ups and chin-ups, in which one's body weight serves as the resistance.

circuit training—A system of training whereby the exerciser performs one set of exercises for each major muscle group.

concentric contraction—A muscle contraction in which the muscle exerts force, shortens, and overcomes the resistance. Also known as a positive contraction.

concomitant—Using both arms or legs at the same time rather than alternately.

controlled movement speed—Lifting and lowering resistance in a slow and controlled manner to maintain a relatively even force output.

dynamic constant-resistance exercise—Training with a resistance that does not change throughout the movement range; for example, using a barbell.

dynamic variable-resistance exercise—Training with a resistance that changes in a predetermined manner throughout the movement range; for example, using a Nautilus-type machine.

eccentric contraction—A muscle contraction in which the muscle exerts force, lengthens, and is overcome by the resistance. Also known as a negative contraction.

extension—Movement that increases the joint angle between adjacent body parts.

fast-twitch muscle fibers—Fibers that prefer anaerobic energy sources to produce relatively high levels of force for relatively short periods of time.

first-class lever—Lever arrangement in which the axis of rotation is between the movement force and the resistance force.

flexion—Movement that decreases the joint angle between adjacent body parts.

free weights—Handheld weights, such as barbells and dumbbells, that may be moved in virtually any direction without restriction.

full movement range—A complete range of joint motion, from flexion to extension and extension to flexion.

high-endurance muscles—Muscles characterized by a large percentage of slow-twitch fibers that are more resistant to fatigue.

hypertrophy—Increase in cross-sectional muscle size.

isokinetic exercise—Training with equipment that automatically matches the resistance force to the muscle force. The amount of muscle force produced determines the amount of resistance force encountered.

isometric contraction—A muscle contraction in which the muscle exerts force but does not change in length. Also known as static contraction, it neither overcomes nor is overcome by the resistance.

isometric exercise—Training in which the muscle force equals the resistance force in a static position. There is muscle tension but no muscle movement.

isotonic exercise—Training with equipment that provides dynamic constant resistance or dynamic variable resistance. The amount of resistive force selected determines the amount of muscle force produced.

low-endurance muscles—Muscles characterized by a high percentage of fast-twitch fibers that are less resistant to fatigue.

momentum—The quantity of motion determined by an object's mass and velocity.

motor unit—A single motor nerve and all of the individual muscle fibers that are activated by the nerve.

multimuscle exercise—An exercise that involves two or more major muscle groups. Linear movements such as bench press and squats are multimuscle exercises.

muscle adaptation—The ability of a muscle to respond positively to a slightly greater training stimulus to become larger and stronger.

muscle balance—Training all of the major muscle groups so that a desirable strength relationship is maintained between opposing muscles.

muscle contractibility—The ability of muscle tissue to shorten when stimulated to do so.

muscle density—The ratio of muscle tissue to nonmuscle tissue within a muscle cross section. High-density muscles are characterized by more protein filaments packed into each muscle fiber.

muscle elasticity—The ability of muscle tissue to return to its normal resting length.

muscle extensibility—The ability of muscle tissue to stretch beyond its normal resting length.

muscle fatigue—The point in an exercise set when a muscle can no longer contract concentrically and overcome the resistance.

muscle fibers—Groups of myofibrils bound into a functional unit and innervated by a motor nerve.

muscle isolation—An attempt to exercise one muscle or muscle group at a time, by single-muscle, single-joint exercises.

muscle length—The actual length of a muscle between its tendon attachments. Relatively long muscles have greater size potential than relatively short muscles.

muscle pump—A temporary increase in muscle cross-sectional size caused by blood and fluid congestion in the muscle tissue during high-intensity training.

myofibrils—Small cylindrical strands that run lengthwise within each muscle fiber and are composed of adjacent sarcomeres.

negative training—Advanced weight training technique that emphasizes the negative (eccentric) phase of exercise to produce greater force output.

Olympic lifters—Athletes who strength train primarily to lift heavier weights in competitive events—the clean and jerk and the snatch.

one repetition maximum (1 RM)—The heaviest resistance that an individual can lift one time; 1 RM is often used as a measure of maximum strength in a given exercise.

overload—Using more resistance than the muscles are accustomed to in a gradual and progressive manner to stimulate strength development.

overtraining—Training that does not allow the muscles to fully recover and build to slightly higher strength levels between exercise sessions. Usually rectified by reducing the training volume or taking longer recovery periods between workouts.

power—The rate of work production; power is the product of muscle force and movement speed.

powerlifters—Athletes who strength train primarily to lift heavier weights in competitive events—the squat, bench press, and deadlift.

preteens—Boys and girls who have not reached sexual maturity, or puberty.

prime mover muscle—The muscle primarily responsible for performing a particular movement. The biceps are prime mover muscles for elbow flexion.

progressive-resistance exercise—A training program in which the exercise resistance gradually increases as the muscles become stronger.

reciprocal inhibition—The blocking of nerve impulses to muscles that oppose a desired movement.

recovery time—The rest period between successive exercise sets (set recovery) or the rest period between successive workouts (workout recovery).

repetitions—The number of times an exercise is performed without interruption. Lifting the barbell from the standards, performing 10 squats, then returning it to the standards constitutes one set of 10 repetitions.

sarcomere—The smallest units of contraction within a muscle, sarcomeres consist of thick myosin proteins and thin actin proteins.

second-class lever—Lever arrangement in which the resistance force is between the axis of rotation and the movement force.

set—The number of separate bouts of exercise completed. Performing 10 curls, resting 60 seconds, then performing 10 more curls constitutes two sets of 10 repetitions each.

slow-twitch muscle fibers—Fibers that prefer aerobic energy sources to produce relatively low levels of force for relatively long periods of time.

spotter—A training partner who provides encouragement, feedback, safety, and reinforcement during strength training sessions. The spotter should be present during high-risk exercises such as bench presses and squats, for safety purposes, and might assist with high-intensity training procedures.

stabilizer muscles—Muscles that stabilize one joint so that the desired movement can occur in another joint. The low back muscles help stabilize the torso during standing barbell curls.

strength—The ability to exert muscle force against resistive force. Strength is typically measured by the amount of resistive force that is overcome.

strength plateau—A situation in which the training program does not result in additional strength gains. Strength plateaus indicate that some aspect of the training protocol should be changed to stimulate further progress.

stress adaptation—The ability of muscle tissue to make positive strength adaptations to progressively greater training demands.

stress intensification—Gradually increasing the muscle demands by training with more resistance, more repetitions, slower movements, high-intensity techniques, or other means for making the exercise more difficult.

superset training—A technique characterized by performing two or more sets of different exercises for a target muscle group; for example, a set of triceps press-downs followed immediately by a set of dips for the triceps muscles.

super-slow training—A technique characterized by 10-second lifting movements to decrease momentum and increase muscle tension.

third-class lever—Lever arrangement in which the movement force is between the axis of rotation and the resistance force.

training duration—The elapsed time for a training set (set duration), or the elapsed time for a training session (workout duration).

training intensity—The degree of effort necessary to complete an exercise set or an exercise session. High-intensity training is characterized by high levels of muscle fatigue.

training principles—Research-based guidelines for developing physical fitness safely and effectively.

training specificity—Training in a particular manner to attain desired results. For example, taking short rests between sets is more effective for developing muscle hypertrophy than muscle strength.

training volume—The total amount of work accomplished (weight lifted) during a training session. One means of estimating training volume is to multiply each exercise weight load by the number of repetitions completed, then summing the totals.

Valsalva response—Holding the breath while working against a resistance. This increases chest pressure, which might restrict blood return to the heart and greatly elevate blood pressure.

work—The product of the resistance force (weight load) times the distance it is moved. Bench pressing 200 pounds two feet produces 400 foot-pounds of force.

Bibliography

American College of Sports Medicine. 1993. *ACSM'S resource manual for guidelines for exercise testing and prescription*, 2nd ed. Philadelphia: Lea & Febiger.

American College of Sports Medicine. 1995. *ACSM's guidelines for exercise testing and prescription*, 5th ed. Philadelphia: Lea & Febiger.

American College of Sports Medicine. 1998. The recommended quantity and quality of exercise for developing and maintaining cardiorespiratory and muscular fitness and flexibility in healthy adults. *Medicine and Science in Sports and Exercise* 30(6): 975-991.

American Council on Exercise. 1993. *Aerobics instructor manual.* San Diego: American Council on Exercise.

American Council on Exercise. 1996. *Personal trainer manual*, 2nd ed. San Diego: American Council on Exercise.

American Council on Exercise. 2003. *ACE personal trainer manual*, 3rd ed. San Diego, CA: American Council on Exercise.

American Dietetic Association. 2000. *Position on nutrition for physical fitness and athletic performance for adults.* Chicago: American Dietetic Association.

American Heart Association. January 15, 1995. Exercise standards: A statement for healthcare professionals from the American Heart Association. *Circulation* 91: 2.

Astrand, P.O., and K. Rodahl. 1977. *Textbook of work physiology.* New York: McGraw-Hill.

Atham, J. 1981. Strengthening muscle. *Exercise and Sport Science Reviews* 9: 1-73.

Borg, G.B. 1982. Psychological basis of perceived exertion. *Medicine and Science in Sports and Exercise* 14: 377-381.

Bouchard, C., R. Shepard, T. Stephens, J. Sutton, and B. McPherson. 1990. *Exercise fitness and health: A consensus of current knowledge.* Champaign, IL: Human Kinetics.

Carlton, R., and E. Rhodes. 1985. A critical review of the literature on the ratings scales of perceived exertion. *Sports Medicine* 2: 198-222.

Charette, S.L., L. McEvoy, G. Pyka, C. Snow-Harter, D. Guido, R.A. Wiswell, and R. Marcus. 1991. *Journal of Applied Physiology* 70(5): 1912-1916.

Decker, J.I., G. Orcutt, and P. Sammann. 1989. *Y's Way to Fitness Walking Leader's Guide.* Champaign, IL: Human Kinetics.

Dishman, R. 1984. Motivation and exercise adherence. In *Psychological foundations of sport*, edited by J. Silva, III, and R. Weinberg. Champaign, IL: Human Kinetics.

Dishman, R., R. Farquhar, and K. Cureton. 1994. Responses to preferred intensities of exertion in men differing in activity levels. *Medicine and Science in Sports and Exercise* 26: 783.

Durstine, L., and R. Pate. 1993. Cardiorespiratory responses to acute exercise. *ACSM's resource manual for guidelines for exercise testing and prescription*, 2nd ed. Philadelphia: Lea & Febiger.

Fleck, S.J., and W.J. Kraemer. 1997. *Designing resistance training programs*, 2nd ed. Champaign, IL: Human Kinetics.

Folinsbee, L. 1990. Exercise and the environment. In *Exercise fitness and health*, edited by C. Bouchard, R. Shepard., T. Stephens, J. Sutton, and B. McPherson. Champaign, IL: Human Kinetics.

Foster, C. 1975. Physiological requirements of aerobic dancing. *The Research Quarterly* 46: 120-122.

Fox, E.L., and D.K. Matthews. 1974. *Interval training.* Philadelphia: Saunders.

Franks, D., and E. Howley. 1989. *Fitness facts.* Champaign, IL: Human Kinetics.

Friedenberg, E. 1967. *The vanishing adolescent.* New York: Dell. Original edition, East Sussex: Beacon Press, 1959.

Gilliam, G.M. 1981. Effects of frequency of weight training on muscle strength enhancement. *Journal of Sports Medicine* 21: 432-436.

Graves, J.E., M.L. Pollack, A.E. Jones, A.B. Colvin, and S.H. Leggett. 1989. Specificity of limited range of motion variable resistance training. *Medicine and Science in Sports and Exercise* 2: 84-89.

Greenberg, J., and D. Pargman. 1989. *Physical fitness: A wellness approach*, 2nd ed. Englewood Cliffs, NJ: Prentice Hall.

Guyton, A. 1974. *Function of the human body*, 4th ed. Philadelphia: Saunders.

Harre, D., ed. 1982. *Principles of sports training: Introduction to the theory and methods of training.* East Berlin: Sportverlag.

Harris, K.A., and R.G. Holly. 1987. Physiological response to circuit weight training in borderline hypertensive subjects. *Medicine and Science in Sports and Exercise* 19(3): 000-000.

Haskell, W.L. 1994. Health consequences of physical activity: Understanding and challenges regarding dose-response. *Medicine and Science in Sports and Exercise* 26: 649-660.

Herbert, W., and D. Herbert. The exercise standards and malpractice reporter, 1987 to present.

Heyward, V.H. 1984. *Designs for fitness.* Minneapolis: Burgess.

Heyward, V. 1998. *Advanced fitness assessment and exercise prescription*, 3rd ed. Champaign, IL: Human Kinetics.

Howley, E., and B.D. Franks. 1992. *Health fitness instructor's handbook*, 2nd ed. Champaign, IL: Human Kinetics.

Howley, E., and M. Glover. 1974. The caloric costs of running and walking 1 mile for men and women. *Medicine and Science in Sports and Exercise* 6: 235-237.

Hunter, G.R. 1985. Changes in body composition, body-build, and performance associated with different weight training frequencies in males and females. *National Strength and Conditioning Association Journal* 7: 26-28.

Hunter, G.P., J. McGuirk, N. Mitrano, P. Pearman, B. Thomas, and R. Arrington. 1989. The effects of a weight training belt on blood pressure during exercise. *Journal of Applied Sport Science Research* 3: 13-18.

Kasch, F.W., and J.L. Boyer. 1968. *Adult fitness: Principles and practice*. Greeley, CO: All American Products and Publications.

Ketner, J.B., and M.B. Mekkion. 1995. The overtraining syndrome: A review of presentation, pathophysiology, and treatment. *Medical Exercise Nutrition Health* 4: 136-145.

Kosich, Daniel. 1996. *Get real: A personal guide to real-life weight management*. San Diego, CA: IDEA Health and Fitness Association.

Kravitz, L., and D. Kosich. 1993. Flexibility: A comprehensive research review and program design guide. *IDEA Today* (June): 000-000.

Martens, R., R. Christina, J. Harvey, and B. Sharkey. 1981. *Coaching young athletes*. Champaign, IL: Human Kinetics.

McArdle, W., F. Katch, and V. Katch. 1991. *Exercise physiology*, 3rd ed. Philadelphia: Lea & Febiger.

McDonagh, M.J.N., and C.T.M. Davies. 1984. Adaptive response of mammalian skeletal muscle to exercise with high loads. *European Journal of Applied Physiology* 52: 139-155.

Mutoh, Y., S. Sawai, Y. Takanashi, and L. Skurko. 1988. Aerobic dance injuries among instructors and students. *The Physician and Sportsmedicine* 16(12): 81-83, 85, 88.

National Dance Exercise Instructor Training Association. 1999. *Fitness manual*. Mineapolis: NDEITA.

National Exercise Trainers Association. 2001. *Personal Trainer Manual*. Minneapolis: National Exercise Trainers Association.

National Strength and Conditioning Association. 1994. *Essentials of strength training and conditioning*. Champaign, IL: Human Kinetics.

Nieman, D. 1990. *Fitness and sports medicine: An introduction*. Palo Alto, CA: Bull.

Nygaard, G., and T. Boone. 1985. *ACEP Coaches guide to sport law*. Champaign, IL: Human Kinetics.

O'Brien, T.S. 1997. *The personal trainer's handbook*. Champaign, IL: Human Kinetics.

Ockene, I., and J. Ockene. 1992. *Prevention of coronary heart disease*. Boston: Little, Brown.

Painter, P., and W. Haskell. 1993. Decision making in programming exercise. In *ACSM's resource manual for guidelines for exercise testing and prescription*, 2nd ed. Philadelphia: Lea & Febiger.

Parker, S., B. Hurley, D. Hanlon, and P. Vaccaro. 1989. Failure of target heart rate to accurately monitor intensity during aerobic dance. *Medicine and Science in Sports and Exercise* 21: 230.

Pollock, M. 1973. The quantification of endurance training programs. *Exercise and Sport Science Reviews* 1: 155-188.

Pollock, M., J. Wilmore, and S. Fox. 1984. *Exercise in health and disease*. Philadelphia: Saunders.

Raglin, J.S. 1993. Overtraining and staleness: Psychometric monitoring of endurance athletes. In *Handbook of Research on Sport Psychology*, edited by R.B. Singer, M. Murphey, and L. Tennant. New York: Macmillan.

Richie, D. 1989. Medical and legal implications of dance exercise leadership: The role of footwear. *Exercise Standards and Malpractice Reporter* 3: 61.

Richie, D.H., Jr., S.F. Kelso, and P.A. Bellucci. 1985. Aerobic dance injuries: A retrospective study of instructors and participants. *The Physician and Sportsmedicine* 13(2): 130-140.

Richie, D.H., and E.L. Washington. 1983. Musculoskeletal problems in aerobic dancers, Part I. *Dance Medicine Health Newsletter* 2: 9-11.

Roberts, S.O., ed. 1996. *The business of personal training*. Champaign, IL: Human Kinetics.

Rockefeller, K.A., and E.J. Burke. 1979. Psycho-physiological analysis of an aerobic dance programme for women. *The British Journal of Physical Education* 13: 77-80.

Saltin, B., et al. 1977. Fiber types and metabolic potentials of skeletal muscles in sedentary men and endurance runners. *Annals of the New York Academy of Science* 301: 3.

Shapiro, U., and D. Seidman. 1990. Field and clinical observations of exertional heat stroke patients. *Medicine and Science in Sports and Exercise* 22: 1.

Southmayd, W., and M. Hoffman. 1981. *Sports health*. New York: Quick Fox.

Sprague, K.C. 1991. *Weight and strength training for kids and teenagers*. Los Angeles: Jeremy P. Tarcher.

Strovas, J. 1984. Aerobic dance instructors are not injury proof. *The Physician and Sportsmedicine* 12: 24.

Thrash, K., and B. Kelly. 1987. Flexibility and strength training. *Journal of Applied Sport Science Research* 1: 74-75.

Vaccaro, P., and M. Clinton. 1981. The effects of aerobic dance conditioning on the body composition and maximal oxygen uptake of college women. *Journal of Sports Medicine and Physical Fitness* 21: 291-294.

Van Camp, S. 1993. Pharmacologic factors in exercise and exercise testing. In *ACSM's resource manual for guidelines for exercise testing and prescription*, 2nd ed. Philadelphia: Lea & Febiger.

Vogel, J., P.B. Rock, B.H. Jones, and G. Havenith. 1993. Environmental considerations in exercise testing and training. In *ACSM's resource manual for guidelines for exercise testing and prescription*, 2nd ed. Philadelphia: Lea & Febiger.

Washington, E.L., S.L. Rosenberg, B. Friedlander, and B. Carlin. 1983. Musculoskeletal problems in aerobic dancers, Part II. *Dance Medicine Health Newsletter* 2: 11-12.

Weber, H. 1974. The energy cost of aerobic dancing. *Fitness for Living* 8: 26-30.

Wells, C., and R. Pate. 1988. Training for performance in prolonged exercise. Lamb, D. and R. Murray, eds. *Prolonged exercise* Vol. 1, 257-389. Carmel, IN: Benchmark Press.

Westcott, W.L. 1974. Effects of varied frequencies of weight training on the development of strength. College Station: Pennsylvania State University.

Westcott, W.L. 1987. Exercise sessions can make the difference in weight loss. *Perspective* 13 (February): 42-44.

Westcott, W.L. 1988. Eliminating myths: Does strength training harm blood pressure? *Perspective* (December): 37-39.

Westcott, W.L. 1991. *Strength fitness: Physiological principles and training techniques.* Dubuque, IA: Brown.

Westcott, W.L. 1996. *Building strength and stamina.* Champaign, IL: Human Kinetics.

Westcott, W.L., and M. Pappas. 1987. Immediate effects of circuit strength training on blood pressure. *American Fitness Quarterly* 6 (October): 43-44.

Whaley, M., L. Kaminsky, G. Dwyer, L. Getchell, and J. Norton. 1992. Questioning the routine use of 220 – AGE heart rate formula. *Medicine and Science in Sports and Exercise* 24: 1173.

Wilmore, J.H., and D.L. Costill. 1999. *Physiology of sport and exercise.* Champaign, IL: Human Kinetics.

YMCA of the USA. 1994. *YMCA strength training.* Champaign, IL: Human Kinetics.

YMCA of the USA. 2000. *YMCA fitness testing and assessment manual.* Champaign, IL: Human Kinetics.

YMCA of the USA. 2004. *YMCA healthy lifestyle principles, 4th ed.* Champaign, IL: Human Kinetics.

YMCA of the USA. 1995. *YMCA prenatal exercise instructor manual.* Champaign, IL: Human Kinetics.

YMCA of the USA. 1996. *YMCA Walk Reebok instructor manual.* Champaign, IL: Human Kinetics.

YMCA of the USA. 2000. *YMCA water fitness for health.* Champaign, IL: Human Kinetics.

Index

Note: The italicized f and t following page numbers refer to figures and tables, respectively.

YMCA OF THE USA HEALTH AND FITNESS RESOURCES

See the YMCA Program Store catalog for details about these additional items for your health and fitness program, or contact the Program store, P.O. Box 5076, Champaign, IL 61825-5076, phone (800) 747-0089. To save time, order by fax (217) 351-1549.

Printed Resources

0-7360-5906-7	YMCA Cardio and Step Aerobics Instructor Manual	$26.00
0-7360-5142-2	YMCA Pilates Instructor Manual	$26.00
0-7360-3316-5	YMCA Fitness Testing and Assessment Manual	$35.00
0-7360-3381-5	YMCA Fitness Specialist Training Workbook	$45.00
1-58518-029-7	Conducting the YMCA Fitness Testing and Assessment Protocol Video	$29.95
0-7360-2214-7	YMCA Fitness Analyst Software	$395.00
0-88011-949-7	YMCA Personal Fitness Program Manual	$32.00
1-887781-00-5	Get Real: A Personal Guide to Real-Life Weight Management	$15.95
0-7360-0146-8	YMCA/IDEA Get Real Weight Management Program Instructor Manual	$19.00
0-88011-899-7	YMCA Walk Reebok Distance/Interval Training Instructor Manual	$16.00
0-88011-543-2	YMCA Walk Reebok Instructor Manual	$50.00
0-87322-629-1	YMCA Healthy Back Book	$14.95
0-87322-717-4	YMCA Healthy Back Program Instructor's Guide	$23.00
0-87322-692-5	YMCA Healthy Back Video	$22.95
0-87322-828-6	Fit for Two: The Official YMCA Prenatal Exercise Guide	$15.95
0-87322-825-1	The YMCA Prenatal Exercise Instructor Guide	$38.00
0-7360-3246-0	YMCA Water Fitness for Health	$39.00
1-890720-01-1	Group Fitness Instructor Manual (ACE)	$41.95
0-88011-942-X	Exercise for Older Adults (ACE)	$36.00
0-99-003272-8	Xerball Instructor Manual	$20.00
0-99-003015-6	YogaBall Instructor Manual	$20.00
0-99-003123-3	Cycle Reebok: Professional Training Manual	$25.00
0-99-003013-X	Rubber Resistance Training Kit (Upper Body)	$30.00
0-99-003014-8	Rubber Resistance Training Kit (Lower Body)	$40.00

Other Resources

The following resources are available at no cost to local YMCAs from the YMCA of the USA, (800) 872-9622 or www.YMCAexchange.org:

YMCA Health and Fitness Programs Starter Kit
YMCA of the USA Medical Advisory Committee Recommendations
YMCA Healthy Kids Day—Annual Promotion and Program Information Packet
Promoting Good Health: A Resource Guide for YMCAs
Youth Health and Fitness Programs: A Resource Guide for YMCAs (vol. I and II)
Diabetes Wellness: A Resource Guide for YMCAs
Mind–Body Programs: A Resource Guide for YMCAs
Collaborations With Hospitals and Other Health Care Facilities: A Resource Guide for YMCAs
Yoga Programs: A Resource Guide for YMCAs
YMCA Personal Fitness Program: A Program Implementation Guide for YMCAs
Automated External Defibrillators (AEDs) in YMCAs: A Technical Assistance Paper

All prices shown are subject to change.